MANAGING

CONSUMER HEALTH INFORMATION SERVICES

EDITED BY ALAN M. REES

ORYX PRESS 1991

The rare Arabian Oryx is believed to have inspired the myth of the unicorn. This desert antelope became virtually extinct in the early 1960s. At that time several groups of international conservationists arranged to have 9 animals sent to the Phoenix Zoo to be the nucleus of a captive breeding herd. Today the Oryx population is nearly 800, and over 400 have been returned to reserves in the Middle East.

Copyright© 1991 by The Oryx Press
4041 North Central at Indian School Road
Phoenix, Arizona 85012-3397

Published simultaneously in Canada

Printed and Bound in the United States of America

∞ The paper used in this publication meets the minimum requirements of American National Standard for Information Science—Permanence of Paper for Printed Library Materials, ANSI Z39.48, 1984.

Library of Congress Cataloging-in-Publication Data

Managing consumer health information services / edited by Alan M. Rees.

    p.   cm.
    Includes bibliographical references and index.
    ISBN 0-89774-622-8
    1. Hospital libraries—Administration. 2. Public health-
-Information services—Management. 3. Consumer education-
-Information services—Management. 4. Medical libraries-
-Administration.   I. Rees, Alan M.
Z675.H7M29 1991
027.6'62—dc20
                                 90-46104
                                 CIP

CONTENTS

PREFACE

Nine years have elapsed since the publication of *Developing Consumer Health Information Services* (Bowker, 1982), the previous incarnation of this book. The earlier version was intended to assist librarians and other health information providers in the development and management of consumer health information programs and services. Although most of the seven programs described no longer exist, these early activities, mainly supported in the late 1970s and early 1980s by LSCA (Library Services and Construction Act) funding, demonstrated and legitimized the library role in providing consumer health information (CHI) services. The programs offered a prescription for the development of collections, reference guidelines, referral procedures, training workshops, and community linkages. The present system involving multi-type library cooperation has evolved from the experience of the past decade. It was clearly recognized that no single type of library could be responsive to the full range of CHI needs.

The objective of this book is to update the earlier work and to provide practical guidance with respect to the development and operation of CHI services for the 1990s in both the community and hospital environments. The book consists of five parts—trends in medical consumerism in the context of the present health care system; descriptions of current CHI library programs; development and operation of programs with respect to the basic functions of collection development and reference/information services; and developments on the international scene that provide comparative insights and validation of the American experience.

This book is intended to complement *The Consumer Health Information Source Book* (Oryx, 1990), which serves as an evaluative guide to the selection of health information resources recommended for the general public. The *Source Book,* with its focus on materials, brings together descriptive evaluations of some 750 books, 79 popular magazines and newsletters, over 700 pamphlet titles, as well as numerous information clearinghouses, toll-free hotlines, and health-related resource organizations.

Part I of this book is devoted to medical consumerism in the 1990s because the context for CHI has significantly changed in recent years. Charles B. Inlander, president of the People's Medical Society, outlines in Chapter 1 some of the current trends in medical consumerism and concludes that from all these changes and alterations, "the bottom line for consumers is the urgent need to be informed and empowered in order to get the most from a system so vital to our well-being." He stresses three necessities for the health care consumer—information, information, information. Tom Ferguson, founding editor of *Medical Self-Care* magazine and prolific medical author, presents in Chapter 2 a profile of health-active, health-responsible medical consumers, who express frustration with their doctors, scrutinize their doctors' qualifications, inquire about hospital mortality rates, seek second opinions, and insist on sharing decision making.

Alan Rees in Chapter 3 reviews the nature of the library response over the past decade and portrays the current scene in terms of programs, services, and technology. He points out that the information service delivery model that has evolved defines the public library as the principal service agent, while complementary and supportive information services are supplied by academic medical center libraries, hospital libraries, medical society libraries, and special libraries.

The five principal types of libraries involved in CHI are well represented in Part II by 13 program descriptions contained in Chapters 4 through 16—public libraries (King County Public Library, Seattle); academic medical centers (Universities of Connecticut, Nebraska, and Miami); hospital libraries (MacNeal, Overlook, Swedish Medical Center, St. Joseph Hospital in Denver, and the VA Hospital in Tampa); medical society libraries (New York Academy of Medicine and the College of Physicians of Philadelphia); and special libraries (Health Education Center in Pittsburgh and Planetree in San Francisco).

The 13 program descriptions provide considerable detail with respect to origins, mode of operation, funding, collections, use of information technology, reference and information services offered, access to online search services and CD-ROM files, staffing, training, relationship to formal patient education activities, marketing, community linkages, networking, and evaluation. A commonality of experience emerges from these descriptions. Although most of the budgets are small, imaginative and creative use is made of limited resources. A clear emphasis is placed upon resource sharing. Networking is either accomplished on a statewide basis, as is the case in Connecticut, Pennsylvania, and Nebraska, or on a more limited geographical basis such as offered by several hospitals.

Part III is devoted to development and operations. Alan Rees in Chapter 17 analyzes collection development policies in terms of quantity and quality considerations, selection criteria, acquisition of materials in alternative medicine, optimal mix of popular and professional publications, and lists recommendations with respect to 13 basic collection categories. Claudia Perry in Chapter 18, drawing upon the extensive experience gained in responding to some 18,000 popular requests annually at the New York Academy of Medicine, discusses the expectations of users, types of requests, reference interviewing, and general reference techniques, and identifies a number of useful print, online, and CD-ROM materials that can be used to improve information services.

Part IV surveys the international scene. Chapters 19 through 22 illustrate the state-of-the-art of CHI programs and services in Canada, the United Kingdom, Australia, and New Zealand. These chapters reflect differences in the organization and financing of health care delivery in the four countries and corresponding differentiation of information needs. Joanne Gard Marshall in Chapter 19 shows how CHI programs have evolved in Canada within the context of the Canadian health care system. Robert Gann in Chapter 20 provides a fascinating glimpse of changes in the British National Health Service that herald the emergence of empowered medical consumers in the United Kingdom. Moira L. Bryant in Chapter 21 describes her pioneering establishment of the first CHI program in Australia, drawing upon the best of both British and American experience. Jill Harris thoughfully portrays in Chapter 22 some of the difficulties encountered in the creation of CHI services in New Zealand in view of the limited resources available and the ambivalence of the medical community.

Of particular interest in relation to the future is the problem of paying for the more extensive use of information technology. The increased availability of online databases and CD-ROM portable databases offer enhanced opportunities for libraries to provide consumers with a sophisticated and enriched blend of bibliographic information, full-text, and reference book information, utilizing user-friendly software and hypertext capability. However, such services are expensive. The challenge will be for libraries to find the resources to pay for such systems. If libraries do not do so, the consumer will be forced to seek and pay for medical information elsewhere.

I wish to take this opportunity to express my appreciation for the cooperation extended by the numerous contributors to this volume. The authors in the five countries represented have shown a patient willingness to overcome the problems associated with the use of multiple word processing programs and computer disks of many sizes and densities. All of the contributors have made creative use of overnight courier services, international phone calls, and FAX machines to facilitate communication. Finally, my thanks to John Wagner of Oryx Press for his insightful, sensitive, and efficient editing.

Alan M. Rees

CONTRIBUTORS

Ralph D. Arcari
Assistant Vice-President for Academic
  Resources and Services
Director, Lyman Maynard Stowe
  Library
University of Connecticut
Farmington, CT 06032

Margaret Bandy
Medical Librarian
St. Joseph Hospital
Denver, CO 80218

Rya Ben-Shir
Manager, Health Sciences Resource
  Center
NacNeal Hospital
Berwyn, IL 60402

Moira L. Bryant
Health Link Librarian
Westmead Hospital
Westmead, NSW, Australia

Mary Campbell
Medical Reference Librarian
King County Library System
Seattle, WA 98109

Tracey Cosgrove, M.L.I.S.
Director, Planetree Health Resource
  Center
2040 Webster Street
San Francisco, CA 94115

Brenda K. Epperson
McGoogan Library of Medicine
University of Nebraska Medical
  Center
Omaha, NE 68105

Tom Ferguson, M.D.
President
Self-Care Productions
Austin, TX 78703

Robert Gann
Health Information Manager
Help for Health
Southampton General Hospital
Southampton, United Kingdom

Jill Harris
Manager, Information Centre
State Services Commission
P.O. Box 329
Wellington, New Zealand

Charles B. Inlander
President, People's Medical Society
462 Walnut Street
Allentown, PA 18102

Kay Johnson
Deputy Librarian for Facilities
  Development
King County Library System
Seattle, WA 98109

Andrea Kenyon
Director of the Library for Public
  Services
College of Physicians of Philadelphia
Philadelphia, PA 19103

Brett A. Kirkpatrick
Director, Moody Medical Library
University of Texas Medical Branch
Galveston, TX 77550

August La Rocco
Associate Professor
Coordinator, Consumer Health
  Information
Louis Calder Memorial Library
University of Miami School of
  Medicine
Miami, FL 33101

Joanne Gard Marshall
Assistant Professor
Faculty of Library and Information
  Science
University of Toronto
Toronty, Ontario, Canada

Lois G. Michaels
Founder and President
Health Education Center
Blue Cross of Western Pennsylvania
Pittsburgh, PA 15222

Kathleen A. Moeller
Medical Librarian
Overlook Hospital
Summit, NJ 07901

Sandra K. Parker
Director of Library and Information
  Services
Swedish Medical Center
Englewood, CO 80110

Claudia A. Perry
Head, Reference/Information Services
The New York Academy of Medicine
2 East 103rd Street
New York, NY 10029

Alan M. Rees
Visisting Professor
Center for the Study of Librarianship
School of Library Science
Kent State University
Kent, OH 44242

Marie A. Reidelbach
McGoogan Library of Medicine
University of Nebraska Medical
  Center
Omaha, NE 68105

Iris A. Renner
Chief Librarian
Securities and Exchange Commission
Washington, DC 20549

Alberta L. Richetelle
University Assistant Librarian
Project Director, Healthnet—
  Connecticut Consumer Health
  Information Program
Lyman Maynard Stowe Library
University of Connecticut
Farmington, CT 06032

Janet M. Schneider
Patients Librarian
James A. Haley Veterans Hospital
Tampa, FL 33612

Carolyn G. Weaver
Health Sciences Library &
  Information Center
University of Washington
Seattle, WA 98105

PART I

Introduction: Medical Consumerism in the 1990s

CHAPTER 1
Trends in Medical Consumerism

Charles B. Inlander

The consumerism movement that was begun in the 1960s, by activists like Ralph Nader, swept through the land with such speed and fervor that by the middle of the 1970s most states and the federal government had passed laws assuring citizens of protection from inferior products, services, and treatments. But, when it came to medical and health matters the laws and the lawmakers remained silent. Today, while change is in the wind, it can be comfortably said that medicine and health care are the last bastions of nonconsumerism in America.

AMERICA'S BIGGEST BUSINESS

Health care in America, according to the federal government, now consumes 12 percent of the gross national product. Health care expenditures are twice that of the total national defense budget. America is a medical mecca with the world's most sophisticated equipment and facilities. America has more doctors per capita than any other nation. While we do not have a national health insurance program, our Medicare and Medicaid programs, which cover the elderly and the poor, respectively, account for a larger expenditure than any other country spends on its entire national health-care program. Close to 36 million operations are performed annually. Consumers receive hundreds of millions of medical tests each year, while Americans are prescribed more drugs than the citizens of any other country. In fact, each year Americans consume more than half of the world's production of pharmaceuticals.

Obviously, medicine in America is big business. The health-care industry itself is becoming the nation's largest employer. In most of our major metropolitan areas, health-care organizations are the biggest employers.

DOES THE SUPPLY CREATE THE DEMAND?

Use of the health-care system overall is growing. While there have been some significant shifts away from inpatient hospital care to ambulatory services, with a reduction in the average length of stay of those who are still hospitalized, overall use of health-care services is increasing. Much of this has to do with the aging of the population in that longer life brings a higher likelihood of medical encounters.

The use of the health-care system is not confined to the traditional medical mainstream. Aside from allopathic medical doctors (M.D.s) in conventional hospital and ambulatory care settings, consumers are using in record numbers what some term nontraditional, alternative, or nonconventional medical services. Chiropractors are flourishing. In fact, the American Chiropractic Association claims one out of every four Americans has seen a chiropractor. Massage therapists, acupuncturists, naturapaths, and a wide range of other medical and health professionals treat an increasing number of "patients" each year. From a health care delivery standpoint, Americans have a wider range of practitioners to choose from than ever before.

Even within the traditional medical disciplines options are greater. The number of specialists grows each year, while the number of specialties is also increasing. At the beginning of the 1980s virtually no one had ever heard of a specialty in sports medicine. Today, there are practitioners who specialize in "sports gynecology." Some observers contend, this author being one, that the medical profession is now creating medical needs where little or no specialization is really necessary.

Yale School of Medicine Professor Lowell S. Levin, contends that the medical profession is making health itself a disease. In an interview in a World Health Organization journal, he pointed out that consumers are "warned" not to exercise, participate in certain activities known to improve health, or alter what might be a poor diet without first "consulting" a physician. Levin notes that in many instances physicians are no more knowledgeable about the planned activity or lifestyle change than their patients.

There is evidence that the expansion of specialties is more related to a glut of practitioners than to medical need. In most urban areas, there are simply more practitioners than necessary. In some ways, this reinforces Professor Levin's observations. The evidence also suggests that the physician surplus will not only continue, but become larger. Physicians are being churned out of medical schools at a rate that far exceeds expected population needs. Such numbers can only suggest the potential for creation of more specialties.

For the typical health-care consumer, the proliferation of practitioners and specialties leads to confusion and frustration. Overspecialization inherently implies consumers being referred from one practitioner to another for the same condition. It means seeing one doctor for one stage of treatment and yet another for the next stage. It also means a whole new set of jargon for the consumer to understand. And, in very practical terms, it tends to make the final stack of bills impossible to comprehend.

WHERE AM I?

But this confusion is not all that confronts the medical consumer. The settings in which health care is delivered are vastly different in the beginning of the 1990s than they were in the early 1980s. Ten years ago, most consumers received their medical care at either a doctor's office or a hospital. Today, a whole new set of facilities exists. Although the doctor's office and hospital still exist, they have now been joined by free-standing surgical centers (surgi-centers), free-standing emergency centers (emergi-centers), other types of outpatient facilities that specialize in such services as lens implants or arthroscopic knee surgery (to name just two), and a variety of other stand-alone services. In addition, consumers today have to choose between a private doctor, a group practice, a health maintenance organization (HMO), a preferred provider organization (PPO), and a whole host of other acronymic organizations that provide some form of health care. The traditional routine of feeling sick and going to the doctor is not as clear-cut or simple as it once was. And if the trends of the past two decades continue, it is not going to become any easier.

SEND CASH!

Another problem facing consumers is their declining ability to afford the cost of health care. Medical inflation over the last 10 years has exceeded almost fourfold that of overall inflation. Consumers are not only faced by an average annual rise of 8 percent to 10 percent per year in hospital and doctor fees, but also have experienced an increase in their insurance premiums. Insurance premiums in the latter part of the 1980s were rising anywhere from 10 percent to 80 percent a year for most payers. Medicare premiums went up 38 percent in 1988 alone for the nation's elderly.

In August 1989, the federal government's Health Care Financing Administration reported these *out-of-pocket* health-care expenses for each man, woman, and child for the year 1987 (the most recent year for which statistics are available):

Doctor Fees	$104
Drugs and Medical Sundries	$101
Nursing Homes	$80
Dentist Fees	$79
Hospitals	$73
Chiropractors, Physical Therapists, and Other Professional Services	$26
Eyeglasses, Contact Lenses, and Accessories	$25

These figures *do not* include any insurance premiums. The sum total of these out-of-pocket expenses is $488 for each person in America. A family of four therefore paid almost $2,000 out-of-pocket for health care *plus* insurance premiums.

Yet in 1990, 37 million Americans were without any health insurance. It is estimated that over half of this number were fully employed! The Pennsylvania Health Care Cost Containment Council, a state-created agency, released a study in 1988 verifying that the uninsured were not necessarily homeless or unemployed persons. The study showed that the majority were the so-called "working poor." Employers could not afford to provide health insurance benefits, or employees could not afford the premium contribution required from their weekly paychecks. Sadly, the numbers of uninsured and underinsured are growing, not declining.

Furthermore, even those with health insurance are faced with higher out-of-pocket expenses. Companies, in an effort to control health-care costs, have altered their health benefits programs. Many have forced employees to pay a larger part of the insurance premium. They have also required employees to pay larger deductibles and copayments when they utilize health services. Some companies have restricted benefits or eligibility for certain services. Thus, as the Health Care Financing Administration noted for 1987, 28 percent of U.S. health-care expenditure was coming from consumers' pockets. Again, that does not include any insurance premium expenditures.

INFORMATION, PLEASE!

From all these changes and alterations, the bottom line for consumers is the urgent need to be informed and empowered in order to get the most from a system so vital to their well-being. This is a new phenomenon in America. Never before have health-care consumers needed, or even felt the need, to have as much health-care information as they do now. However, information about the health-care system and world of medicine is often hard for the consumer to access. Information about doctors, hospitals, and other service organizations is often not in the public domain. Vital information about the quality of the personnel who provide medical care in a given community and the facilities in which they work is often nonexistent or exempted from public disclosure.

Accurate and reliable information about health and medical conditions, treatments, and other services related to a person's health-care needs often are difficult for consumers to acquire. People have traditionally not worried about health-care service provision and have historically "trusted" their doctor and hospital. The average consumer has been a passive user of medical services; the typical health-care customer is not only uninformed about his or her condition, but also lacks the ability to actively seek out relevant information.

Even the most highly educated members of our society are generally poorly informed about health and medical matters. It is not unusual for CEOs of major corporations to be uninformed or misinformed about their company's health insurance benefits or Medicare's provisions upon retirement. It is even more interesting to see many of our "Titans of Industry" become passive and childlike at the hands of the medical system. The average American consumer is still ignorant about health and medical matters, but this situation is rapidly changing.

THE COMING REVOLUTION

Not unlike eastern Europe, the winds of change have buffeted American medicine. Over the coming decades, we are likely to see the most important revolution in medical history. Unlike medical revolutions of the past, which involved new drugs, nutritional knowledge, medical equipment, or surgical techniques, the coming revolution will center on the empowered consumer.

No longer will medical and health knowledge be solely in the hands of the providers. No longer will the language of medicine be a cryptic code. No longer will the treatment and care of people be in the hands of a small group of practitioners who own the machines and control the journals. Indeed, the wave of the medical future involves the informed customer. Of course, this is not a new concept. Thirty years ago consumerism arrived in such areas as automobile repair and safety, mortgage and lending disclosure, funeral disclosure requirements, and environmental issues. As a result, today every state has laws that require automobile service departments to provide written estimates of work with limits on charges in excess of a cost estimate, or laws that mandate the return of used parts upon customer request. In banking, the consumer revolution brought about federal and state lending disclosure requirements that permit the consumer a "look see" period, full information about overall interest rates and payments, and other safeguards.

Yet, until recently, the world of health care has been a dark secret—a medical Albania. And, in many ways, it still is. "Peristroika" has yet to fully materialize in matters of health and medicine. Less than two-thirds of our states have statutes that require physicians and hospitals to give consumers copies of their own medical records upon request. Most states do not require courts that have found physicians guilty of medical malpractice to report the verdict to the state medical licensing boards—the only entities authorized to revoke or suspend licenses. There are no federal laws that require inserts detailing contraindications and cautions in prescription medication packages dispensed to consumers. And medical equipment, with the exception of X-ray inspection, generally goes unchecked by regulators once in the hands of physicians or hospitals. While most states require that butcher scales be inspected at least once a year for accuracy to protect the consumer, not a single state requires physicians' blood pressure cuffs to be inspected for calibration.

In 1989, a federal law went into effect establishing a National Practitioner Data Bank. The Data Bank stores information on actions (including malpractice settlements) taken against every physician, and other practitioners, by hospitals, licensing boards, and courts. The purpose of the Data Bank is to protect the consumer from bad practitioners who jump from one state to another either just before or after disciplinary actions. Hospitals and licensing boards are required to look at the data on a prescribed basis. The theory is that by so doing they will not employ or allow bad providers to practice medicine. However, the law only requires that they examine the data, not that they take any course of prescribed action. Furthermore, and even more heinous, the law excludes public access to the data. Obviously, the medical industry overwhelmed the interests of the consumer. However, there is now a growing public outcry about this failure of our legislators to protect the public.

The above example illustrates what is beginning to emerge in medical consumerism. The consumer backlash over the Catastrophic Health Care Act of 1988 and its subsequent revocation by Congress is another illustration. For the first time in history, the public's desire to be involved in health policy and medical matters is being demonstrated.

At a more practical level, consumers are demanding to know more about their health conditions and the procedures and treatments they are receiving. Letters to the editor of prestigious medical publications, such as *The New England Journal of Medicine* and the *Journal of the American Medical Association,* document physicians' awareness that consumers are demanding more information about not only the treatment they receive, but about the training and competence of the practitioners themselves.

Because of this growing demand for provider accountability, there is clearly a friction developing between that segment of the medical profession that is reluctant to change and a citizenry that will no longer accept the *status quo.* As a result, consumers are seeking alternate ways of accessing the information they need to make informed medical decisions. In several locations across the country, consumer health libraries have emerged, such as at the Center for Medical Consumers in New York City, and the Planetree Health Resource Center in San Francisco. Many hospitals have opened their captive, in-house medical libraries to patients and their families. This step was taken because of public demand.

Bookstores do a brisk business in their health sections and the nonfiction bestseller lists usually have one or two "health" books in the top 10. Only a decade ago such bestseller status for health books did not exist.

Consumer organizations, such as the Public Citizen Health Research Group and my own People's Medical Society, have emerged as strong and viable sources of consumer health information over the past decade. Since the People's Medical Society was founded in the early 1980s, there have been weeks when over 3,000 letters and phone calls have been received from consumers seeking information about their health rights, medical conditions, and actions they can take to make the system work better for them.

As a result of this demand, the People's Medical Society has produced over 100 books and pamphlets, some self-published and others by major trade publishers. The prepublication demand for these books has been so great that all of our books have more than broken even before the first copy was ever mailed.

What makes these medical consumer publications different from medical books in the past is their empowering nature. No longer is a book valid simply because the initials "M.D." follow the author's name. In addition, the new publications are documented. For example, in *Medicine on Trial* (Prentice Hall, 1988; paperback, Pantheon, 1989), a People's Medical Society book, there are more than 700 references cited from the medical literature. Interestingly, the editors questioned the need to provide references, thereby expressing a long-standing commercial publishing fear that references and citations scare away the general public. We held fast to our position that sources are important and that readers can make up their own minds about how to use the references. The book has been highly successful with the general public.

Public libraries, of course, offer the single greatest source of information to the public on matters of health and medicine. We have received thousands of requests from libraries not only for our publications, but also for ways of assisting their patrons by making medical and health information more useable or accessible. Some libraries have reorganized their health- and medical-related books, putting them into sections that are free-standing or self-contained. In 1983, the People's Medical Society published a booklet detailing how to start a People's Medical Library. With the assistance of individuals who had created small community collections of a wide range of medical books, we outlined the steps required to make such an entity a reality. To our surprise, the greatest request for the booklet came from public librarians. Many later reported using the booklet to help reorganize their own facilities. This has proven to be beneficial for both libraries and their users.

WHAT DID YOU SAY?

One of the dilemmas the medical consumer faces when trying to access medical and health information is medical jargon. The words of the trade are alien to most consumers. Even trying to look them up in a dictionary is difficult, since many of the terms and phrases are rooted in Latin or Greek. And even if the definition is found, trying to understand it is often a further excursion into medical confusion.

For example, we can only sympathize with the consumer who has been told that her spouse has suffered a myocardial infarction. Looking up "myocardial" will tell her it has something to do with the heart. But what does the definition of "infarct" mean: "a neocrotic area of tissue resulting from failure of local blood supply." If the doctor had merely said, "Your husband has had a heart attack," she would have immediately understood. If the dictionary had provided a simple definition, the problem would have been solved. If an easily accessible glossary of medical terminology written purposely for the consumer were in her home, considerable frustration could have been avoided. The point is simple: consumers are demanding easily understood and clear definitions of medical terminology.

THE FACTS . . . NOTHING BUT THE FACTS

Consumers are also seeking full disclosure. Today, we know virtually nothing about the hospitals and physicians that serve us. The small amount of information that is disclosed in published sources reveals virtually nothing that can help assess the quality of the services we receive. For example, studies show that being board certified or graduating from a highly respected medical school are not valid indicators of a practitioner's competence. The type of data that reveal competency, e.g., complication rates and number of procedures performed, is generally not in the public domain.

The clamor for outcome-based data about practitioners and hospitals is growing. It stems from both consumers and businesses who are paying for the services through corporate benefits programs. Both groups are seeking quality information so that maximum value is received from the vast expenditures on health care. Pennsylvania, responding to this demand from both businesses and consumers, passed a law (Act 89) in the late 1980s which established the Pennsylvania Health Care Cost Containment Council. But don't let the name fool you. While saving money on health care is the goal, the legislation, and now the Council itself, recognize that the primary means of saving money is through information, and that information takes a number of forms.

One form is merely cost comparing a procedure from hospital to hospital. Another way is to take the same data, factor in morbidity and mortality data, and make comparisons. Yet another way is to add the severity of the person's condition to the previous data to achieve further insight into quality.

In Pennsylvania, all of the above and much more is now being produced about every hospital and soon every practitioner. It will revolutionize the data the public has about hospitals, practitioners, and the health-care system in general. It is destined to spread across the nation. This will surely spark a medical data revolution that will benefit consumers. The demand for data will grow as the public becomes more sophisticated in its understanding and potential use of medical information.

EVEN A COMPUTER YOU CAN USE

Another major development that will surely aid the consumer in the coming years is information-based technology. Today, a consumer with a home computer can log on to databases with information that only medical personnel could access in the past. Consumer health organizations are already utilizing these databases and translating that information into understandable language for general consumer consumption.

On the horizon are even more exciting technological trends that consumers will be able to utilize. These trends will change forever the way medicine is practiced. They start with the computer. The advances now being made in computer technology and software development are phenomenal. The individual consumer using such technology will be able to wake up in the morning, type or call a symptom into their own personal computer, which will be immediately matched against the system's database and the person's individual medical record. The computer program, utilizing a "diagnostic" tree, will indicate a possible diagnosis, recommend steps that should be taken, professional services that can be accessed, medications that should be used or avoided, and more.

The September 16, 1985, issue of *The Wall Street Journal,* noting what was on the horizon, ran a feature article entitled "Computer Aided

Healing," which suggested the need for physicians to have computer-assisted decision support systems for diagnosis and treatment. The article went on to suggest that ultimately such diagnostic support could be put into the hands of consumers. Thus, the potential for consumer access to medical information has been known for quite a while, and it is unlimited. Much is already reality.

LEARNING FROM THE PAST—MAKING THE FUTURE

Clearly, the future of medicine will rest more and more in the consumer's hands. And, yet, as difficult as it may be to fully appreciate such a future, a look to the past shows that most health care has always been delivered by consumers themselves. It has been estimated that 85 percent of all health care is self-care, such as treating cuts and bruises, soothing a sore throat, and taping a sprain. Such self-cure constitutes the majority of the medical encounters we deal with over a lifetime. The 15 percent of the medical treatment that we seek from others is not only expensive, but exists primarily because most consumers do not have the expertise or training to deal with the problem. Yet, much of that expertise is now coming to us through technology. Today, consumers can take their blood pressure at home and test themselves for pregnancy and certain types of cancer. Each year, more and more "home" tests are coming to the marketplace that just a decade or two ago were only available in a physician's office or at a hospital. The technology of the future will give us the tools to be educated self-care practitioners.

Of course, trained practitioners and health-care facilities are not going to disappear. But, they will be different. They will primarily handle the more difficult and technologically sophisticated cases. Hospitals, whose case mix has already been drastically altered, will see the mix altered again as traditional acute-care facilities will only be used for longer term, complicated procedures. Nurses will be featured more prominently, not because of the growing shortage, but because of their new role as primary caregiver. Today, doctors are doing many things nurses can, should be, and eventually will be doing.

People with health-care needs will be congregating in living arrangements that can easily meet those needs. Such housing facilities are already beginning to appear with nurses on staff and physicians and allied health professionals on call. Home care will be a major site of medical care delivery. Like the old-fashioned house call, medical personnel will be assisting persons to cope with disabling and chronic conditions in their homes, thus avoiding costly hospitalization and unnecessary disruption of personal lifestyle. The late Claude Pepper was probably the nation's leading advocate for home-based care, realizing that medical facilities in and of themselves are not necessarily beneficial to the treatment of a person with a chronic or degenerative condition. His last piece of legislation, introduced just prior to his death in 1989, would have amended the Social Security Act to create a new section under Medicare that would have dealt strictly with home care.

INFORMATION . . . INFORMATION . . . INFORMATION

Real estate professionals say the smart investor must consider three things: location, location, and location. For the health-care consumer, three things are also necessary: information, information, and information. If the future is going to place more demands on the individual health-care customer, the need for knowledge and information will be paramount. The ability to find useful and easily understandable data about conditions, practitioners, facilities utilized, medications used, and all the matters associated with paying for such services must be present.

Consumers are already demanding information from their health-care providers. Doctors report that the number of patients asking questions is growing. They also note that the number of questions is growing per visit. Many people are now bringing a written list of questions to their medical appointments.

Some consumers, on the advice of consumer organizations, are setting up interview appointments with prospective practitioners. At these meetings, potential customers/patients are asking many probing questions not only about the background of the practitioner, but about his or her philosophy concerning certain treatment modalities. In other words, consumers are starting to do their homework.

The women's health movement helped open the doors to hospitals in certain ways. Now, most hospitals provide tours of maternity and delivery services for would-be parents. This type of activity is encouraged by birthing education organizations. Some hospitals are even marketing such "tours."

More such activities are going to occur as consumers become more active and involved in their own health care. Government will also be playing a larger role in helping the consumer use the system. Congress has mandated numerous studies into health-care services over the past few years, and each year they are authorizing more. The Health Care Financing Administration, the agency that runs Medicare, has an extensive Peer Review Program that annually inspects every participating hospital in the country. Other government agencies are looking at nursing homes, home-care programs, and health maintenance organizations to assess the quality and cost of medical services. Each of these studies and reviews culminates in written reports, many of which are now available to the public.

While most of these reports and studies are written in medical jargon, or are laden with statistics that go beyond the level of the average individual's understanding, consumer pressure is now being exerted to publish the information in language more understandable to the layperson.

IT CAN BE SO MUCH BETTER

But what about the advances of medicine itself? Have I intentionally ignored them? The art of medicine and the sciences supporting it will continue to progress. Each year new and more advanced technology and treatments arrive and will continue to do so. Some are beneficial, others are not. Some will last, others will disappear. Certain practitioners will hail a new procedure, treatment, or discovery, others will debunk it. But, in the course of time, only the informed and knowledgeable consumer will actually receive the full benefit.

Many consumers look at the current health-care system with skepticism and disgust. They are skeptical of all the claims made by medical hucksters and disgusted by the way they are often treated by health-care providers. A recent poll shows that public confidence in medical institutions has dropped from 73 percent to 33 percent in the last 30 years. Data published in medical journals also suggest that the quality of medicine is not all the public relations arm of organized medicine claims it to be. America, while the leader in numbers of physicians, medical services, and money spent, does not lead the world in health status. We do not have the longest life span, we lag in infant mortality, and we have higher rates of heart disease and cancer than many other countries.

Also, we suffer from very disturbing trends in medical delivery. Recent studies show that the quality of medical care varies from location to location within the country, even though medical education and services are relatively uniform. We see wide regional variations in outcomes which physicians say is "normal," but which other experts say is possibly bad medicine. These same regional studies also show a wide range of outcomes within a given region and even between hospitals located only blocks from one another and serving similar populations.

One recent study, reported by the Rand Corporation, demonstrated that the closer one lives to a high-volume medical center the more likely one is to lose an organ. The Rand report found that of those who lived near one of these centers, by age 20, 68 percent had their tonsils removed versus 6 percent for those who lived far from such facilities; by age 70, 75 percent of the women would have lost their uterus versus 20 percent who lived away; and, by age 80, 60 percent of the men would have lost their prostate versus 20 percent who lived away. As more such data become available, and more are published annually, consumers' needs for information and analysis services will continue to grow.

There is no question that the future of medicine and health care is going to be an exciting one. What physicians and hospitals do today will undoubtedly be obsolete in just a few years. Much of what we were doing in 1980 is already obsolete. Clearly, we are moving ahead at a breakneck pace. New discoveries and new technologies are announced almost daily. The speed itself makes it almost impossible for the provider to keep up with all that is new. Empowered consumers, persons who know where to turn to find the answers to their medical questions, will be increasingly prevalent in the future. Medical consumerism, now in its infancy, will blossom quickly.

While medicine may be the last bastion of nonconsumerism, the changes that we will see in the decades ahead will be so dramatic that health-care delivery in the early 1990s will look archaic. And while the future is exciting, the road will be bumpy, because both providers and consumers are not accustomed to it. But the die is cast. Medical consumerism is the wave of the future and, from this author's perspective, is arriving none too soon.

BIBLIOGRAPHY

Carver, Cynthia. *Patient Beware.* Scarborough, Ontario: Prentice-Hall, 1984.

Inlander, Charles B., Levin, Lowell, and Weiner, Ed. *Medicine on Trial.* New York: Pantheon Press, 1989.

Inlander, Charles B. and Pavalon, Eugene. *Your Medical Rights.* Boston: Little, Brown & Company, 1990.

Inlander, Charles B. and Weiner, Ed. *Take This Book to the Hospital with You: New and Revised.* New York: Pantheon Press, 1990.

Preston, Thomas. *The Clay Pedestal.* Seattle, WA: Madrona Publishers, 1981.

Starr, Paul. *The Social Transformation of American Medicine.* New York: Basic Books, 1982.

Thomas, Lewis. *The Youngest Science: Notes of a Medicine-Watcher.* New York: Viking Penguin, 1983.

CHAPTER 2
The Health-Activated, Health-Responsible Consumer

Tom Ferguson, M.D.

A TYPOLOGY OF MEDICAL CONSUMERS

Market researcher John Fiorillo of New York's Health Strategy Group has described three categories of health consumers:

- Passive patients
- Concerned consumers
- Health-active, health-responsible consumers

When I recently shared a podium with my old teacher, Yale cancer surgeon (and bestselling author) Bernie Siegel, I was fascinated to hear that he divides his cancer patients into the same three groups.

Passive Patients

These consumers regard their health with a grim resignation. They feel that there is little they can do to improve their health or to manage illness. When passive patients get cancer, they often give up without a fight.

"On some level they welcome their cancer as a way to escape their problems through death or disease," Siegel explains. He finds that when they get cancer, passive patients tend to deteriorate and die even more quickly than their physicians predict. As you might expect, passive patients rarely come to the library seeking health information.

Concerned Consumers

Concerned consumers are the "A-students" of medical practice. While they sometimes ask questions and may occasionally seek out a second opinion, they will almost always go along with whatever their doctor recommends. Concerned consumers see themselves as operating under the umbrella of the physician's authority.

Concerned consumers demonstrate childlike obedience, hanging on their physician's every word and rarely questioning their doctor's decisions. But concerned consumers may become overly dependent on their doctors. Thus while they may seek medical information, they will do so only if they feel their physician approves. In meeting the information needs of these consumers, librarians will do well to emphasize conservative resources: AMA publications, the *Harvard Medical School Health Letter,* the *Columbia University Complete Home Medical Guide,* and other official or quasi-official books and periodicals. And since concerned consumers are sometimes so intimidated by their physicians that they may never raise the questions that concern them the most, it is always a good idea to ask concerned consumers whether their physician ordered any medical tests or prescribed any drugs. You may then wish to suggest that they can become a more responsible patient and help their doctor by reading up on that drug or that test.

Concerned consumers respond to a diagnosis of cancer by becoming "model patients." Indeed, they sometimes act as if they were more interested in pleasing their doctor than with getting well. According to Siegel, concerned consumers are obedient to the end, living just about as long as their doctors predict.

Health-Active, Health-Responsible Consumers

These highly motivated men and women are determined to play an active role in their own health. They will not hesitate to disagree with their health advisors, and they frequently choose to explore alternative and holistic therapies. They will frequently express to librarians their frustration with their doctors. They understand that medical treatments involve substantial costs and hazards as well as potential benefits. If they are not satisfied with a doctor's recommendation, they may seek a second, third, or even a fourth or fifth opinion. These are the consumers who will benefit most from a consumer health information library, such as the one pioneered by San Francisco's Planetree Health Resource Center (*see* Chapter 13).

The publications they will find most useful fall into several categories:

- Materials produced by self-help groups, (e.g., Alcoholics Anonymous), consumer advocacy groups, (e.g., People's Medical Society), and self-help clearinghouses (e.g., the National Alliance for the Mentally Ill, The National Self-Help Clearinghouse).
- Medical textbooks written for the primary practitioner (e.g., *Current Medical Diagnosis and Treatment* and others in the Lange series).
- Popular health and psychology books (e.g., *The AMA Family Medical Guide; The Road Less Traveled;* and *Love, Medicine, and Miracles.*)
- Alternative periodicals (e.g., *Yoga Journal; New Age; East-West Journal;* and *Medical Self-Care*).

When faced with a health problem, they will frequently search out additional information, ask the advice of their more experienced friends, consult an alternative practitioner, or simply wait and watch.

These consumers refuse to play the victim, even when they discover that they have cancer. They regard their diagnoses as a provocative challenge, as an invitation to examine their lives. When they or a family member develops an illness, they will read anything that might help them get well again. These are the most enthusiastic and tireless seekers of health information.

They do not share the concerned consumer's self-imposed limitations. Indeed, they refuse to relinquish control of the key decisions having to do with their own care. They express their emotions freely, ask lots of questions, and do not hesitate to question their physicians' suggestions or to criticize their physicians' actions. But it would be a mistake to assume that these individuals are "anti-doctor." "They question the doctor because they want to understand their treatment and participate in it," Siegel explains. "And they demand dignity, personhood, and control no matter what the course of the disease."

The characteristics of these three types of medical consumers are listed in Table 2-1.

TABLE 2-1: Three Kinds of Medical Consumers

	Response to Illness	*Clinicians See Them As*	*Outcomes*
Passive Patients	Resignation	Unmotivated	Worst
Concerned Consumers	Obedience	Cooperative but overly dependent	Average
Health-Active, Health-Responsible Consumers	Intense self-directed involvement	Motivated and demanding	Best

And while the numbers of passive patients are on the decrease, those of the other two groups are on the increase, as illustrated in Table 2–2.

TABLE 2-2: Three Kinds of Medical Consumers: Numbers

	1975	*1987–88*	*2000*
Passive Patients	85–95%	55–65%	30–40%
Concerned Consumers	5–10%	30–35%	40–50%
Health-Active, Health-Responsible Consumers	1–2%	5–8%	20–25%

Source: Health Strategy Group, New York.

MEDICAL CONSUMERS AND CLINICAL NEGOTIATION

While passive patients and concerned consumers come to the doctor's office prepared to follow "doctor's orders," health-active, health-responsible persons prefer to use their physician as a consultant. They want their physician to join with them in a joint process of *clinical negotiation,* in which health professional and client take turns stating their opinions and preferences. Each has a chance to hear and respond to the other's point of view. The discussion continues until both parties agree on a proposed course of action.

Today's sophisticated medical consumers can almost instantly tell when a physician is *not* open to clinical negotiation. Such physicians act as if their time is precious. They look hostile if anything they say is challenged. They interrupt their clients constantly, while refusing to let themselves be interrupted. They may dismiss a client's heartfelt questions with "Let me worry about that," or "You needn't concern yourself with that." Physicians who bypass the negotiation process and rely on moral authority, intimidation, or other manipulative techniques may not see the health-active, health-responsible consumer a second time.

Physicians skilled in the art of clinical negotiation will invite their clients to join them in an atmosphere of privacy and comfort, without distracting interruptions. They listen to their clients carefully and will respond directly—both to spoken and to implied questions. They make every effort to make the client feel trusted, respected, and valued. As the proportion of health-active, health-responsible consumers increases, clinical negotiation will gradually replace authoritarian pronouncements as the new standard of physician-client communications.

THE PATIENT AS HERO

Probably the most famous health-active, health-responsible consumer is Norman Cousins, who has described his medical experiences in such books as *Anatomy of an Illness, The Healing Heart,* and *Head First: The Biology of Hope.* Cousins started a revolution by making himself the hero of the medical drama. Ten years ago it was very difficult to chart your own course through the medical world. It is now becoming much easier. Progressive health workers are encouraging their clients to take higher levels of self-responsibility, and a variety of new medical institutions are springing up to support this new, competent medical consumer. Some examples of this trend are described below.

Planetree's Patient-Centered Hospital

You are on the second floor of a modern medical center, but you would never know it. The Planetree Model Hospital Unit does not feel, look, or sound like a hospital. Classical music plays softly in the background. Patients wear their own robes and pajamas, sleep on flowered sheets, and are encouraged to sleep in as long as they like.

There is no nurse's station; it has been replaced by a convenient study area where patients are encouraged to read and write in their own charts. There are no visiting hours; friends and family are welcome at all times. Family members cook for their ailing loved ones in a special patients' kitchen. Interested family members are trained to serve as active care partners, changing dressings, flushing out permanent IV lines, and performing other vital nursing services. Family members who learn these techniques in the hospital can continue them at home after the patient is discharged.

At the Planetree Model Unit, it is clear from the very beginning that things are arranged for the convenience of the patient, not the medical staff. The patient-centered model is spreading. Planetree recently opened its second site at the San Jose Medical Center. A nurse on the Unit explains why: "Once patients get a taste of the Planetree model, they simply won't permit themselves to be admitted anywhere else."

The Commonweal Cancer Help Program

This is a program for people with cancer who are receiving the best of available medical care but want to do something more. Founder and director Michael Lerner, the recent recipient of a MacArthur Foundation "genius" grant, used the fellowship to visit 30 of the world's best-known alternative cancer treatment centers. He returned from his research convinced that a common characteristic of many of the best centers was a high concentration of health-active, health-responsible patients seeking to integrate the best of conventional and alternative cancer therapies.

Lerner and his colleagues at the Commonweal Cancer Help Program now offer a week-long seminar eight times a year at Commonweal's rural, coastal retreat center in Bolinas, California, one hour north of San Francisco. Participants are invited to involve themselves in imagery, meditation, gentle yoga stretching, vegetarian diet, massage, art therapy, guided support groups, and classes on informed choice in both conventional and alternative cancer therapies.

Participants are encouraged to develop their own highly personalized approaches to recovery, which often include elements of a psychological or spiritual quest. Goals for healing that emerge from the program may include changes in diet, lifestyle, relationships, living arrangements, or work. Participants often report that as a result of the seminar they are able to develop a less frightening and more hopeful relationship with their illness. As one recent participant commented: "The retreat experience was one of the richest experiences of my life. I learned to see healing in a whole new way: as an effort to discover who we really are."

The New Jersey Self-Help Clearinghouse

This clearinghouse was originally set up as a telephone switchboard to help New Jersey residents find local self-help groups in their areas of concern. Over the past several years, it has become something more.

Edward J. Madara, the Clearinghouse's director, has become a leader in the movement to help interested people start their own self-help groups.

Callers on the Clearinghouse's helpline are given information about the specific groups in their area. If there is no group in their area of interest, the Clearinghouse helps callers find like-minded people in the same community and consults with them to help them establish their own mutual support group. The Clearinghouse staff and volunteers have been responsible for the formation of an estimated 550 new groups over the past eight years. The Clearinghouse also publishes the best national directory of self-help groups (*Self-Help Source Book, 1988–1989,* $8.00, 2nd ed., 123 p.). The free brochure, *Ideas and Considerations for Starting a Self-Help Group* is available on request from the Clearinghouse at St. Claire's-Riverside Hospital, Pocono Road, Denville, NJ 07834.

A MEDICAL REFORMATION

The health-active, health-responsible consumer is leading us into a sort of medical reformation which has a great deal in common with the religious reformation of the sixteenth century. Before Martin Luther's time, the Catholic Church dominated religion, and it was considered unthinkable for an individual to have his or her own religious opinions. Luther and his contemporaries decided that priests did not possess a monopoly on religious knowledge and that motivated individuals were capable of making their own religious choices.

Today, nearly 450 years later, health-active, health-responsible individuals are proving that doctors do not have a monopoly on health knowledge. These confident, assertive, informed health consumers are changing health care by demanding a more active role. Medical librarians can learn a great deal from them.

Where do we go from here? Looking into my crystal ball I see several important trends:

- **Encouraging Innovation, Responsibility, and Frugality in Health Care.** We must develop new ways of financing health care that provide us all with built-in incentives to keep ourselves healthy, manage our own illness problems, and raise health-responsible children. This may include health IRAs, a medical voucher system, or a shift from licensing individuals to licensing health-care institutions.
- **The Health Information Explosion with More and More Health Information Becoming Available.** There will be an increasing need for experts: writers, teachers, and advisors who can identify areas of great promise and who will work with other experts to process data into consumer-accessible, consumer-digestable knowledge. (Our company, Self-Care Productions, attempts to do exactly this. Please write or call for a listing of our present and future publications: Self-Care Productions, 3805 Stevenson Avenue, Austin, TX 78703, (512) 472-1333. We would also welcome your suggestions

of the most-needed publications for the intelligent health consumer.)

- **The Self-Care Computer.** The explosive growth of microprocessors and communications networks will open up new ways for people to take care of themselves through on-line self-help groups, psychological software, health by 800- and 900-numbers, and voice-interactive health information on demand. Over the coming decades, we will develop new forms of health media that we can now only dimly imagine.

A CASE STUDY OF THE HEALTH-ACTIVE, HEALTH-RESPONSIBLE CONSUMER

I would like to conclude this chapter by telling you about a very special friend of mine. Three years ago, at age 70, Helen developed mysterious pains in her legs and shoulders. She visited her doctor and accepted without question the prescription he gave her. The drug produced unpleasant side effects. Her doctor substituted another medicine, which produced a different set of side effects. A third drug produced similar results—some relief, accompanied by annoying side effects. After three months of medical treatment, Helen's condition was still undiagnosed, although her pain was markedly reduced. Her medical expenses for that period were: doctor's visits, $215; medical tests, $92; and drugs, $86, for a total of $393.

Earlier this year the pain returned. But by this time Helen resolved not to leave things totally up to the doctor. She was ready to take her health care into her own hands. She began, again, by visiting her physician. "We're *still* not sure exactly what it is," he told her. But when he reached for his prescription pad, Helen held up her hand to stop him. "Please write down what my choices are," she told him. "I want to consider *all* my options."

Her doctor wrote down the names of three drugs, the same three she had taken before. Helen went to her local hospital library and read up on each of them. She was surprised to learn that high-dose aspirin often produced equal results at considerably less cost and with fewer side effects. She began treating herself with aspirin.

A friend suggested acupuncture. She visited an acupuncturist and had a short course of treatments, with good results. However, the improvement lasted only a few days after each treatment. She subscribed to two health magazines and began taking a multiple vitamin/mineral insurance formula. A friend from church loaned her a relaxation/healing tape. She listened to it every night at bedtime. It eased the pain and helped her to sleep.

At a friend's suggestion, Helen began an early morning exercise class at the local municipal swimming pool, and this seemed to help. She ordered a book on rheumatism and an information packet on rheumatic conditions from a consumer health information center. Another friend recommended a heating pad that supplied moist heat. Helen found it extremely helpful. This time her medical expenses were: physician's visits, $45; acupuncturist, $60; aspirin, $4; self-care information (three books, two magazine subscriptions, one information packet, one cassette tape), $71; self-care tools (heating pad), $36; for a total of $216.

At the end of three months her symptoms had improved remarkably, and Helen had become a health-active, health-responsible consumer. Helen's experience reinforced my sense of the rapid and important changes that are currently taking place in our health-care system. Helen Ferguson is my mother.

CHAPTER 3
Medical Consumerism: Library Roles and Initiatives

Alan M. Rees

CONSUMERS AND HEALTH INFORMATION

The information needs of medical consumers must be viewed within the context of the total national health-care system. In the United States, medical consumers have been forced by the system to assume a greater role in personal decision making than, for example, in Australia or the United Kingdom. The American consumer has the additional burden of making judicious decisions in regard to costs, access, and quality of health care. In many other countries, medical consumers have very limited choices with respect to when, where, and how often they receive health care. Moreover, individuals in those countries have little control over cost or quality since these are governmental rather than personal responsibilities.

A prominent feature of contemporary American society is the element of choice. While in many ways desirable, this can be onerous. The existence of more than 100 VCR models, 150 types of breakfast cereal, 50 kinds of toothpaste, and 30 brands of dogfood forces consumers to study labels and prices in order to make intelligent and cost-conscious choices. Similarly in health care, multiple choices confront the consumer. In Chapter 1 Charles Inlander points to the existence of free-standing surgi-centers, emergi-centers, and outpatient facilities, all of which provide specialized services, and argues that the consumer must also choose between a private doctor, group practice, HMO, PPO, and a host of other agencies providing some form of health care. He concludes that never before have health-care consumers "needed, or felt they needed, to have as much health care information as they have now." Dr. Louis W. Sullivan,[1] Secretary of Health and Human Services, makes the same point, "We need to move toward equal health opportunity for our citizens, including the good health information and the family and community support that will help every American make the right choices for healthy and productive lives."

Another element of medical consumerism relates to widespread dissatisfaction with the present health-care system. A recent Louis Harris/Harvard School of Public Health survey showed that while Americans are reasonably satisfied with the quality of health care, they are highly dissatisfied with both access and cost.[2] This discontent stems from the high cost of health care; the excessive amount of dollars consumed by bureaucracy (marketeers, advertisers, public relations specialists, utilization review managers); the amount of unnecessary, inappropriate, and marginal care given patients; and the inequities in access demonstrated by 31 million Americans without health insurance.

Yet another concern is related to the quality of health care. Consumers have good reason to be concerned. A recent Harvard Medical School study of 31,000 patients hospitalized in New York State in 1984 revealed that 3.7 percent experienced injury that was the result of medical intervention and not of the underlying disease. In about 1.7 percent of patients, an injury was caused by medical negligence and sometimes resulted in permanent disability or death. Peter Miloch, general counsel of the New York State Health Department, argues that "consumers of health have a right to know as much about their doctors as they know about the products they buy at Grand Union or Sears."[3] The Public Citizen Health Research Group[4] insists that consumers need to know the "very real differences between hospitals and physicians, in terms of deaths, injuries, and other medical statistics."

Medical consumerism is also driven by the notion that more individual responsibility is desirable and necessary. Much of contemporary disease and disability can be avoided by preventive measures. Improved self-care and personal responsibility can significantly reduce the incidence of heart disease, cancer, and other diseases. This requires access to relevant and accurate information, with the result that many consumers actively seek reliable information on nutrition, exercise, weight control, and other preventive practices.

It is, of course, simplistic to think in terms of "generic" medical consumers. Tom Ferguson suggests a typology of consumers—passive patients; concerned consumers; and health-active, health-responsible persons. He argues that the number of health-active, health-responsible persons is growing. These are the people who are determined to play an active role in their own health. These are the people who express frustration with their doctors, scrutinize the qualifications of their physicians, inquire about hospital mortality rates, question their doctors, demand to see their medical records, explore alternative therapies, and seek second opinions. They are also active seekers of information and heavy library users.

Today's medical consumer seeks information for a variety of reasons: to determine what is wrong and how serious it is; to seek reassurance that a diagnosis is accurate and that the recommended treatment is most appropriate; to investigate alternative treatments; to explore the ramifications of treatment in terms of future lifestyle; to seek information on topics that lie outside of a physician's specialty; to confirm that a medical problem is incurable or untreatable; to find a consultant or specialist; to check qualifications; and so on. No longer is a physician the sole conduit for the dissemination of medical information.

Rya Ben-Shir offers in Chapter 9 an alternative to Ferguson's classification of medical consumers; she categorizes those with "the terrible diagnosis," problem and repeat callers, confused and rambling callers, persons contemplating lawsuits, and practical jokers. Although considerable humor underlies such a typology, there is an implicit reality and Ben-Shir gives some fascinating examples of such users. Health has become a preoccupation and consumers pursue health for many different reasons.

EVOLUTION OF THE LIBRARY RESPONSE

The library response to the growing demand for consumer health information has evolved over the past decade. Beginning in the mid-1970s, under the leadership of medical librarians such as Eleanor Goodchild and Ellen Gartenfeld, libraries became increasingly involved in providing organized health information services to the general public. The earliest initiative came from a small cadre of medical librarians who perceived the need to create more extensive health information services for the community. While health professionals had ready access to a multiplicity of health information products and services, members of the public requiring medical information were forced to accept whatever was available through their local public libraries. In general, both medical school and hospital libraries denied access to nonprofessional users. It was evident, however, that public libraries had neither adequate resources nor trained staff to respond to the full range of information requests.

The earliest funding for making medical information more available to the general public came through a series of Library Services and Construction Act (LSCA) grants provided by state libraries in the late 1970s and early 1980s in California, Nebraska, Massachusetts, Ohio, Illinois, Connecticut, and Pennsylvania. Typically, these grants involved a cooperative effort on the part of medical and public libraries. The funding provided support for the preparation of lists of recommended materials, development of model collections and purchase of materials to improve library collections, formulation of reference guidelines, provision of backup reference services, conduct of training workshops, creation of linkages with health organizations in the community, sponsorship of Tel-Med (dial-up recordings of medical information), organization of health fairs, sponsorship of health education programs in library community rooms, and development of multi-type library networking.

LSCA funding also resulted in a refinement and definition of the library role in providing health information to the community. The LSCA demonstration grants produced a clearer identification of both the nature and extent of health information needs in the general community. Library staff became sensitized to the need to improve health information services. To improve collections, recommended lists of quality materials were compiled to supplement the resources available in many library settings and substantial sums of money were spent in collection improvement. These purchases reflected well-defined criteria. Grant support also led to a definition of a realistic library role in offering extended information services. As Andrea Kenyon notes in Chapter 8, LSCA programs legitimized the dissemination of health information to the public. A clear differentiation was made between medical information and medical advice and most librarians became more confident and comfortable in providing health information services. Above all, it was recognized that no one type of library could be responsive to information needs. Consequently, networking arrangements were established to provide the pooling of abilities and resources necessary for delivering health information services to the community.

Multi-Type Library Involvement

Five major types of libraries are now involved in Consumer Health Information (CHI) services: *academic medical centers*—for example, at the Universities of Connecticut, Miami, and Nebraska; *medical society libraries*—the New York Academy of Medicine and the College of Physicians of Philadelphia; *public libraries*—King County Public Library System (Seattle); *hospital libraries*—Overlook Hospital, (Summit, NJ), MacNeal Hospital (Berwyn, IL), Swedish Medical Center and St. Joseph Hospital (Denver); and *special libraries*—Planetree in San Francisco, the Health Education Center in Pittsburgh, and, in the federal sector, Veterans Administration libraries such as the one at Tampa.

In all these types of libraries, the information services provided are similar. Differences do exist, however, with respect to the motivation for making such services available and the conditions and limitations under which services are provided. By and large, academic medical centers, especially those supported by state funds, provide CHI as a public service to the community. The principal objective has been to provide educational and consultation support to nonhealth sciences libraries which would enable them to deliver enhanced services at the local level. One medical school devotes resources to providing lay health information to friends of the library, alumni, and medical center benefactors, in addition to the community at large. Hospitals have launched CHI services to provide a community service, to improve their public relations, and to assist the marketing activity in their institutions. An investment is made in CHI services to extend market penetration and increase market share.

The information service delivery model universally adopted defines public libraries as the prime service agent, while supportive services are provided by medical libraries. The supportive services are supplied in some instances by a statewide source such as in Pennsylvania, Nebraska, and Connecticut, or on a local basis such as at MacNeal Hospital, where the HealthAnswers program provides reference services to patrons of 12 public libraries in the Hospital's target market area. Overlook Hospital in Summit, New Jersey, provides under contract supplemental and referral services to libraries in two neighboring counties. In Seattle, the King County Consumer Health Information Network (KCCHIN) links two public library systems (King County and Seattle Public) with an academic health sciences library (University of Washington Health Sciences Library), and 18 hospital libraries (members of the Seattle Area Hospital Library Consortium).

The Health Education Center in Pittsburgh is a unique library service. The Center, now an affiliate of Blue Cross of Western Pennsylvania, makes library services available to the more than 2.7 million Blue Cross subscribers. The emphasis is on health promotion, disease prevention, risk reduction, and the dissemination of information as a catalyst for healthy behavior. Lois Michaels describes in Chapter 14 Tel-Aid (a dial access health information system) and the Consumer Health Library as component elements of HealthPLACE, a health education and information resource for consumers. The Consumer Health Library provides information services to health professionals, students, teachers, and the lay public. Services offered include telephone reference, interlibrary loans, audiovisual lending, and on-site usage of the Library's collection.

THE DEMAND FOR HEALTH INFORMATION

The basis of the library response lies in the attempt to cater to a perceived demand for health information in the community. There is a dearth of data that measures the extent of the popular demand for health information. Anecdotal evidence indicates that between 5 and 10 percent of all reference requests in public libraries are health-related. Joanne Marshall,[5] in her excellent study of consumer health information services public libraries in Ontario, estimates that 8 percent of all reference requests are health-related. The data gathered by the libraries represented in this volume indicate that a large demand exists for disease-related and drug information together with information required for coping with chronic disease. Marshall reports that a mean of 41 percent of questions received by the public libraries studied in Ontario related to disease or treatment, while a mean of 23.9 percent related to health promotion and prevention. Moira Bryant notes that for Health Link at Westmead Hospital in Australia, 59 percent of a total of 14,468 specific requests were classed as "information for coping with an illness," while 41 percent were categorized as "information for a healthier lifestyle." Ralph Arcari and Alberta Richetelle note that of a total of 99 questions referred to Healthnet in a one-year period, 54 related to diseases and syndromes and 18 to treatments and surgery. Marie Reidelbach et al., in their study of users of the CHIRS program in Nebraska, found that 92 percent of the respondents were "seeking information about a disease, treatment, diagnosis, drug, or outcome of a condition or treatment." Most consumers appear to be more interested in diseases and treatment than in wellness and prevention.

Typical topics requested have been identified by a number of the programs. The "top ten" topics identified by Bryant—cholesterol, cancer, diabetes, nutrition, coronary heart disease, stress management, pregnancy/childbirth, weight reduction, stroke, and arthritis—do not differ significantly from similar lists reported by other programs. Kenyon cites examples of specific topics such as Alzheimer's disease, balloon angioplasty, and sex predetermination.

However, in recent years the number of information requests related to quality, cost, and access information has increased. Persons want to know more about the qualifications of medical providers; hospital mortality rates, and other indicators of quality; comparative costs of medical services and alternate modes of financing health care, such as HMOs and PPOs; health insurance; and Medicaid and Medicare.

INTERNATIONAL SIMILARITIES AND DIFFERENCES IN CHI SERVICES

There is also a commonality of interests on the part of Australian, Canadian, British, Kiwi (New Zealand), and American users. Despite differences in the health-care systems, library users require similar kinds of information. The major difference in information usage relates to the growing American preoccupation with quality, cost, and access to health care. Such concerns are not relevant to most users in those countries where there is a nationalized or semi-nationalized health service. The authors of the chapters on CHI in countries outside of the United States provide some illuminating commentary on such differences.

The problems faced by consumers in Australia, New Zealand, and the United Kingdom relate more to the frustrations imposed by limited availability of high technology equipment and procedures, the long distances that must be travelled for treatment at regional or national centers, restrictions on access to specialists imposed by general physician gate-keepers, long waiting lists for elective procedures, and a medical establishment experiencing considerable difficulty in adjusting to shared decision making with more militant and demanding patients.

Bryant notes that in Australia there is still a low level of complaints against doctors. Information needs relate usually to information that is useful in improving health, understanding an illness and its treatment, or coping with chronic conditions. Similarly, Robert Gann observes that only recently have British patients started to behave like empowered health consumers. There is still no legal basis to informed consent in Great Britain. However, the recent White Paper, *Working for Patients,* recommends the introduction of limited competitive market forces into the National Health Service. The British White Paper outlines a program of action with two objectives: to give patients better health care and greater choice of the services available; and to produce greater satisfaction and rewards for National Health Service staff who successfully respond to local needs and preferences.[6]

Jill Harris provides evidence for an increasing demand for health information in New Zealand and a willingness on the part of the public and medical librarians to respond. Lack of financial resources within the government-run New Zealand health-care system and a large measure of what appears to be ambivalence on the part of the medical establishment have limited the development of CHI services in New Zealand. There is a lingering suspicion that what works in the U.S. or the U.K. will not necessarily be applicable in New Zealand.

PROBLEMS IN DELIVERING CONSUMER HEALTH INFORMATION SERVICES

The response by libraries has been limited by a number of factors. Marshall, in her survey of public libraries in Ontario, pinpoints a number of problems reported by library staff in responding to patrons' questions. These include patrons presenting an incomplete or unclear query, library does not own the source, librarian fears about giving a wrong answer or advice, librarian is unsure about conflicting sources, and so on.[7]

The major problems encountered in a number of libraries appear to be:

1. Difficulties of specialized medical terminology
2. Problems in evaluating quality materials for purchase
3. Difficulties in defining what is authoritative medical information
4. Limitations of staff expertise in handling health information requests
5. Absence of reference guidelines in dealing with health requests
6. Constraints in terms of staff time available to respond to reference requests
7. Restrictions in budget for the purchase of specialized reference materials
8. Unreasonable patron expectations regarding what can be provided
9. Threats of censorship in the hospital library setting
10. Patron confusion over the librarian's role

1. Difficulties of Specialized Medical Terminology

This has produced problems for public librarians who have had to learn a specialized vocabulary. One solution has been to hire a medical librarian to handle reference requests. This has been possible in large library systems but is not feasible in smaller libraries. Hospital and academic medical librarians have the advantage of knowing the vocabulary and the specialized reference collections in this area. Limitations in terminology do not, however, appear to have been an insurmountable problem.

2. Problems in Evaluating Quality Materials for Purchase

The difficulty of sifting through the morass of popular medical publications to separate the accurate and reliable from the ephemeral and the trash is well known. The basic problem is not, however, discriminating between the obviously valuable and the evident trash at two extreme ends of a spectrum but rather evaluating materials in the gray area in between. Many popular medical books are authored by persons who have no evident qualifications and the publishers are often equally unknown. Most libraries have created criteria for dealing with such publications. The cost of selection errors varies from a mere $19.95 for a popular medical book to more than $150 for a specialized medical text. Selection problems and criteria are discussed in more detail in Chapter 17.

Considerable assistance has been extended to improve collections through the development of subject bibliographies and lists of recommended medical reference materials. Topical bibliographies on subjects such as AIDS, cancer, mental health, and nutrition have been compiled, for example, by Healthnet, CHIRS, and the College of Physicians of Philadelphia. Claudia Perry, Ralph Arcari and Alberta Richetelle, and Mary Campbell and Kay Johnson include lists of recommended reference publications as appendixes to their chapters in this volume.

3. Difficulties in Defining What Is Authoritative Medical Information

Many readers are engaged in the quest for certainty. They seek definitive and authoritative information on which they can rely for decision-making purposes. Unfortunately, in science and medicine one deals with probability and not certainty. There is no one definitive treatment or one best drug for many diseases and conditions. On many medical topics there is no clear consensus. Many users are disturbed by conflicting evidence and published opinion on issues such as the treatment of breast cancer or cholesterol. There can be no one "best" book on premenstrual syndrome or nutrition.

4. Limitations of Staff Expertise in Handling Health Information Requests

Many staff members are uncomfortable in responding to health requests and lack the depth of knowledge of the terminology and content of medicine to enable them to deal with many health-related questions. Moreover, many requests deal with highly personal and often emotionally charged topics. Embarrassment and discomfort often ensue. Training programs have focussed attention on methods of dealing with confused, distraught, or angry patrons. The training video in the form of a trigger tape produced by the King County Library brilliantly illustrates such problems by means of simulated scenarios at the reference desk and suggests sensitive ways of responding.

5. Absence of Reference Guidelines in Dealing with Health Requests

Considerable progress has been made in establishing adequate guidelines. Specific guidance has been given with respect to reference interviewing techniques, question negotiation, matching the level of the requester to available resources, use of indexing and abstracting services and specialized reference materials, and bibliographic instructional techniques. Perry in Chapter 18 summarizes the essential points involved and offers helpful guidelines in dealing with a wide variety of users and information requests. Arcari and Richetelle provide in Chapter 4 a set of 11 specific guidelines, including question clarification, conducting reference interviews, checking terms in a medical dictionary, avoiding diagnosis, and making referrals. Likewise, Tracey Cosgrove in Chapter 13 lists seven basic interview questions to ask of patrons.

6. Constraints in Terms of Staff Time Available to Respond to Reference Requests

Responding to medical information requests can be most time-consuming. Consequently, some type of control must be exercised to limit the amount of time. In many public libraries, this problem is solved by fitting health information requests into the same policy guidelines as other types of requests. The amount of staff time required in an academic medical center or medical society library to respond to referrals can be considerable and special funding has been secured to free the necessary staff time. In Pennsylvania, at the College of Physicians of Philadelphia, an annual appropriation of $100,000 from the state allows the staff to respond to requests from some 756 state-supported libraries, answer more than 500 questions each year, and fill more than 2,000 document requests. Similarly, in Nebraska the McGoogan Library of Medicine at the University of Nebraska answers some 360 requests and provides photocopies of about 1,703 articles each year. The New York Academy of Medicine has been offering telephone service to the public in New York City and has responded to as many as 18,000 requests in one year. Since no external funding exists, it is not surprising that the decision has been made to curtail this service.

7. Restrictions in Budget for the Purchase of Specialized Reference Materials

The cost of acquisition is not particularly burdensome with respect to popular medical materials. However, the average cost of a professional medical book in 1989 was $80.87, while the average cost of a journal subscription was $102.[8] In many instances, textbooks, such as the *Cecil Textbook of Medicine,* can cost as much as $125. Consequently, there is a severe limitation in the purchase of such professional-level materials. Several excellent lists of recommended purchases have been compiled by Arcari and Richetelle, Perry, and others.

8. Unreasonable Patron Expectations Regarding What Can Be Provided

As Perry aptly points out in Chapter 18, "Most health information consumers do not know the medical literature or the tools to use it effectively . . . few, if any, have the ability to think in terms of, or derive meaning from, statistical probabilities, ranges of normal values . . . . and very few individuals seem to grasp the concept that a wide range of factors combine to produce unique health situations for unique individuals possessing the same general problem." In short, many users want simple answers to complex questions, and they expect the answers during a quick trip to the library during the lunch hour. This lack of realism forces library staff to explain what can reasonably be expected.

9. Threats of Censorship in the Hospital Library Setting

In some hospital settings, pressure exists from the medical staff to review and approve purchases of materials for the patients' library. This has been stoutly resisted and there are few reported cases of such intimidation. However, close attention is usually paid to acquiring only those materials that fall within the medical mainstream. Very few alternative medicine publications are purchased for hospital libraries. Such materials are more likely to be found in public libraries or at Planetree (*see* Chapter 13), where particular attention is paid to extending the range of choice available to library users.

10. Patron Confusion over the Librarian's Role

It is not surprising that many lay users do not clearly understand the librarian's role in providing health information in view of the fact that many librarians have an incomplete comprehension of their own role. The line between information dispenser and information interpreter is somewhat blurred and it is often difficult to spell out clearly the limitations imposed by law on what a librarian can do with information. Many users expect active assistance in applying information to self-diagnosis. Confronted by difficult and complex choices in terms of treatment options, users wish to engage the librarian in personal decision making. Considerable frustration ensues in this connection when the librarian explains that this is not possible.

The role and professional responsibilities of librarians in delivering CHI services is well defined by August La Rocco in Chapter 6. He offers a checklist of valuable prerequisites or performance standards that should dominate the role of CHI staff. These include being cognizant of findings and developments across the entire spectrum of medicine; designing strategies for optimal collection development; being conversant with the latest technologies in information transfer; acquiring capabilities in the marketing of information; establishing community linkages with other health information agencies; and conceptualizing the flow of health information in terms of a triage structure where smaller libraries can turn to larger libraries for information they lack.

CONSUMER HEALTH INFORMATION AND PATIENT EDUCATION

It is important to conceptualize the difference between consumer health information and patient education. *Consumer health information* is information on health and medical topics that is relevant and appropriate to the general public. By way of contrast, *patient education* is the process of influencing patient behavior to produce changes in knowledge, attitudes, and skills calculated to maintain and improve health. In this manner, patient education has defined behavioral objectives such as smoking cessation and obesity control, while the behavioral change resulting from the educational intervention is usually measurable. Library services do not have defined and measurable behavioral objectives. Although there is a clear distinction between simply supplying information and producing behavioral change, the informational materials used are often identical. Information is a necessary but not sufficient ingredient in patient care.

This interface between consumer health information services and patient education has been creatively explored and developed within the Veterans Administration Library System (VALNET). The Patient Health Education (PHE) Program of the VA has seven regional PHE coordinators who serve as consultants to the 46 facilities with local PHE coordinators. At the local level, the PHE coordinators, as Iris Renner and Janet Schneider explain in Chapter 16, enjoy "a collegial relationship with the librarians identifying, providing, and disseminating information and educational resources while the PHE coordinators develop and teach others how to develop high quality PHE programs." Renner and Schneider explain their role in the management of the Patient Education Resource Center (PERC) established at the Tampa VA library. PERCs contain classrooms and areas within the library for viewing audiovisual programs at individual study carrels.

This innovative library role within the VA involves the broadcasting of patient education videos through the hospital's closed-circuit television system, and the acquisition of books, audiovisual hardware, software, and anatomical models. Specifically, the hospital librarian has forged clearly defined roles: as resource provider to both patient educators and patients, as member of the patient education committee, as liaison with medical center staff who need to contact the committee, as reality orientation group leader helping patients prepare for discharge, as developer of patient communication skills, as closed-circuit television system coordinator, as publicity manager for PE programs, and as editor of a quarterly newsletter distributed to patients by the PE committee.

The major thrust of CHI activity seems to have shifted in recent years from the public library to the hospital setting. Most public libraries have over the past decade incorporated health information services to consumers into their routine reference operations. In this connection, LSCA grant support has been highly successful. In the hospital setting, a significant increase can be observed in the number of libraries now involved in providing information services to patients, their families, and the general community. This growing interest in CHI on the part of hospitals stems from two factors: the potential impact of community health information services on hospital marketing, as described by Ben-Shir; and as an adjunct activity to patient education. Sandra Parker describes such cooperative endeavors with patient and nursing educators at Swedish Medical Center, while Kathleen Moeller refers to her cooperative activity with the director of community health education. Margaret Bandy outlines in detail the drafting of a successful proposal to the St. Joseph Hospital administration as a result of a cooperative effort between the medical librarian and the patient education coordinator. Their joint proposal quoted from the AHA Policy and Statement on the Hospital's Responsibility for Patient Education: "patient education/information services (should) be provided as an integral part of care to assist patients in making informed decisions about their use of health care services, managing their illnesses and implementing follow-up care."

The development of cooperative activity between medical librarians and patient educators along the lines described by Bandy, Parker, Moeller, and Renner and Schneider in this volume is likely to increase. It can be argued that providing health information service to patients and their families, and to the community at large, is central to the mission of the parent institution (the hospital) and critical to the future of the library. Moeller cogently comments that "adding consumer health information services is one of the best survival strategies for hospital libraries."

THE FUTURE

In the near future, the resources available to libraries for delivering CHI services will be improved and extended. A number of relevant online services already exist: the Combined Health Information Database (CHID), PDQI (Physician Data Query Patient Information File) of the National Cancer Institute, and the Consumer Drug Information Database of the American Society of Hospital Pharmacists. In addition, menu-driven CD-ROM versions of Medline are now available for end-user searching by consumers. *The Consumer Health and Nutrition Index* is a quarterly publication that offers relatively inexpensive access ($89.50 annual subscription) to some 90 popular health magazines and newsletters.

Health Index Plus recently introduced by Information Access Company (IAC) supplies on compact disc the indexing of core health publications including professional journals, consumer magazines, and newsletters together with the full text of some 80 titles. The cost of a basic subscription to *Health Index Plus,* with hardware and 12 monthly updates, is $6,000 per year. IAC's *Health Reference Center* on compact disc provides a more extensive range of information services by linking bibliographical references with the full text from professional and consumer journals, a medical dictionary, authoritative medical and drug reference texts, and *The Consumer Health Information Source Book,* containing book reviews and further information sources, together with background information on 300 diseases and medical conditions. The price of the *Health Reference Center* is $12,000.

By the end of 1990, the *Consumer Health & Nutrition Index,* 1985-present (Oryx Press), and *Consumers' Index* (Pierean Press) will be available on one CD-ROM—*The Consumers Reference Disc, 1985-Present,* available from National Information Services Corporation. The annual subscription with quarterly updates is $795. MDX (Medical Data Exchange) has most recently introduced the *MDX Health Digest,* a consumer health database consisting of some 5,000 abstracts of articles drawn from a number of popular health magazines and newsletters, newspapers, and medical journals. The abstracts of articles in the professional journals are derived from the Medline database and are not especially prepared for consumers. The introductory price for an annual subscription delivered in the form of floppy disks is $1,850, which includes monthly updates. Online and CD-ROM versions are planned.

Also available to libraries and individuals is the BRS Colleague Comprehensive Core Medical Library—the complete text of 90 medical reference works and textbooks such as the *Merck Manual* and *Scientific American Medicine,* and journals such as the *New England Journal of Medicine, Lancet* and *Annals of Internal Medicine.*

Consumers will also have at their disposal a range of diagnostic software that will enable them to have the same type of clinical decision support available to physicians. Such computer-supported, clinical diagnosis systems have been demonstrated to operate with a high degree of accuracy. Similar systems, developed for use by consumers with personal computers, will guide users along a detailed branching network of logical decisions to reach definitive diagnostic conclusions and recommendations.

Another form of consumer assistance offers a great potential. This consists of the software for clinical reference and patient advice. If one has a sore throat accompanied by fever and swollen glands, one enters the symptoms into a microcomputer. Then, a decision tree prepared by medical consultants, pinpoints the problem, indicates its severity and whether to seek professional advice, and suggests possible home remedies. Modules along these lines presently available from Clinical Reference Systems include Patient Advice Adult, Patient Education Pediatric, and Patient Medication Advisory. Although designed for use by health-care professionals, these computerized files permit the generation of handouts for patients on a multiplicity of topics. The Patient Education Pediatric Module, for example, contains information on over 500 infant, child, and adolescent health problems and can print definitions, descriptions, symptoms and their causes, guidance on when to seek treatment, recommendations for home care, and preventive measures. The franchised Ask-A-Nurse service offered by many hospitals utilizes similar protocols in performing telephone triage and referral.

Robert Rodale[9] speculates that "customized, personalized health information" will be possible utilizing advanced print technology, so that a subscriber to *Prevention* magazine who is susceptible to cancer will be able to call a hotline number and receive in his or her next subscription copy a personalized insert with information on suggested risk-reducing modifications in lifestyle. Also planned for consumers is dial-up 900-number telephone service for obtaining information with respect to drugs, physicians' qualifications, and disease descriptions.

The library has defined and demonstrated its vital role in disseminating health information to the community. Further advances will depend on the financial resources available for the purchase of print, microform, online, and CD-ROM products and specialized information services. The major problem confronting libraries in offering an extended line of services is cost. Providing a full range of health information services in libraries lies beyond the means of many library systems. It is most likely that some form of fee-for-service will be required or possibly the cost will be underwritten by hospitals, clinics, insurance companies, or health maintenance organizations as a public service. If these extended services are not provided by libraries, consumers will be forced to purchase information from companies that will deal directly with consumers.

REFERENCES

1. "U.S. Health Gap Is Getting Wider." *The New York Times.* March 20, 1990. A8.

2. Brody, Jane. "Personal Health: The Malpractice Crisis." *The New York Times.* April 26, 1990. B7.

3. "What Americans (and Other Countries) Think of Their Health Care System." Remarks by Humphrey Taylor, President, Louis Harris and Associates. *Health Letter.* 5 (12), December 1989. 1–5.

4. "354,000 Injuries, Including 89,000 Deaths, Caused by Negligence in American Hospitals." *Health Letter.* 6 (4), April 1990. 4–5.

5. Marshall, Joanne et al. *Health Information Services in Ontario Public Libraries. Final Report of a Research Project.* Toronto: Faculty of Library and Information Science, University of Toronto, August 1989.

6. *Working for Patients: A Summary of the White Paper on the Government's Proposals Following Its Review of the NHS.* Department of Health, 1989. 12p.

7. Marshall, Joanne et al. *Health Information Services in Ontario Public Libraries.* 26.

8. Brandon, Alfred N. and Hill, Dorothy R. "Selected List of Books and Journals for the Small Medical Library." *Bulletin of the Medical Library Association.* 77 (2), April 1989. 143.

9. Rodale, Robert. "Health Facts in the Year 2000." *Prevention.* 42 (1), January 1990. 23–24.

PART II

Program Descriptions

CHAPTER 4
Healthnet: Connecticut Consumer Health Information Network: An Administrative and Operational Perspective

Ralph D. Arcari and Alberta L. Richetelle

ORIGINS

Healthnet (Connecticut Consumer Health Information Network) began in January 1985 as an outreach program of the University of Connecticut Health Center (UCHC) Library. This program was partially funded for its first three years with Library Services and Construction Act (LSCA) grant support through the Connecticut State Library.

The University of Connecticut Health Center Library had always served in a cooperative role with the public libraries in its immediate area. Staff of the Health Center Library had been active in the Capitol Region Library Council (CRLC), the library cooperative in the greater Hartford area serving over 60 public, academic, and special libraries. The director of the Health Center Library has been a member of the CRLC board and president of this council in 1981–1982. Workshops on health information for CRLC members were presented by members of the UCHC Collection Management and Information Services departments. However, it was apparent that an actual consumer health information program rather than irregular presentations would be more beneficial to the library community and patrons.

The need for a consumer health information program was reinforced by a report prepared by the Connecticut State Library in 1984, "Assessment of Connecticut Citizens' Information Needs and Library Use Study." According to this study, health information ranked third as a topic of concern of those surveyed by a telephone poll. Consumer issues and money matters ranked first and second; jobs, housing, and education ranked fourth, fifth, and sixth. As a result, an LSCA grant proposal was prepared by Ralph D. Arcari, Director of the UCHC Library, and Sandra K. Millard, then Head of the UCHC Library Information Services Department. The proposal was submitted to the State Library in the fall of 1984. The priorities for LSCA funding were the disadvantaged populations of urban areas. The Healthnet grant proposal was targeted toward the communities of Hartford, New Haven, Bridgeport, New London, New

Britain, and Waterbury, and letters of endorsement from the directors of the public libraries in these cities were included in the grant proposal. The grant received funding and approval and Alberta L. Richetelle was hired in January 1985 to be the Healthnet coordinator.

Three considerations were important in the development of the Healthnet proposal. First, public libraries were perceived to be neutral sources of information with the librarian neither advocating nor advising on an individual's health. This neutrality was viewed as an asset in the development of a program that would encourage library patrons to view their public libraries as a primary source for health information. Second, the University of Connecticut Health Center would serve as a technical information resource to back up public libraries for information that was not available in their collections. Third, the public libraries would serve as focal points for information from public and private health agencies and from self-help groups. A request for information would result in the patron not only receiving a direct answer to a question but also a referral to, and possibly publications from, the American Heart Association, the State Department on Aging, the local chapter of Mended Hearts, or other organizations. The program objective for the first year of Healthnet in 1985 was to develop public libraries as important access points for consumer health information. Program services would be:

- Training for public librarians
- Consultation on collection development
- Newsletter
- Resource sharing
- Community health forums
- Subject bibliographies
- Identification and evaluation of health information resources
- Development of promotional programs and materials

In order to have public librarians feel confident and comfortable in answering consumer health questions, it is necessary to provide a level of understanding of the medical reference literature. To impart this insight, a series of workshops on medical reference service were initially scheduled for the staffs of the six urban public libraries. In addition to medical reference works, the workshops covered guidelines for answering consumer health questions.

A core collection of medical reference materials was also necessary before public libraries could adequately provide consumer health information. Each of the participating libraries was visited and evaluations were made to determine how their collections could be developed to ensure that each library had a basic medical reference collection. The urban libraries with which the Healthnet program worked in its first year were brought up to a minimum collection standard. A core medical reference bibliography was developed against which these collections were reviewed. This bibliography, as most recently updated, is included in Appendix I to this chapter.

In order to publicize Healthnet, health professionals and representatives of health associations were scheduled to speak on health topics at meetings held in a library's community room. At these meetings, attendees were provided with examples of consumer health information from the library's collection or from a health agency or association. Sickle cell disease, for example, was the subject of a community room discussion held in the Bridgeport Public Library branch located in a minority neighborhood.

Publicity was also obtained for Healthnet through press releases and public service announcements on the radio. One feature story published by the Bridgeport *Post* resulted in a subsequent story on Healthnet in the Connecticut section of *The New York Times* in August 1986.

In preparing the grant proposal, one concern of specific interest which the public librarians requested be addressed was that of collection development. Uncertainty exists with respect to which books should be acquired out of the plethora currently published on health in a society in which the medical profession has been substantially demythologized. The subject bibliographies prepared to provide assistance for selection purposes resulted in an immediate and positive response on the part of public librarians. Subject bibliographies have been prepared on AIDS, women's health, mental health, cancer, chronic illness, pregnancy, childbirth, infertility, and health information for older adults. Each citation is annotated and the bibliographies are updated regularly.

THE NETWORK CONCEPT

The network concept in Healthnet focuses on the public library as the locus for information derived from multiple sources. Healthnet was not intended to be a one-way transmission of information from the state's medical school library to the state's public libraries. Rather, it was envisioned as a program that allowed participants and existing agencies and associations to share information and reach a larger population.

At the end of the first year of operation, the decision was made to expand the Healthnet program to all public libraries in the state. The success of the program in the six urban libraries provided the encouragement to serve the other 163 towns in the state. Because Connecticut is only 5,000 square miles, the distances the Healthnet coordinator must travel to visit public libraries are not unreasonable. Moreover, the state of Connecticut has no county government. For library cooperative purposes, Connecticut is divided into six Cooperating Library Service Units (CLSUs). Each CLSU has a regional office and staff that can assist in program development and the preparation of material for regional presentations. The grant proposal for year two (1986) consequently emphasized the ability of the Healthnet program to rely on this regional structure to provide Healthnet services to the entire Connecticut public library community. Healthnet proposals for continuation of grant funding on a statewide basis were successful for 1986 and 1987.

Because LSCA funding is designed to initiate programs rather than provide for long-term support, it was necessary to seek other funding sources to continue Healthnet. It quickly became apparent that the program could not be financed as a self-supporting enterprise relying on payments in proportion to budget size from Connecticut's public libraries. There were just too many small libraries for which even a modest payment of several hundred dollars was not feasible. At this point, the Connecticut Library Association (CLA) approached the UCHC Library and offered to make Healthnet a component of its legislative program for 1987 when CLA approached the State General Assembly for financial support for library programs. The University of Connecticut Health Center administration, library director, and CLA legislative liaison reached agreement on the priority for continuation of Healthnet. CLA then began the process of obtaining legislative support. As a result, Healthnet has successfully made the transition from a grant-supported program to a continuing, operational outreach program of the UCHC Library.

During the years in which Healthnet was supported through LSCA funds, its total budget varied between a first year high of $45,000 to a third year low of $30,000. After becoming a part of the UCHC Library operation, Healthnet received two other LSCA grants for specific consumer health projects. One was to provide a set of audiovisuals to each of the six CLSUs on health care for the senior citizen and the aged; the other was to provide printed materials on nutrition for Connecticut's public libraries.

Healthnet is an example of cooperation between a state medical school library, public libraries, a library association, and health agencies. There is a mutual respect between those participating in Healthnet. The UCHC Library serves as a resource for public libraries but does not itself attempt to collect consumer health information in depth for the state. This function is left to the public libraries. In short, Healthnet represents a partnership between the medical and public library communities, each of which has an interest in consumer health from a separate but cooperative perspective.

HEALTHNET OPERATIONS

During the first year of operation (1985) an advisory committee consisting of public librarians and health professionals was established and given the task of providing direction to the planning process for programs and services during the first three years of the program. The committee outlined three broad goals as the basis for program development: 1) to help public libraries develop comprehensive, up-to-date consumer health reference and general collections; 2) to train librarians to effectively use these collections to meet a wide variety of health information needs; and 3) to make the public aware of the health information resources of their local public libraries.

An informal survey was conducted in 1985 of the six urban libraries and their branches. The needs assessment included the completion of a questionnaire and on-site visits. The survey resulted in a compilation of the specific objectives of the program:

1. Collection development—core lists of consumer health information books, pamphlets, and audiovisuals

2. Training in consumer health reference tools and techniques
3. Identification of sources of consumer health information— government agencies, health associations, etc.
4. Assistance in developing a consumer health resource file
5. Evaluation of print and nonprint materials
6. Planning and presenting consumer health forums at public libraries

Collection Development

One of the first tasks of Healthnet was to develop a core list of consumer health reference books for use by participating libraries in developing reference collections capable of answering a wide variety of health questions. The librarians in the Information Services Department of the Health Center Library assisted in developing the initial list by recommending titles from the Library's reference collection that they determined to be most useful in answering consumer questions. Public librarians from the six urban libraries were also consulted for recommendations. The core list was revised over the next few years during the time it was used in the training workshops on medical reference tools and techniques. The list eventually evolved into three separate categories: First Priority, including titles essential for a basic collection in any size library; Second Priority, including titles important for medium to large libraries; and the Third Priority, including additional recommendations for titles suitable for large libraries with extensive reference collections identifying health and medical information as a priority. This tripartite format for the core list proved to be very useful when the network was expanded in the second year to include libraries in large urban areas as well as small rural libraries. The core reference list is included in Appendix I.

A survey of reference questions asked at the six urban libraries was conducted towards the end of the first year of the program. It was hoped that the results of the survey would provide some direction to the development of appropriate services by Healthnet, such as the compilation of subject bibliographies on topics of high interest to library patrons. A sample was taken of health-related reference questions asked during four randomly selected weeks. During the sampling period, a total of 195 health reference questions were recorded. These questions represented the following major subject categories:

SUBJECT	% OF TOTAL
1. Diseases, Disorders, Syndromes	30
2. Prescription and OTC Drugs	17
3. Nutrition	14
4. Pregnancy and Childbirth	8
5. Health Care Facilities	7
6. Mental Health	6
7. Health Professionals/Biographical	4
8. Surgery	4
9. General Health Information (questions involving more than one topic)	4

10. Alternative Therapies	3
11. Medical Tests	2
12. Environment	1
	TOTAL 100%
	N = 195

The data showed that 63 percent of the questions were asked by females, and our rough estimations of the ages of the patrons showed that 39 percent of the questions were posed by persons judged to be young adults, 36 percent by older adults, 12 percent by seniors, 10 percent by teenagers, and 1 percent by children. The age category of the remaining 2 percent was not recorded.

During Healthnet's third and fourth year of operation (1987 and 1988) funds were earmarked to assist public libraries to enhance their medical and health reference collections. A project was developed to determine the titles owned by libraries and to evaluate where deficiencies existed. The plan was to bring all reference collections up to a level whereby each would be able to answer very basic consumer health questions. One hundred twenty libraries, including large urban libraries and small libraries in rural areas, surveyed their reference collections using the core list developed by Healthnet as a checklist. Each library's collection was evaluated as to whether it contained the basic titles listed in the first priority, and purchases were then made to remedy deficiencies. It is interesting to note that approximately 50 percent of the libraries participating in this survey did not have all of the titles in the first priority.

One other important collection development service provided by Healthnet is the compilation of subject bibliographies on various consumer health topics for librarians to use as purchasing guides for their collections. Topics of these annotated bibliographies include: Acquired Immune Deficiency Syndrome (AIDS); cancer; chronic illness; mental health; nutrition; health information for older adults; and pregnancy, childbirth, and infertility. The compilation of these bibliographies is a cooperative effort between Healthnet and those public librarians with a special interest in a particular topic, as well as local and statewide health organizations and agencies. Titles evaluated for these bibliographies are restricted to those in print at the time of publication of the bibliography.

A bibliography was also developed using recommendations from statewide self-help/mutual-support groups. These groups were sent a questionnaire asking for recommendations of specific books, pamphlets, and audiovisuals that group members felt most helped them cope with their specific health concern. This represented a different approach to developing a bibliography in that actual library users rather than librarians were providing recommendations of specific titles. Once the data from the survey were compiled, a bibliography was developed that included the name of the self-help/mutual-support group recommending the specific titles. The bibliography was distributed to public libraries throughout the state as well as to the self-help groups who made recommendations.

Two collection development grant proposals were written by the Healthnet director and subsequently funded with Library Services and Construction Act (LSCA) grants through the Connecticut State Library.

Both proposals were developed as a result of recommendations from public librarians as to identified and documented needs. The first project involved the identification, evaluation, and acquisition of a collection of videocassette programs on topics of interest to older adults. Representatives of health organizations concerned with the health of elderly persons were surveyed to determine general subject areas of importance to be considered. Subjects identified included Alzheimer's disease, use of medications, nutrition, communicating with health professionals, sexuality, fitness, long-term care issues, stress management, and handling grief and loss. Following identification of the topics, over 40 videocassette programs were previewed for purchase consideration. Eleven titles were selected and copies of each were purchased and distributed to the six regional library cooperatives (CLSUs), which in turn made them available to their public library patrons. In addition, a general mailing announcing the availability of the videocassette programs was sent to senior centers, community service agencies for older adults, and other health professionals throughout the state.

The other collection development project involved the identification, evaluation, and acquisition of a basic collection of books and pamphlets on a variety of nutrition topics. Registered dieticians served as consultants for this project by identifying important nutrition topics and assisting in the development of a basic list of 100 titles to be considered for purchase. The *Surgeon General's Report on Nutrition and Health* was consulted in order to identify nutrition topics to consider. Libraries interested in participating in the project were asked to survey their collections and to indicate which titles on the basic list they already owned. Once the survey information was compiled, titles were then ranked in order of priority for purchase. One hundred and forty libraries participated in this project with each receiving anywhere from 10 to 28 titles on the list. In addition, each library received pamphlets and fact sheets on such topics as food safety, fiber, nutrition and PMS syndrome, calcium and osteoporosis, food allergies, and nutrition for children and teenagers. Participating libraries also received posters on nutrition, a bibliography of the nutrition books, and a sample press release to be used in developing displays and publicizing the availability of the nutrition information.

Training

Training workshops for librarians in the network have covered medical reference tools and techniques and the identification of sources of consumer health information. Sixteen reference workshops (including one advanced medical reference workshop), and five workshops on identifying sources of consumer health information, were conducted during the period January 1985 through December 1989.

The reference workshop format offered includes a discussion of guidelines for providing medical information to consumers, as well as a "hands on" evaluation of titles included in the core list. Participants in these sessions have welcomed the opportunity to learn firsthand which titles are more suitable for answering specific kinds of questions. Librarians unfamiliar with any of the titles on the core list have commented that the hands-on evaluation was valuable and afforded them the opportunity to determine whether to purchase specific books for their collections. A copy of the reference guidelines presented at the workshops for answering consumer health questions is included in Appendix II to this chapter.

The other workshop offered on a regular basis covers the many sources of consumer health information and includes a discussion of the information resources of public and private, local, state, and federal agencies. The purpose of this workshop is to encourage public librarians to use the resources of these organizations to answer consumer health reference questions. Librarians are also encouraged to acquire pamphlets, fact sheets, and similar literature from these organizations and organize them to make the information accessible to library patrons. The information resources and services of such organizations as the local chapters of the American Heart Association, American Cancer Society, and the Arthritis Foundation, as well as the federal health information clearinghouses and national health organizations, are discussed. Publications lists and sample publications from these organizations are distributed. Many of these organizations have Spanish-language publications, and a few have literature in other languages, such as Chinese and Vietnamese, which are of interest to libraries in large urban areas with diverse populations.

The Healthnet librarian maintains regular contact with the major statewide health associations as well as with the federal health information clearinghouses and the National Health Information Center to keep informed about any new publications and services that may be of interest to public librarians. Information about new publications and services available from these organizations is included in the Healthnet newsletter and discussed in training workshops.

The organization and maintenance of the Health Topics File of the Health Center Library is also discussed in the consumer health resources workshop and tips for organizing a similar file in public libraries are also covered. The Health Topics File is a collection of news clippings, pamphlets, fact sheets, journal articles, and other similar materials arranged by subject and maintained in two four-drawer file cabinets. This file is used by the Information Services staff and Healthnet to answer consumer health reference questions as well as by patients, the general public, and health center professionals.

Healthnet publishes a newsletter several times during the year and distributes it to network libraries and state health agencies and associations. The newsletter is also mailed for a nominal annual subscription fee to health sciences libraries and out-of-state public libraries. The newsletter keeps librarians informed about new consumer health resources and services, as well as recently published books, pamphlets, and audiovisuals, and serves as a vehicle for public librarians and statewide health organizations to share information about various programs and services related to the provision of health information to the general public.

Reference Services

One of the services provided by Healthnet is backup reference service for consumer health questions from public libraries. Our approach is to work with librarian intermediaries who refer the question rather than deal directly with patrons. This is done for a variety of reasons, the most important of which is that public library patrons may view the Health Center Library, rather than their local public library, as a primary source of health information. Such a situation would be counterproductive to the goals of the Healthnet program. Working with the public librarian is also much more efficient since the Healthnet librarian can determine exactly what has already been consulted, thus eliminating any duplication of effort. Written guidelines for reference referrals to Healthnet are discussed and distributed at each of the reference training workshops. The referral guidelines are included in Appendix III to this chapter.

For the most part, questions referred to Healthnet are those requiring very specific information, such as latest treatments for diseases. About 100 consumer health reference questions are referred to Healthnet each year. For the period July 1988 to June 1989, these questions represented the following subjects:

SUBJECT	NO. OF QUESTIONS
Diseases, Disorders, Syndromes	54
Treatments, Therapies, Surgery	18
Health Care Services, Facilities, Clinics, Professionals	10
Medical Tests	5
Nutrition	4
Pharmaceuticals: Prescription and OTC	3
Environmental/Occupational Health	3
Dental	1
Other (multiple subjects)	1
	TOTAL 99

Many of the reference referrals present unique problems, one of which may be the general lack of appropriate information for the lay public on a specific topic. By the time the question reaches Healthnet, most of the standard references and resources, including those that are lay oriented, have been checked. These questions may also come from patrons who are not satisfied with the very basic information supplied in such reference sources as the *AMA Family Medical Guide* or *The Columbia University College of Physicians and Surgeons Complete Home Medical Guide*. For the most part, answers to the referred reference questions can be found in the professional medical literature, which is often complex and technical. The Healthnet librarian will review several different sources of information on the topic in question and make a decision as to what is understandable to someone with little or no medical background.

Promotion

Healthnet has used a variety of methods to encourage people to associate health information with their local public libraries. Bookmarks with a short bibliography and a brief list of community agencies providing information on the topic were designed and distributed by the six network libraries during the program's first year. The topics for these bookmarks included cancer, stress, alternative therapies, and the informed health-care consumer. In addition, programs on consumer health topics presented by local health professionals have been held in the community rooms of several libraries, with information provided about books and other sources related to the topic that are available at the sponsoring library. Topics for these community health programs have included nutrition for older adults, sickle cell disease, nutrition and weight management, and how to talk to your doctor. The community program on sickle cell disease was held in the branch library of a predominately minority neighborhood and included free sickle cell trait testing for attendees.

Healthnet assisted four network libraries to develop month-long health information observances to highlight the wide variety of health information resources available at each of the libraries. Displays of colorful health-related posters and books and pamphlets on health topics were featured, and subject bibliographies on selected topics were distributed to library patrons. Two of the libraries sponsored health talks presented by local health professionals. Public service radio announcements were also developed during Healthnet's first year as another means of informing the public about the health information resources of their local public libraries. The Health Center's Department of Institutional Relations and Department of Biomedical Communications assisted in the development of the messages and distribution of the audiotapes to local radio stations. Six tapes were produced, one for each of the six original network libraries. The taped message included the following:

"My friend has scleroderma . . . what is it?"
"Where can I find information on weight loss diets?"
For answers to these and other kinds of health questions, call or visit (name of local library inserted).

Future Development

Future goals for Healthnet include the continuation of the basic services of collection development, training, reference services, and publicity. In addition, several other areas of development need to be explored, one of which is to encourage health professionals to be more involved in the network's activities. This can be achieved by developing formalized educational programs informing doctors, nurses, and other similar groups involved in community health education and preventive medicine of the consumer health information resources and services of their local public libraries. The goal will be to request that health professionals refer their patients to public libraries for treatment-related information. One can easily imagine physicians using tear-off prescription pads to refer their patients to the local public library for specific health information about a particular disease, or for information on preparing low fat recipes.

Other areas that need further attention are Healthnet's involvement in statewide efforts to educate Connecticut's residents about such critical topics as AIDS, cholesterol, drug and alcohol abuse, and maternal and child health issues. Connecticut has one of the highest per capita income levels of any state in the U.S., while three of its cities have higher than average infant mortality rates and are listed in the top 10 poorest cities nationwide. Another future challenge will be to devise effective ways to reach those residents who are not traditional library users and provide them with appropriate health information to meet their interests and concerns. This can be accomplished by bringing the public library to neighborhood health clinics, public health screening programs, nutrition sites, and other similar health-related community activities. More formal arrangements with the Connecticut Department of Health Services Health Education Division as well as with the Connecticut Department of Environmental Protection need to be explored for possible cooperative informational programs that will reach more of Connecticut's residents. Another concern is focused on an exploration of how new informational technologies can be used to provide more efficient delivery of information to public library patrons and the expansion of the network to include more local, state, and national resources able to meet the growing diversity of demands for consumer health information.

APPENDIX I:
Core Bibliography of Consumer Health Reference Books

The following are recommended titles for health and medical reference collections for public libraries. Titles in the **First Priority** include those books that are essential for a basic collection in any size library. **Second Priority** titles include those that are important for medium to large libraries. Purchase of second priority titles would depend on the size of the library with respect to collection, population served, and budget. Titles in the category of **Additional Recommendations** should be considered for purchase by large libraries with extensive reference collections and/or those that identify health and medical information as a priority service to their community. The titles are *not* listed in rank order in each of the priorities. When ordering any of these titles, check current availability and price in *Books in Print*.

FIRST PRIORITY

Dictionaries/Directories/Bibliographies

Connecticut Directory of Self-Help/Mutual Support Groups. 1985–1986. New Haven, CT. Connecticut Self-Help/Mutual Support Network. Free to public libraries upon request. Contact: Roxanna Simmons, (203) 789-7645.

Consumer Health Information Source Book. 3rd ed., pbk. By Alan Rees and Catherine Hoffman. Oryx Press, 1990. (ISBN 0-89774-408-X) $39.50.

Dorland's Illustrated Medical Dictionary. 27th ed. Saunders, 1988. (ISBN 0-7216-3154-1) $35.95 text ed.

Folio's Medical Directory of Connecticut. Folio Associates, 1988. (ISBN 0-934684-11-1) $34.00. Annual. A Medical Directory of Massachusetts is also available. Order from: Folio Associates, Inc., 111 Perkins St., Boston, MA 02130.

Health Care, U.S.A. By Jean Carper. Prentice Hall Press, 1987. (ISBN 0-13-609686-7); (ISBN 0-13-609694-8, pbk.).

Learning AIDS: An Information Resources Directory. 2nd ed. American Foundation for AIDS Research, distributed by R.R. Bowker, 1989. (ISBN 0-9620363-1-5) $24.95.

Medical and Health Information Directory. Vol. 3. Edited by Karen Backus. Gale Research, 1986. (ISBN 0-8103-2522-5) $165.00.

Anatomy

The Johns Hopkins Atlas of Human and Functional Anatomy. 3rd ed. Revised and updated. Johns Hopkins Press, 1986. (ISBN 0-8018-3282-9); (ISBN 0-8018-3283-7, pbk.) $18.50.

Diseases, Diagnosis, Treatment

American Cancer Society Cancer Book: Prevention, Detection, Diagnosis, Treatment, Rehabilitation, Cure. Edited by Arthur Holleb. Doubleday, 1986. (ISBN 0-385-17847-6) $24.95.

The American Medical Association Family Medical Guide. Revised and updated. Edited by Jeffrey R. Kunz. Random House, 1987. (ISBN 0-394-55582-1) $29.95.

Merck Manual of Diagnosis and Therapy. 15th ed. Edited by Robert Berklow. Merck, Sharpe, & Dohme Research Laboratories, 1987. (ISBN 0-911910-06-09) $19.75. Published every 5–6 years.

Patients' Guide to Medical Tests. 3rd ed. Revised and expanded. By Cathey Pinckney and Edward Pinckney. Facts on File, 1987. (ISBN 0-8160-1292-X) $21.95.
OR

People's Book of Medical Tests. By Tom Ferguson and David Sobel. Summit Books, 1985. (ISBN 0-671-44172-8) $24.95; (ISBN 0-671-55377-1, pbk.) $12.95 pbk. (New edition to be published this year.)

Professional Guide to Diseases: An Up-to-Date Encyclopedia of Illnesses, Disorders, Injuries and Their Treatments. 2nd ed. Edited by Helen Hamilton and Barbara McVan. Springhouse, 1986. (ISBN 0-87434-035-7) $24.95.

Drugs (Prescription and Over-the-Counter)

Handbook of Non-prescription Drugs. 8th ed. American Pharmaceutical Association, The National Professional Society of Pharmacists, 1986. (ISBN 0-917330-54-4) $70.00. Published every 2–3 years.

United States Pharmacopeia Drug Information for the Consumer. Consumer Reports Books, 1987. $25.00. May be substituted for *USPDI Vol. 2: Advice for the Patient.* Exact same format and information as following entry.

USPDI: United States Pharmacopeia Dispensing Information. U.S. Pharmacopeia Convention, 1985. *Vol. 1: Drug Information for the Health Care Provider,* $99.00; *Vol 2: Advice for the Patient,* $37.50; 2 vol. set, $120.00. Order from: U.S. Pharmacopeial Convention, Inc., Order Processing, P.O. Box 2248, Rockville, MD 20852.

Nutrition

Food for Health. By M.E. Ensminger. Pegus Press, 1986. (ISBN 0-941218-0704) $49.50. A one-volume condensed edition of *Foods and Nutrition Encyclopedia.*

Foods and Nutrition Encyclopedia. 2 vols. By Audrey Ensminger et al. Pegus Press, 1983. (ISBN 0-941218-05-8) $99.00.

OR

Mayo Clinic Diet Manual: A Handbook of Dietary Practices. 6th ed. Saunders, 1988. (ISBN 1-55664-032-3) $34.95.

SECOND PRIORITY

Dictionaries, Directories

ABMS Compendium of Certified Medical Specialists. 1st ed. 1986–1987. American Board of Medical Specialists, 1986. 7 vols. with supplement. $200.00.

OR

Directory of Medical Specialists. 22nd ed. 3 vols. Marquis, 1985. $235.00

American Hospital Association Guide to the Health Care Field. American Hospital Association, 1987. $72.50. Annual.

American Medical Directory. 29th ed. 4 vols. American Medical Association, 1985. $350.00

The Best in Medicine: Where to Get the Finest in Health Care for You and Your Family. By Herbert J. Dietrich and Virginia H. Biddle. Harmony Books, 1986. (ISBN 0-942036-07-7) $12.95 (pbk.).

Dictionary of Medical Syndromes. By Sergio Magalini. 2nd ed. Lippincott, 1981. (ISBN 0-397-50503-5) $56.00.

Directory of Nursing Homes 1990–1991. 4th ed. Edited by Sam Mongeau. Oryx Press, 1990. (ISBN 0-89774-614-7) $225.00.

Diseases, Diagnosis, Treatment

Cecil Textbook of Medicine. 18th ed. Edited by James B. Wyngaarden and Lloyd H. Smith. Saunders, 1988. (ISBN 0-7216-18480, 1 vol. ed.); (ISBN 0-721-61851-0, 2 vol. set) $96.25, 1 vol.; $124.25, 2 vols.

Conn's Current Therapy, 1989. Edited by Robert E. Rakel. W.B. Saunders, 1989. (ISBN 0-7216-2581-9) $50.00.

Current Medical Diagnosis and Treatment. 26th ed. Edited by Marcus Krupp, et al. Lange, 1987. (ISBN 0-8385-1344-1) $32.50. Published annually.

Current Obstetric and Gynecological Diagnosis and Treatment. 6th ed. Edited by Ralph C. Benson. Appleton Lange, 1987. $34.50.

Current Pediatric Diagnosis and Treatment. 9th ed. Edited by C.H. Kempe et al. Appleton Lange, 1987. $31.50.

OR

Nelson Textbook of Pediatrics. 13th ed. By Richard E. Behrman and Victor Vaughn. Saunders, 1987. $79.00.

Current Surgical Diagnosis and Treatment. 7th ed. By Lawrence W. Way. Appleton and Lange, 1985. (ISBN 0-87041-196-9) $34.50.

Diagnostic and Statistical Manual of Mental Disorders (Third edition—Revised) (DSM-III-R). American Psychiatric Association, 1987. (ISBN 0-89042-019-X) $22.95.

Diagnostics. 2nd ed. By Matthew Cahill and Minnie B. Rose. (Nurses Reference Library) Springhouse, 1985. (ISBN 0-916730-89-1) $23.95.

Harrison's Principles of Internal Medicine. 11th ed. Edited by Robert Petersdorf and Raymond D. Adams. McGraw, 1987. Available in one-volume edition at $85.00 (ISBN 0-07-007261-2) and a two-volume edition at $95.00 (ISBN 0-07-079454-5). Published every 3 years.

Report of the Committee on Infectious Diseases (Red Book). 20th ed. American Academy of Pediatrics, 141 Northwest Point Boulevard, P.O. Box 927, Elk Grove Village, IL 60007.

Nutrition

Food Values of Portions Commonly Used (Bowes and Church's) 14th ed. By Jean A.T. Pennington and Helen Nicols Church. Harper & Row, 1985. $17.95; $8.95 (pbk.) (ISBN 0-06-181679-5).

ADDITIONAL RECOMMENDATIONS

Dictionaries, Directories

American Dental Directory. American Dental Association, 1985. Annual. Probably not essential for public libraries, but important to know it exists.

Psychiatric Dictionary. 6th ed. Edited by Robert Campbell. Oxford University Press, 1989. (ISBN 0-19-505293-5) $45.00.

Saunder's Health Care Directory. 1984–1985. Saunders, 1984. (ISBN 0-7216-6866-6) $89.00.

Health Statistics

Health United States, 1985. National Center for Health Statistics, DHHS. Publication PHS 89-1232. $10.00.

Statistical Handbook on Aging Americans. Edited by Frank L. Schick. Oryx Press, 1986. (ISBN 0-89774-259-1) $42.50.

Drug/Alcohol Use

Encyclopedia of Drug Abuse. By Robert O'Brien and Sidney Cohen. Facts on File, 1984. (ISBN 0-87196-690-5) $40.00.

Handbook of Abusable Drugs. Edited by Kenneth Blum. Gardner Press, 1984. (ISBN 0-89876-036-4) $79.95.

Roads to Recovery: A National Directory of Alcohol and Drug Addiction Centers. Macmillan, 1985. $17.95.

Poisoning

Handbook of Poisoning: Prevention, Diagnosis, and Treatment. 12th ed. By Robert Dreisbach and William Robertson. Appleton Lange, 1987. (ISBN 0-8385-3643-3) $16.50.

APPENDIX II:
Guidelines for Providing Medical Information to Consumers

1. Be aware of the patron.

The typical consumer health question comes from someone who has just returned from a doctor's office or has just learned that a family member is ill. The person may be upset and may not be clear about the information needed.

2. Conduct your best reference interview.

Ask the patron how much information is needed. If the need is not readily apparent, determine if the person needs the information because of a personal health concern or if the question is related to research for a school paper. The most nonthreatening way to find this out is simply to ask "Do you need this information for a school project?" If the person responds with a "No," assume it is a personal health question. This probing is necessary even though it may be the opposite of your usual practice. Most patrons freely relate their real problem at this point.

It is important to differentiate between health questions of a personal nature and those related to school reports because answering each kind of question involves a different approach. Often the person with a personal health concern may phrase the question in a very general way because of uncertainty about the information needed. Usually the information needed for a personal health concern is very specific. The person who is writing a paper, on the other hand, most often needs information that is broad in scope.

3. Always ask if the patron has checked with a physician or pharmacist.

This should not be asked to imply that you are not willing to help, but to remind patrons to check with their physician or pharmacist. Many patrons do not realize, for example, that many pharmacists will assist them with drug information questions.

4. Always check terms in a medical dictionary.

If the patron is uncertain about a medical term and you are also uncertain, always check the spelling in a medical dictionary. A good medical dictionary is the best first-line reference tool for answering health questions. Be sure to check variants of spelling, and if you've done a thorough search and still can't find the word in a medical dictionary, suggest that the patron check with a health professional for the correct spelling.

If the patron is uncertain about the spelling of a drug name, variants should *not* be checked because this could lead to inaccurate information. Many drugs have similar sounding names but are prescribed for very different reasons. Ask the patron to get the correct spelling of the drug name from his or her physician or pharmacist before attempting to answer the question.

5. Do not interpret medical information.

For telephone reference, always begin by letting the caller know you are reading the information from a printed source; state the title, author, and year of publication. Definitions for terms unfamiliar to the caller can then be checked and read from a standard medical dictionary; again, give the full bibliographic citation. For lengthy material, suggest that the person come into the library or offer to mail a photocopy of a page or two. Be sure to write the title of the book, publisher, and publication date on the photocopy.

6. Do not give medical advice, opinion, or make recommendations. Describe your role as a provider of information.

Many patrons begin a question with "Do you think I should . . . ? or "What's the best . . . ?" Be very clear with the patron that you cannot interpret the information, that you have no medical training and are not a doctor. If there are additional questions or more information is needed, tell the patron that you will be happy to search further. If the person is persistent about wanting advice or recommendations, suggest that he or she discuss this with a health professional.

7. Understand that the specific information the patron wants may not be available anywhere in the medical literature and describe the limitations of medical information.

Many people believe that every cause, cure, treatment, or explanation for everything remotely connected with health and disease has been written about in the medical literature. It is important to understand that this is not the case and that there will be times when a patron with a specific health information need will have to be satisfied with an incomplete answer.

Be aware, however, that in many instances, the effective reference interview can result in a reformulation of the original request and an improved chance of finding information. Often the reformulated question is what the patron wanted to ask in the first place.

Understand and explain to the patron the limitations of medical information, in particular that such information becomes quickly outdated and that medical professionals often disagree about the diagnosis and treatment of a specific disease.

8. Do provide answers to drug information requests.

Answers to requests for side effects or general information about drugs can be carefully handled by referring the person to the *USPDI* (*United States Pharmacopeia Dispensing Information*). When possible, always add a referral to the patron's physician or pharmacist.

9. Do not provide a diagnosis.

Many patrons may recite a variety of symptoms and ask if these mean they have a specific disease. You may know the answer without checking in a medical text because your aunt may have had the very same symptoms, but be aware that you would be providing a diagnosis and illegally practicing medicine without a license. Once again, describe your role as a provider of information only.

10. Do not recommend a specific practitioner.

This is a question that comes up frequently and even if you're convinced that your surgeon, pediatrician, etc. is the best in the world, **never** make a recommendation. If a patron is looking for a recommendation for a specific kind of physician, suggest that he or she call a local hospital. Many hospitals have physician referral services, but these kinds of services do not give information about the physician's competence; they only give three or four names of physicians who have privileges at that particular hospital. You may also suggest the patron consult the *Directory of Medical Specialists* or the *AMA Medical Directory*, but once again these will only provide very general information.

11. Provide the best and most complete information needed to answer the patron's request.

This is the ultimate goal of all reference librarians; however, certain medical questions present unique problems. A patron may have a question about the diagnosis, treatment, and prognosis of a specific disease that you know or later find out is usually fatal. What should you do? If you feel uncomfortable about giving the information over the telephone, phototocopy what you found and send it to the patron. If the patron is in the library, be sure there is quiet place for the patron to read the information (you should do this anyway). You should not, under any circumstance, withhold the information since this can be considered a form of censorship. Many patrons wanting information about a serious disease may already suspect the prognosis.

12. Always provide either an answer or a referral or both.

There is no excuse for not being able to provide a patron with a referral to another resource, association, or agency if you are unable to answer the question. If you have exhausted your library's resources and have not been able to find the information the patron wants, please call HEALTHNET for assistance.

Keep in mind two excellent referral sources—the Cancer Information Service, (800-4-CANCER), and local and statewide self-help groups. The Cancer Information Service will answer questions from someone who has cancer or from a family member or friend. CIS will provide information on the latest treatments for different kinds of cancer and will make referrals to physicians.

Self-help groups can be an excellent source of information. Members in a self-help group can share information about specific physicians they found to be most helpful in treating a specific disease or condition and usually know all about the latest treatments and support services available. Be clear with the patron that you are recommending a self-help group as an information resource, lest the patron think you are suggesting a need for emotional support. Consult the *Connecticut Directory of Self-Help/Mutual Support Groups* for a listing of these groups.

APPENDIX III: Guidelines for Reference Referrals to HEALTHNET

One of the many services provided by HEALTHNET is reference support for public libraries. Many consumer health questions can be routinely handled by most public libraries, depending upon the breadth and scope of their reference collections. Occasionally, however, there are questions that need to be referred to HEALTHNET for one or more of the following reasons:

1. The resources of the local public library have been exhausted.
2. The patron wants the most comprehensive and current information about a new treatment, drug, etc.

3. The patron wants a copy of a specific article from a medical journal referred to in a news story.

In order to help HEALTHNET provide this reference service, public librarians should adhere to the following guidelines: (1) Only *consumer health* questions should be referred to HEALTHNET. Consumer health questions are defined as those that relate to a personal health concern or that of a family member or friend. Questions from students (high school, college, etc.) doing school projects *should not* be referred to HEALTHNET nor should questions from health professionals (including nurses, mental health counselors, etc.). Reference questions from health professionals should be directed to Information Services at the Health Center Library—their telephone number is 679-2942. Contacts can be made by either the health professional or the librarian. Students who are seeking health information for school projects will usually find more appropriate information related to their topic at large public libraries. Although the Health Center Library is open to the public seven days a week, much of the information is very technical. Students doing school projects should be directed to large public libraries for their health information needs. (2) Public library patrons *should not* be referred directly to HEALTHNET. Contacts should be made by the librarian. Often the public librarian may have already completed a preliminary search for the information and this would be important for the HEALTHNET librarian to know before proceeding further with a search. This not only prevents a duplication of effort, but may also result in an exchange of information related to the topic which may be helpful to the public librarian and HEALTHNET as well. Information related to the reference question will be sent to the public library which in turn will pass it on to the library patron.

HEALTHNET hours are 8:30 a.m. to 4:30 p.m., Monday through Friday.

When reference questions are referred to HEALTHNET, we will provide an answer with one or more of the following:

1. Photocopy of up to six (6) pages from one or two books.
2. A free, brief, online database search (when appropriate) to find the most current journal article(s) that will provide the information needed. The HEALTHNET librarian will select one journal article identified from the search and send a photocopy, along with a copy of the search. The search, which will usually include abstracts, will also be sent with instructions that copies of additional articles may be available for a fee. As a general rule, patrons will be told to check with the public library about their ILL policy and whether or not there is a fee for ILL requests for journal articles. (See note below for UCONN Health Center Library's ILL policies.)
3. For more extensive information needs, the titles of one or more books in the UCHC collection will be given with instructions that they may be obtained through interlibrary loan from the patron's public library. (See note below.). When appropriate, the HEALTHNET librarian will also recommend specific titles that may

not be in the UCHC Library, but may be available from another public library in the state.

4. Copies or originals of any brochures, fact sheets, etc., which may provide the information needed.
5. Names, addresses, and telephone numbers for additional resources. Public librarians are encouraged to contact HEALTHNET not only for reference support and back-up, but for collection development purposes as well. We can assist you by recommending titles in a specific subject area or by identifying other sources of information. Occasionally, we can supply copies of pamphlets or fact sheets that you can add to your vertical file.

Note: ILL policies for the UCONN Health Center Library, Farmington, CT are:

- No charge for book loans to public libraries.
- $7.00 fee for journal articles (up to 50 pages); an additional $5 is charged for one-day rush service.
- ALA ILL forms must be used; OCLC may also be used for ILLs; requests may be faxed (679-4046); please indicate whether you want the request returned to you via fax, since we charge extra for this service.

CHAPTER 5
CHIRS: Consumer Health Information Resource Services for Nebraska Residents

Marie A. Reidelbach, Carolyn G. Weaver, and
Brenda K. Epperson

HISTORY

The Consumer Health Information Resource Services (CHIRS) for Nebraska Residents was initiated in January 1985 as a cooperative project between three independent agencies and groups: the Leon S. McGoogan Library of Medicine at the University of Nebraska Medical Center, the largest health sciences library in the state; the Nebraska Library Commission; and the more than 70 public and academic libraries affiliated with the statewide information network managed by the Commission. These three groups, with different sources of funding, goals, and constituencies, have worked together for the last five years toward a single objective—to provide all Nebraska residents, regardless of physical location, with access to information that will allow them to make informed decisions about their own health care.

Nebraska is considered to be a rural state, with 60 percent of the population concentrated in the eastern one-third of the state, in the two major metropolitan areas around Omaha and Lincoln. Health practitioners and hospital libraries are thinly scattered outside the metropolitan areas, and they rely heavily on interlibrary borrowing through the Biomedical Communication Network to obtain professional information that is not available locally.

Under the auspices of the Nebraska Library Commission, the state is divided into six library service regions. The Commission fully supports an electronic mail network for all libraries in the state, and any library in Nebraska, regardless of type, is eligible to receive net lender reimbursement from the Commission for interlibrary loans provided to other network participants. Smaller libraries in each region receive backup support from a designated regional resource library, with special libraries such as the McGoogan Library accepting referrals for interlibrary borrowing or reference services in their subject specialty. Health practitioners lacking other access to a medical library are in fact encouraged to refer professional requests to McGoogan via their local public library.

The mission of the McGoogan Library, as a state-supported academic health sciences library, is to provide information support for patient care, teaching, and research needs of University of Nebraska Medical Center (UNMC) faculty, staff, and students. The Library is both headquarters to, and a resource library for, the Midcontinental Regional Medical Library Program (MCRMLP). This mission is extended to include service to unaffiliated Nebraska health professionals and others with a need for professional-level health science information. Approximately 16 percent of all reference services provided by the reference staff in the mid-1980s were to persons not affiliated with UNMC.

By 1984, the need for consumer health information services in the state was clear. Public libraries were receiving increasing numbers of health-related questions which they were reluctant to handle both because of inadequate training in the subject matter and because of a lack of authoritative materials in their collections. As a result, increasing numbers of questions from laypersons were being referred to the McGoogan Library, which often found it difficult to respond appropriately, since the collection contained virtually no materials at the nonprofessional level. Laypersons approaching McGoogan directly were often referred back to the local public library, only to be told that the information had to be obtained from McGoogan!

OBJECTIVES

In 1984, the McGoogan Library decided to break this information impasse by seeking LSCA Title III funding from the Library Commission to develop a consumer health information program for the state. The design of the program was shaped by a number of environmental factors: (1) the need to provide service to an entire state; (2) the existence of a statewide library network in which resource libraries routinely provide backup services for needs that cannot be met locally; (3) a small reference staff at McGoogan which would not be able to cope with a large increase in workload; and (4) a high probability, based on preliminary conversations with Commission staff, that additional professional staff for CHIRS would not be funded.

It was therefore decided that CHIRS would follow the pattern established for the Biomedical Communications Network. This approach assumed that the ability of local libraries to cope with health information requests would be improved through collection enhancements and training of staff, that most consumer health information services would be delivered through the local public library, and that the McGoogan Library would continue to respond to questions primarily upon referral from another library.

The original objectives of CHIRS, as stated in the grant application, were:

1. To work within the structure of the Nebraska Library System to improve the delivery of consumer health information to Nebraskans.

2. To provide educational and consultation services to nonhealth science librarians which would enable them to deliver enhanced first-line services.
3. To serve as a health information resource library for the state of Nebraska by providing information services beyond the capacity of the local library.

The CHIRS concept won easy acceptance from public libraries in the state primarily because it is based on an enhancement of local library services, rather than the creation of a new health information delivery system in addition to that already in existence. The program focused on improving the quality and quantity of authoritative health information available through local libraries, rather than striving to create a highly visible role for McGoogan. The McGoogan Library consistently remains in the background as a provider of health information to laypersons, with the local public library serving as a transparent interface between the consumer and McGoogan for services actually provided by the resource library.

A heavy emphasis was placed on training nonhealth science library staff to respond appropriately to consumer health information requests. Both written guidelines and a full-day workshop for nonhealth science librarians were offered to improve the ability of local libraries to deal with health-related questions. The enhancement of local collections was encouraged by providing training in the evaluation and selection of consumer health materials and through the distribution of core lists and other selection aids. However, no funding was provided by CHIRS to local libraries for the purchase of consumer health materials. This approach was taken in order to encourage self-reliance in the library network in Nebraska, so that health information would continue to be delivered to consumers even if McGoogan could no longer participate.

A collection of consumer health materials, both circulating and noncirculating, was established at McGoogan so that the reference staff would have access in responding to questions referred through the network to both the professional collection and to materials at a level appropriate for the general public. By fully exploiting existing service patterns, the consumer would receive information at the point most convenient for him or her—the local public library—while having access to the more specialized resources of an academic medical library when local resources proved inadequate to meet his or her information needs.

STAFFING AND GOVERNANCE

Unlike many other consumer health programs, nonhealth science libraries were not involved in the writing of the CHIRS grant or the initial design of the program. The grant request was drafted by the associate director for public services at McGoogan, reviewed internally with appropriate library staff, and discussed informally with Library Commission staff, who agreed that the service was worthy of support. The request was submitted in the spring of 1984 and funding was received in August 1984, with services to begin in January 1985.

The first task of the CHIRS program was to involve nonhealth science libraries in its future development. A 10-member CHIRS Advisory Council was established immediately, with representatives from all six library systems, the Nebraska Library Commission, and the Nebraska Department of Health. The associate director for public services and the head of reference at McGoogan served as *ex officio* members. The charge of the Advisory Council was to ensure that the program recognized the needs and limitations of all types of libraries in the state, and to provide input into the development and direction of the program. It was at the Council's suggestion that the schedule of workshops was accelerated, and that audiovisuals not be acquired for the CHIRS collection at McGoogan. In addition, Council members provided valuable suggestions for marketing, influenced the Commission to provide direct funding for medical reference collections to resource libraries (apart from funding for the CHIRS program), and individually and as a group acted as advocates for the program across the state.

FUNDING

CHIRS was initially funded by a LSCA Title III grant of $19,000 from the Nebraska Library Commission to the McGoogan Library. Although it was recognized that LSCA projects are normally funded on a year-to-year basis, CHIRS was designed as a three-year project. The first year established the framework for the program through the acquisition of the basic collection, the development and testing of workshops, and the establishment of protocols for the provision of backup information services. The two subsequent years concentrated on the offering of additional workshops, promotion of the program, and increased delivery of information support services, with evaluation, refinement, and incorporation of the program into regular state-supported library operations expected by the end of the third year.

Since the beginning of the program, the McGoogan Library has contributed space, supplies, and a substantial amount of personnel time to the project. Although it is difficult to place a dollar amount on personnel contributed to the ongoing project, statistics show that the average subject request takes roughly two hours to complete. As indicated in Table 5-1, the library currently processes an average of 37 requests a month, requiring approximately 74 hours of effort by the reference staff, plus the time required by other library staff to photocopy and mail materials to the user. The statistics also clearly indicate that the requests are increasing each year. If the trend continues, additional library personnel will be needed to keep up with the growing demand.

CHIRS received approximately $64,000 in LSCA Title III funds during the first three years of operation. The grant supported the initial collection, document delivery, travel for workshops and advisory committee meetings, publicity, and printing expenses. With the termination of the grant in 1987, funding for the continuation of CHIRS was a major

TABLE 5-1: Yearly Breakdown of CHIRS Requests Received

	YEAR 1 Jan 1985 to July 1985	YEAR 2 Aug 1985 to July 1986	YEAR 3 Aug 1986 to July 1987	YEAR 4 Aug 1987 to July 1988	YEAR 5 Aug 1988 to July 1989
T O T A L REQUESTS	196	399	361	396	447
AVERAGE REQUESTS PER MONTH	28	33	30	33	37

TOTAL REQUESTS FOR 5 YEAR PERIOD = 1799 requests
AVERAGE NUMBER OF REQUESTS PER MONTH FOR
5 YEAR PERIOD = 32 requests/month

concern for the Library. A one-time grant of $1,100 was awarded by the Eastern Library System in 1987 for collection support. Since 1988, the collection has received only minimal funds from the McGoogan Library's materials budget, with less than $1,500 designated for the CHIRS collection during the past two years. Presently, a grant is being written to acquire additional funding from the Nebraska Library Commission. The dollars received would be used only for acquiring materials for the collection.

Document delivery for subject requests continues to be funded by the Nebraska Library Commission, both because the program enhances the services offered by all libraries in the state and because McGoogan does not otherwise participate in net-lender reimbursement for document delivery through the state network. Table 5-2 indicates the number of items mailed since the inauguration of the project, with an average of 4.8 items provided for each subject request. These items come from both the CHIRS and the professional collection, with the latter being the more heavily used.

COLLECTION DEVELOPMENT

A prime objective of the CHIRS project was to acquire a state-of-the-art collection of consumer health materials to use in responding to consumer requests. The materials needed to be authoritative, timely, and written at a lay level. Standard bibliographies such as *Consumer Health Information Source Book* were used as initial selection tools. Although

TABLE 5-2: CHIRS Requests Filled by Year and Collection Type

	TOTAL REQUESTS FILLED	TOTAL ITEMS SENT	ITEMS FROM CHIRS COLLECTION	ITEMS FROM PROFESSIONAL COLLECTION
YEAR 1 Jan 1985 to July 1985	196	595	169 (28%)	426 (72%)
YEAR 2 Aug 1985 to July 1986	399	1916	714 (37%)	1202 (63%)
YEAR 3 Aug 1986 to July 1987	361	1766	745 (42%)	1021 (58%)
YEAR 4 Aug 1987 to July 1988	396	1950	622 (32%)	1328 (68%)
YEAR 5 Aug 1988 to July 1989	447	2290	707 (31%)	1583 (69%)
TOTAL	1799	8517	2957 (35%)	5560 (65%)

Total number of pages photocopied: 58,751.   Total number of originals sent: 418.

NOTE: To successfully fill a majority of the subject requests received requires the full or partial use of materials from the professional collection.

these proved to be an effective way to quickly acquire an initial collection, we found that a number of items were already out-of-print due to the ephemeral nature of many consumer health publications. We realized that ordering two copies of each book was advantageous, and it became standard policy to order both a circulating and a reference copy of each title.

Selection decisions were made by the head of the Reference Department and the collection development officer, relying heavily on book reviews for selection purposes. These include *Consumer Health Information Source Book, Booklist, Library Journal, Consumer Connections* (the newsletter of the Consumer and Patient Health Information Section of the Medical Library Association), and *Medical Self-Care*. In addition, *American Libraries* and subject bibliographies of established consumer programs were used as supplementary selection tools. Consultations with health professionals identified additional items for purchase.

Questions have been monitored over the years as an aid in collection development. Questions for which no information in the CHIRS collection was available were recorded. The collection development officer was informed and consumer health materials were eventually purchased to help fill these gaps in the collection. Unfortunately, there will always be topics not addressed in lay material because of the rarity of the disorder or the experimental nature of the treatment. For these requests, materials are extracted and sent from the professional collection and the requestors are encouraged to discuss the information with their health professionals.

The professional collection of the McGoogan Library has provided a major information resource for the CHIRS program. It often contains the only material available to address the consumer's question, since questions often deal with rare syndromes or new or experimental treatment. Obviously a local public library cannot afford to maintain collections that address such clinical questions. By referring the question to the CHIRS program, the local library can provide an information service to the consumer that would not otherwise be available locally. Table 5-2 shows that of the total number of requests filled over the last five years, 65 percent of the materials sent were from the professional collection, whereas only 35 percent came from the CHIRS collection. This is not surprising in that the questions that can be easily answered through the lay literature are screened out and answered at the local level.

Reference and circulating copies of pamphlets are either purchased or obtained free from various health care organizations. The journal *Medical Times* has proved to be an especially useful selection source for pamphlet material, since it contains a patient education section which lists a variety of pamphlets available on selected topics. The CHIS collection on microfiche also provides access to pamphlets on a wide variety of topics.

Journal subscriptions are an essential component of the CHIRS print collection. Consumer health journals are shelved with the CHIRS collection rather than with the professional journals, since this makes it much easier for patrons and librarians to access all the consumer materials in one location. Contrary to the practice of other consumer health programs, audiovisual materials have not been considered for purchase for the CHIRS collection. Although it was initially planned that a limited number of nonprint items would be acquired, the CHIRS Advisory Committee recommended that this option be dropped due to the limited funds available.

A file of materials to be ordered is maintained by the Reference Department. This file contains book reviews, pamphlet titles, and newspaper clippings for potential orders. Developing a state-of-the-art collection means monitoring what is being published and purchasing the best materials available. Due to limited collection funding since the termination of the grant, items purchased included new editions, outstanding new works, and materials to fill subject gaps in the collection.

SERVICES

The CHIRS program emphasizes two basic services: 1) the provision of support services to nonhealth sciences libraries in order to enable them to deliver enhanced first-line health information services to their patrons; and 2) the establishment of a collection of health science materials written for the layperson that is available at the McGoogan Library for on-site use or borrowing via interlibrary loan.

Making consumer health information easily accessible to on-site and off-site patrons of the McGoogan Library is a primary goal of the CHIRS project. Pamphlets are kept in the vertical file in the Reference Department, while the books and journals are located in a clearly designated section of the reference area and identified with a special CHIRS book plate.

All titles purchased for the CHIRS collection were listed in a bibliography published regularly during the time the project received LSCA funding. The bibliography and its supplements were distributed free to all public and high school libraries in Nebraska and to individuals upon request. A nominal fee was charged to requesters outside the state. The bibliographies were intended both as an aid for collection development in libraries and as a means of identifying and requesting specific items from the collection. We learned from the Advisory Committee and from participants in the various workshops that the bibliographies were rarely if ever made available to library users. For this reason, after publication of the third edition of the bibliography in 1987, it was decided that a fee would be charged for future bibliographies to cover printing and distribution costs and that it would be sent to libraries only upon request.

Consumers are encouraged to use their local public libraries instead of contacting the McGoogan Library directly. If the local library cannot supply enough information, the request is referred to the McGoogan Library via phone, mail, or electronic mail. Libraries may request any title from the UNMC collection. Items in the CHIRS collection are loaned at no charge to the user (with reimbursement provided by the Library Commission), while titles from the professional collection are assessed the usual interlibrary loan fee. For subject requests, a UNMC reference librarian scans the collection and sends whatever books, pamphlets, or articles best answer the request. There is no charge for filling a subject request for a consumer, even if professional materials are used.

Although it is preferable for patrons to initiate their requests through their local libraries, some patrons do contact the McGoogan Library directly. As can be seen in Table 5-3, 62 percent of the CHIRS requests were received from libraries, while the remaining 38 percent came directly from requestors. We do respond to direct inquiries, but requestors are encouraged to use their local public libraries for future health information requests.

CHIRS has truly proved to be a service for all Nebraska residents. Statistics maintained since the start of the program indicate that the number of requests received from areas in the state correlate closely with the area populations. The state of Nebraska covers a land area of 76,644

TABLE 5-3: Comparison of Library Referral Requests and Direct Inquiries from Individuals

TYPE OF REFERRAL		TOTAL NUMBER OF REQUESTS PER YEAR
YEAR 1 No statistics available		N/A
YEAR 2 Library referred:	282 (71%)	399
Directly requested:	117 (29%)	
YEAR 3 Library referred:	198 (55%)	361
Directly requested:	163 (45%)	
YEAR 4 Library referred:	243 (61%)	396
Directly requested:	153 (39%)	
YEAR 5 Library referred:	266 (60%)	447
Directly requested:	181 (40%)	
TOTAL REQUESTS* Library referred:	989 (62%)	1603
Directly requested:	614 (38%)	*total is for Year 2 through Year 5 (August 1985 through July 1989)

square miles and is divided into 93 counties, served by six library systems which vary in size from seven to 20 counties. The total population in 1984 was 1,605,971, with an average population density of 20.5 persons per square mile. Some counties in the western part of the state have less than two people per square mile, while in the Eastern System, where Omaha is located, the population density is over 1,190 persons per square mile. As Figure 5-A shows, the distribution of requests received since the program began closely parallels the distribution of the state's population.

FIGURE 5-A: CHIRS Requests by Location, January 1985–July 1989

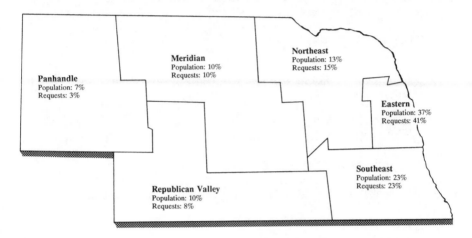

Total Population: 1,605,971
Total # Requests Filled: 1,799

Source: *Nebraska Statistical Handbook 1986–1987,* 9th ed.
(Lincoln, Nebraska: The Nebraska Department of Economic Development, 1987), 13–19.

CHIRS was originally established to serve Nebraska residents only and continues to receive funding from the Nebraska Library Commission to support document delivery within the state. For this reason, services to nonresidents are limited. Nonresidents may use the collection in the Library, and photocopies of materials will be sent to out-of-state patients at the request of a Nebraska health professional. Anyone may use the collection on-site. Any Nebraska resident may borrow materials from the CHIRS collection by showing two pieces of identification or a letter of referral from a health professional.

CHIRS WORKSHOPS

In the first year of the program a full-day workshop entitled *Consumer Health Information and the Non-Health Sciences Librarian* was developed and presented to nonhealth science librarians at various locations throughout the state. The workshops provided a thorough introduction to the delivery of consumer health information by nonhealth science librarians. Guidelines were presented for evaluating and selecting consumer health materials; the legal aspects of providing consumer health information to laypersons were explained; and medical reference techniques and tools were introduced. By the end of the day, participants not only understood how and why medical reference differs from general reference, but also gained sufficient confidence to offer such services to their patrons. One hundred twenty-two people participated in 11 workshops provided during the first two years of the CHIRS program.

MARKETING AND PUBLIC RELATIONS

Promotion of CHIRS has been targeted toward three different audiences: 1) nonhealth science librarians; 2) health information consumers; and 3) health professionals. A series of brochures and posters highlighting the project were distributed to network libraries to inaugurate the program. All brochures featured the unique CHIRS logo, using a different color of ink to highlight its contents. The brochures included: 1) an overview of the program; 2) access procedures; and 3) a patron brochure. The main thrust of the publicity campaign was to familiarize librarians with the program while encouraging requestors to continue to rely on the public library as their primary resource for all types of information.

Health professionals were targeted by an active publicity campaign during the second year of the grant. A new brochure was specifically designed and mailed to all physicians in the state, emphasizing the collection as a resource for patient education materials. Once again the campaign stressed the local public library as the access point for consumer health information.

The CHIRS bibliography continues to be distributed as a public relations tool to patient educators at the University of Nebraska Medical Center. Encouraging the use of CHIRS materials for patient education has further strengthened the educators' positive opinion of this project. Planning is underway to provide a computerized listing of the CHIRS collection to the UNMC clinical staff as a part of the current Patient Information System. Physicians and nurses may search this electronic database to select materials for use with their patients, with the documents delivered directly to the health professional.

A tabletop display entitled "Information . . . The Key to Decisions for Health Care for You and Your Family" has been used extensively. It is intended for use by libraries at health fairs, meetings, or anywhere library services are promoted. It may be borrowed for up to two weeks by any library in the state. Exhibit users are provided with a sign containing their library's name and phone number as the sponsor of the exhibit. To date, the exhibit has been used by more than 36 libraries in the past five years.

An additional promotional product for CHIRS is an 11-minute continuous playing slide/tape presentation which can be used alone or with the CHIRS display. This can also be borrowed for up to two weeks by any library in the state.

Future marketing plans include both a new poster promoting the CHIRS program and an updated CHIRS bibliography. Although the project continues to be well received, constant marketing is vital to promote the service as we continue to seek collection funding and to justify the continuation of "free" document delivery to consumers.

EVALUATION

Since the inauguration of the program in January 1985, a user evaluation form with an attached postage-paid envelope has been mailed along with each subject request. Of the 1,799 forms mailed to date, 665 (approximately 37 percent) have been returned. Responses indicate that 89 percent of consumers considered the quantity of material sent to be appropriate, while 80 percent were satisfied with the level of materials. Overall, 52 percent were completely satisfied, while 44 percent were partially satisfied.

Ninety-two percent of the respondents were seeking information about a disease, treatment, diagnosis, drug, or outcome of a condition or treatment, and 63 percent of the users had discussed their condition or treatment with a health care provider before requesting information from the library.

A concern in starting up and continuing a program is determining how effectively system mechanics are working. Evaluations clearly indicated that 59 percent of the users had obtained CHIRS services through their public libraries, confirming that the referral process is working and overall users are satisfied with the process.

The evaluation form has been a tremendous validation of the success of the program. It is used by the McGoogan reference librarians to assess their ability in answering consumer questions and provides written documentation that the program merits continuing support by the Library and the Library Commission. In addition, it allows the consumer to comment on the information received and request additional materials if necessary. A sample of the evaluation form is shown in Appendix I.

THE FUTURE

The McGoogan Library of Medicine is committed to the continuation of the CHIRS program, and is actively striving to obtain permanent funding. More than 1,800 Nebraska residents have benefited from the CHIRS program during the past five years of its existence, and those consumers have shared their positive experiences with their local public libraries. Statewide enthusiasm for the program has fostered a closer working relationship between the academic medical center and public libraries. Without doubt, the program has become a vital information resource for health-care consumers in the state.

BIBLIOGRAPHY

Consumer Health Information Service. Ann Arbor, MI: University Microfilms International, 1983, 1985, 1987–1989.

Rees, Alan M. and Hoffman, Catherine. *The Consumer Health Information Source Book.* 3rd edition. Phoenix: Oryx Press, 1990.

Tappana, Kathy. "CHIRS Assists Nebraska Public Libraries." *MCMLA Express.* 7 (2) May 1985. 5+.

Weaver, Carolyn G. "Consumer Health Information: As Close as the Nearest Public Library." *Nebraska Library Association Quarterly.* 16 (1) Spring 1985. 16–18.

━━━━━━━━━━━━━━━━

APPENDIX:
CHIRS: Consumer Health
Information Resource Services

Leon S. McGoogan Library of Medicine
University of Nebraska Medical Center

Information on the subject of _____ has been provided for you through the CHIRS Program, a grant funded by the Nebraska Library Commission under the Library Services and Construction Act. CHIRS is administered by the McGoogan Library of Medicine, working in cooperation with your local library. Please help us evaluate the CHIRS program by completing this questionnaire and returning it as soon as possible in the postage-paid envelope which has been provided. All responses will be held in strict confidence.

THANK YOU VERY MUCH FOR YOUR ASSISTANCE.

1. Please check the one response which best describes the *type* of information which you were seeking:
   ____ General, nontechnical information about a health- related topic such as exercise, diet, child-care, drug abuse, etc.
   ____ Specific information about a disease, treatment, diagnosis, drug, outcome of a condition or treatment, etc.
   ____ Patient education materials. (Health professional requestors only.)
   ____ Other (please describe):
2. If your request was for specific information about a condition, treatment, etc., have you discussed the subject with a health-care provider?
   ____ Yes, before requesting information from the Library.
   ____ Yes, since receiving this information.
   ____ No, but I intend to talk to my health care provider about the subject.
   ____ No. My question has been fully answered.
   ____ I am a health-care professional. Materials were requested for patient education.
3. How many items (books, photocopies, or audiovisuals) did you receive from the McGoogan Library in response to your request? _____
4. Please evaluate the *quantity* of the materials which you received.
   ____ Too much material sent.
   ____ Not enough material sent.
   ____ Quantity was just right.
5. Please evaluate the *level* of the materials which you received: (*Health Professionals:* Please respond from the viewpoint of the ultimate user of the information.)

_____ Materials were too technical.
_____ Materials were too general or elementary.
_____ Materials were at just the right level.
_____ Other (please explain):

6. How completely did the materials provided satisfy your information needs?

_____ Completely _____ Partially _____ Not at all.

7. How did your request for information reach the McGoogan Library? (Check only one response, please.)

_____ I went to my local library for information, and they referred the request to the McGoogan Library. (Materials were picked up at my local library.)

_____ My local library referred me directly to the McGoogan Library.

_____ My physician or other health-care provider referred me to the McGoogan Library for information.

_____ I learned about CHIRS from _____ and contacted you directly for services or information.

_____ I requested information directly from the McGoogan Library without being referred by anyone else.

PLEASE RETURN THE QUESTIONNAIRE TO:

CHIRS Project Coordinator
McGoogan Library of Medicine
University of Nebraska Medical Center
42nd and Dewey Avenue
Omaha, Nebraska 68105
THANKS AGAIN FOR YOUR ASSISTANCE.

Request filled by _____

CHAPTER 6
The Ellen Gartenfeld Health Information Network (EGHIN)

August La Rocco

DETERMINANTS OF NEED

When Americans are polled, they are most likely to list health as their number one concern, choosing physical well-being over anything else, including love, as their chief source of happiness.[1] This, no doubt, is a major factor in accounting for what Alan Rees[2] refers to as, "the public's voracious appetite for health information." Moreover, when questioned, the public lists print media as their main source of health information.[3] This focus of interest is not without its reward to the consumer, for it has been demonstrated that high health knowledge is associated with positive health habits.[4] Further, as D.R. Seibold et al.[5] observe, "The more people understand and can cope with health related issues, such as nutrition, disability, disease early warning signs, and risk factors for chronic disease, the more the entire health care system is strengthened." Being *au courant* with diverse and rapidly changing health knowledge is an enormous task for consumers and those who are instrumental in keeping the public informed. Consequently, the librarian's role in facilitating the flow of health information from the source to the end-user is a most significant one.

Information for the consumer on health care tends to be scattered, diverse, and not ordinarily part of any system. Any of several types of libraries may contain the information needed by the the the consumer—public libraries, hospital libraries, academic libraries, or information centers on categorical diseases. A design for coordination and the mapping of pathways to consumer health information awaited leadership.

RISE OF LIBRARIES ON THE SCENE IN PROVIDING HEALTH INFORMATION

As in any health context, in the field of librarianship there are certain leaders who challenge the status quo and, through their efforts at innovation, point to new directions. Their accomplishments with respect to consumer health information are well documented in Alan Rees' book, *Developing Consumer Health Information Services.*[6] Among these leaders were Ellen Gartenfeld and Eleanor Goodchild. A definitive narrative of the consumer movement in America is yet to be written, since enough time is yet to pass to afford the necessary historical perspective.

With the awakening interest in consumer health information, the first two federally funded programs, begun in 1976–77, were CHIPS, in California, and CHIN, in Massachusetts. These two programs were in many respects models for future programs in this field. CHIPS, the Consumer Health Information Program and Services, began in 1976 as the result of a contractual arrangement between the Los Angeles County Harbor-UCLA Medical Center Libraries and the Carson Branch of the Los Angeles County Library to provide consumer health information services.[7] The administrator of the program was Eleanor Goodchild. The two libraries are one mile apart and serve more than two million people of multi-ethnic backgrounds.

The major aim of the project was to coordinate and share findings and activities associated with the CHIPS goal of establishing a network involving different kinds of libraries as well as health agencies. The fact that this was a network involving multi-type libraries was particularly significant, since until that time networks of health information resources were essentially of one type of library. This bridging of the gap between public and health science libraries constituted an innovation in networking.

Shortly after CHIPS was begun in 1977, CHIN, the Consumer Health Information Network, was initiated in Massachusetts. This project was jointly funded under the Library Services and Construction Act and the National Library of Medicine. Like CHIPS, CHIN was a cooperative endeavor comprising the Mount Auburn Hospital in Cambridge and the six public library systems of the hospital's catchment area.[8] The late Ellen Gartenfeld secured the original funding and was the project's coordinator. She later secured the additional funding which by 1982 amounted to $277,000.[9] CHIN's purpose, as with CHIPS, was to bring together the skills and resources of public and health science libraries in order to make health information more available to residents in the community. Under this program, public libraries were conceived as the primary access points for consumers and community-based professionals. At the same time, it committed Mount Auburn Hospital to providing the ongoing support that the public libraries require in order to fulfill this role. Assistance from the Hospital included the overall administration of CHIN, the production of a union list of books, assistance in collection development, in-service training for public libraries, and guidelines for evaluation of input. The pioneering work of Goodchild and Gartenfeld served as an impetus for consumer health services in libraries in other parts of the country.

ELLEN GARTENFELD HEALTH INFORMATION NETWORK

The Ellen Gartenfeld Health Information Network was started in 1985. Its beginning has somewhat different roots from programs elsewhere. The impetus for its development came from patients and family members of financial support groups of the medical school at the University of Miami. Members of these groups increasingly turned to the Louis

Calder Memorial Library of the medical school for health information. The Library has always regarded these benefactors as primary users and, therefore, offered its fullest assistance. In handling these information requests, the Library staff learned that while the Library had the resources to meet the needs of health-care professionals, the collection of popular materials was inadequate. Further, the materials it did have were not organized into a structured body of information. It was decided, therefore, to establish consumer health information services in the Library as a distinct unit. The Medical Auxiliary, one of the support groups, generously provided the funding for start-up costs. This enabled the Library to proceed with a program of development of the network in successive stages. Formal networking of consumer health information services throughout South Florida, with the Calder Library serving as a focal point, was determined to be the ultimate goal. Due to the modest funding at hand, it was necessary to start on a small scale in terms of expenditures and staff, with the aim of gradually expanding operations. By small scale is meant the acquisition of 100 books, 10 periodicals, and a pamphlet collection on microfiches.

The first step in this program called for the naming of this division of the library, which became the Ellen Gartenfeld Health Information Network (EGHIN) in honor of the coordinator of the highly successful CHIN program, and the daughter and niece of two of the Medical Auxiliary officers. EGHIN represents an application of Gartenfeld's concept to the design and implementation of a long-range program to meet the needs of the larger and more diverse community of South Florida.

The next step in planning and implementation of EGHIN was the designation of space within the Library and the obtaining of equipment and supplies. The area chosen was the former browsing room, consisting of 1,600 square feet. The patron area includes bookcases, periodicals shelving, divans, chairs, and a display case. The overall effect is one of informal and comfortable surroundings.

COLLECTION DEVELOPMENT

The next step in the implementation of EGHIN was the acquisition of a basic working collection. The contents of the collection were to reflect the health needs of the general population. Particular emphasis was placed upon collecting literature on the elderly, due to the demographics of South Florida with its high proportion of elderly and the fact that seed money for establishing the Library collection was provided by a group of senior citizens (Medical Auxiliary).

Although books and periodicals are essential components of any biomedical library, there is another dimension to consumer health libraries. Whereas pamphlets are a relatively insignificant part of a medical library for professionals, they assume a much more important role in a consumer health collection. Many consumers seek brief, succinct, authoritative information, which need is often met by pamphlets. Consequently, emphasis was placed on acquiring a pamphlet collection in addition to books and periodicals.

The publication of *CHIS, Consumer Health Information Service* was fortuitous.[10] It allowed us to acquire for EGHIN 1,200 pamphlets on microfiche. The entire corpus is well indexed, and each pamphlet is summarized in a printed manual with insertions for the fiche. The basic collection consists of publications up to 1983. We have subsequently acquired the 1985 supplement of 380 additional pamphlets. Printouts of fiche can be made with a projection-printer, which was also acquired. The latest edition of *CHIS* was published in 1989.

Along with the acquisition of *CHIS*, we proceeded with building a books and periodicals collection. Expenditure restraints encouraged careful and judicious evaluation of materials. Various selection tools were employed, among the most valuable being Rees' *Consumer Health Information Source Book.*[11] This work provided critical evaluations of books and recommendations for purchase. Starred items are noted for a core collection. Other sources used in collection development were *The New York Times Book Review, Library Journal, American Journal of Public Health* and *American Journal of Nursing.*

Beyond the recommendations contained in these sources, certain criteria were established for book purchase. The author of any book considered must have a terminal degree (M.D. or Ph.D.). If not, then the book must be sponsored or bear the imprint of a recognized health organization, e.g., the American Public Health Association. This rule is not inflexible, however, and exceptions are made. For ongoing building of the book collection, CATLINE may also be employed. Despite the fact that it is a database primarily intended for health professionals, there are over 1,000 entries on consumer health. By creating an SDI profile employing relevant MeSH descriptors, new items in CATLINE can be identified. Since books cited in CATLINE bear no assessment criteria, they should generally be ordered on an approval plan.

Utilizing these sources and criteria, 100 books were initially ordered. The book collection has since grown to more than 200. Books are cataloged on OCLC. Two sets of cards are produced. One set of cards is entered in the Library's main catalog, just as it appears in OCLC; the second set is filed in the office of the coordinator.

The selection of periodicals requires even more careful evaluation than books, since subscription costs involve a continuing, long-term expenditure. There is also an appreciable quantity of editorial content of a questionable nature. A survey by the American Council on Science and Health of 30 popular journals showed that a significant percentage contained unreliable health information.[12] Periodicals chosen for EGHIN were among those highly recommended by Rees. Ten periodicals were chosen for subscription, which number has remained stable.

INFORMATION RETRIEVAL

Implicit in any contemporary concept of networking is computer access. Theoretically, libraries are no longer dealing with owned materials, but with available ones. As R.G. Schuman puts it, "Users need what they need when they need it. They don't care who owns what; they expect libraries to not only identify resources, but to provide resources."[13] It should be possible in a maximally functioning network to tap into any system anywhere. EGHIN, as part of the Calder Library, has capitalized on this capability through Docline and other interlibrary loan systems.

Online bibliographic resources of consumer health information are now fairly extensive. By way of example, the Consumer Drug Information Index or CDIF offers online descriptions of more than 250 of the top generic drugs marketed in the United States. This represents more than 50,000 brand names, comprising 95 percent of the prescriptions in the United States. Descriptions are written in simple lay language. Particularly helpful is the combined Health Information Database or CHID. It consists of a number of subfiles, such as Arthritis, Diabetes, Health Education, Digestive Diseases, and High Blood Pressure. One can search all of the subfiles at once, or any of them separately. CHID is a multi-media database, including printed materials and audiovisuals.[14] A search can be limited to format, such as large print, pamphlets, newspaper articles, videotapes, motion pictures, filmstrips, or slides. One can further restrict a search to availability, such as free documents on a subject. Especially useful is the audience level parameter. Each citation indicates if the item is aimed at the general public, health professionals, patients, or health-care providers. One can search by any of these access points. Also included in many of the citations is an evaluation notation. CHID is the result of a project comprising a number of federally funded agencies.

Other databases not specifically directed to the consumer, but which contain information of this kind are the GPO Monthly Catalog, Public Affairs Information Service or PAIS, Health Planning and Administration, Nursing and Allied Health Literature, National Information Sources on the Handicapped, and the National Clearinghouse on Mental Health.

Consumer health librarians are quite often asked questions pertaining to articles that have recently appeared in newspapers, such as a new drug being tested for arthritis. Online newspaper indexes can quickly identify such information. Vutext (Knight Ridder), to which the Calder Library subscribes, indexes newspapers of major cities. Each issue of a newspaper is textword indexed and as up-to-date as the preceding day of publication. One can search newspapers, such as the *Miami Herald,* and obtain not only the citation of the article in question, but full or partial text retrieval.

USAGE FEEDBACK

As a means of evaluating services provided, a log was devised with a format for recording patron affiliation, title of queries, whether a manual or computer search was performed, manner in which the information was transmitted (phone, mail, or in-person), and, finally, the time needed to fill the request.

Our statistics indicate that the time required to fill requests has ranged from five minutes to five hours. The average time per request is 36 minutes. The median time is 20 minutes per request.

In terms of the users of EGHIN, the statistics are compiled in terms of affiliated and unaffiliated users. Affiliated users consist of faculty, staff, and students of the University, and voluntary organizations supporting the Library (Medical Auxiliary, Friends for Life, Charity Mrs.). Unaffiliated users are the general public, hospitals, and other libraries. There is no specific breakdown for each of the two categories of affiliated and unaffiliated. Of 114 users in the last annual report, 73 or 64 percent were affiliated users, while 41 or 36 percent were unaffiliated.

The most frequent type of request has been for assistance in choosing a physician. In this regard, the University of Miami's *Directory of Clinical Services* has been most helpful.[15] Marquis' *Directory of Medical Specialists,* used by most libraries, is arranged by broad specialty category. Patients, however, are more likely to be interested in physicians in clinical subspecialties, such as those who are not only board certified, but who specialize in corneal transplants. The University of Miami *Directory* addresses this type of request.

As to type of request, 42 percent fell into the physician category. The next highest (31 percent) was for information on a particular disease, followed by 21 percent for information on medications. The remaining 6 percent may be broadly categorized as nondisease related, such as preventive health care and exercise. Clearly, most people are less interested in health maintenance than in immediate problems involving illness. These statistics reveal the paucity of questions on health maintenance and prevention.

NETWORKING

Network operation of EGHIN may be considered as triage structured. While requests to Calder by consumers in person, by mail, or via telephone are invariably honored, EGHIN was never intended to totally displace health information services at community libraries. Indeed, community libraries are expected to maintain viable collections in consumer health. Librarians at such libraries should mediate requests and endeavor to provide the necessary information within the limits of their library's resources and acquired skills in health information retrieval. If a given question cannot be answered, then Calder can be called upon through EGHIN to draw upon its resources and personnel training in health sciences librarianship. EGHIN may thus be perceived as the apex of a triaged system.

While EGHIN markets its services to primarily volunteer support groups, it should be stressed that its policy is to answer any question regardless of who submits it. Our aim is to keep referrals at a minimum. EGHIN will honor such requests rather than refer them. The users of EGHIN are drawn from the community at large and, as it becomes better known, on a statewide and regional basis. While there is no formal linkage with the state or region, this is an ultimate goal.

The CLASSIC network (Calder Library Access to Service System/Information Consortium) affords an added dimension to consumer health information transfer via a separate track. CLASSIC is a fee-based, cost recovery, extramural service whose members are given the status of primary clientele (faculty, staff, or students). Members, thereby, have full library privileges and are entitled to all services at in-house rates.[16] While membership is open to anyone in the community, hospitals are preponderant in number—21 of a total of 41 as of 1989. Through the instrumentality of CLASSIC, EGHIN has become increasingly engaged in the growing involvement of hospitals in patient education and presentation to the lay community of wellness programs. Health educators and physicians call upon EGHIN for needed materials in preparing their presentations. While such materials are, ultimately, of intrinsic benefit to the consumers, hospitals have recognized their value in public relations.

PERFORMANCE STANDARDS

In the course of the administration of EGHIN, certain principles or standards of professional performance have emerged. These have been incorporated into a Procedure Guide written for the Library, certain elements of which are suggested as paradigmatic. The administrator or coordinator of consumer health information services should perform the following:

1. Be cognizant of new findings and developments across the entire spectrum of health and medicine. This aspect of consumer health information librarianship bears particular emphasis as it has ethical implications. Patrons seeking information on a particular health matter are in effect putting themselves in the hands of a librarian who may well influence their health outcomes. Let us assume that a patron is seeking information on the effects of smoking. If the librarian provides the patron only with publications of the Tobacco Institute, it is conceivable that the patron may well make a decision to smoke or continue smoking, thus adversely affecting the patron's health. Scenarios of this kind can be multiplied manifold. As another example, consider the ongoing question of cholesterol. A recent article in *Atlantic Monthly* has had widespread impact.[17] The author denies that the risk of heart disease is lessened by low cholesterol diet or special drugs. On the other hand, the National Heart and Lung Institute and the American Heart Association argue to the contrary.[18] A patron who wishes to learn about cholesterol should not simply be shown the *Atlantic Monthly* article, but should be presented with literature on both sides of the issue. It may fairly be argued that a precept of the Hippocratic Oath has a bearing on the consumer health librarian's calling—above all do no harm.[19]
2. Design strategies and programs for optimal collection and dissemination of health care information to the consumer. This means engaging in systematic collection development in accordance with defined criteria for materials selection. The librarian must acquire competence in evaluating books, journals, pamphlets, and other media.

3. Contribute to the corpus of professional literature on consumer health information. This may be accomplished by means of bibliographies, issuance of specialized directories, descriptions of innovative practices, or state-of-the-art studies.
4. Be conversant with the latest technologies in information transfer by engaging in planned and systematic reading and analysis and appraisal of library literature and information science.
5. Understand the health implications of providing health information to the layperson. The librarian recognizes that one ought not withhold information, as long as it exists in published form. But under no circumstances should the librarian comment on the efficacy of therapy prescribed by a physician.
6. Acquire capability in the marketing of health information available in the library. Brochures on services should be written together with newsletters.
7. Establish community linkages to health information services. The librarian must be thoroughly knowledgeable as to the scope, diversity, and breadth of community referral resources, and forge working relationships with individuals involved in health-care delivery.
8. Play a role in the fostering and development of continuing education. To this end, the librarian should assist in coordinating workshops, seminars, and symposia for other librarians.
9. Demonstrate a thorough knowledge of unit routines and procedures, conduct statistical and other studies, and recommend more efficient procedures and services.
10. Have a positive attitude toward reference work and exhaust all sources in the library before turning to other sources. Be objective in helping the patron and regard everyone as important regardless of the question.
11. Conceptualize the flow of health information in terms of a triage structure where smaller libraries can turn to larger libraries for information they lack.
12. Interpret library regulations and policies in a uniform and just manner so all patrons and staff receive equal treatment.

PROMOTION OF EGHIN

In order to promote the marketing of EGHIN services, a brochure was written and 5,000 copies were printed.[20] The brochure describes EGHIN's goals and services, and invites user support by way of contributions towards an endowment fund. This brochure was sent out to health agencies throughout South Florida and to support groups of Calder.

To further promote awareness of consumer health services, an exhibit was offered. This is in the nature of a tribute to Ellen Gartenfeld. It consists of a selected display of her publications, a portrait, pottery she collected, and a fond remembrance by the library director of his professional association with Ms. Gartenfeld as published in the *Bulletin*.

EDUCATION

EGHIN regards as its mission not only the provision of health information but also active participation in the education of librarians to acquire knowledge to improve their competence in this field. To this end, it cosponsored an all-day workshop at the Calder Library given by Alan Rees in 1987. Topics covered were strategies for collection development, communications skills, and knowledge of relevant information resources. It was well attended both by public and hospital librarians in the region.

As may be seen, the duties of a consumer health librarian are quite diverse, and include the gathering of information on community resources. In the course of work at EGHIN, it was evident that there was no referral directory on Alzheimer's disease for the area. As a consequence, a "Guide to Caregiving Resources in Greater Miami" was compiled. This consists of information on day-care centers, full-time nursing facilities, and support groups offering assistance on this illness to residents in Dade, Broward, and Palm Beach counties.

THE FUTURE

It is hoped that EGHIN will play an increasing role in advancing the cause of medical consumerism and, in so doing, help South Floridians take greater responsibility for their own health through better access to health information. This involves employment of the newest information technologies, collection development in greater depth, refinement of performance standards, enhancement of networking operation, more intensive marketing, and wider education activities.

REFERENCES

1. Ignatieff, M. "Modern Dying." *The New Republic.* 199 (6) December 26, 1988. 28–33.

2. Rees, A.M. "Characteristics, Content and Significance of the Popular Health Periodicals Literature." *Bulletin of the Medical Library Association.* 15 (4) October 1987. 317–22.

3. Connell, C.M. and Crawford C.O. "How People Obtain Their Health Information—A Survey of Two Pennsylvania Counties." *Public Health Reports.* 103(2) March-April 1988. 189–95.

4. Kivela, S.L., Nissinen, A, Pekka P. "Dimensions of Health Behavior among the 65-74 Year-Old Population in Eastern Finland." *Functional Neurology* 3(3) 1988. 309–35.

5. Siebold D.R., Myers, R.A., and Willinganz, S.C. "Communicating Health Information to the Public: Effectiveness of a Newsletter." *Health Education Quarterly* 10(3/4) Fall/Winter 1984. 263–86.

6. Rees, A.M., ed. *Developing Consumer Health Information Services.* New York: Bowker, 1982.

7. Goodchild, E.Y., Furman, J.A., Addison, B.L., and Umbarger, H.N. "The CHIPS Project, a Health Information Network to Serve the Consumer." *Bulletin of the Medical Library Association.* 66(4) October 1978.

8. Gartenfeld, E. "Community Health Information Network (CHIN), Boston." in Rees, A.M. *Developing Community Health Information Services.* New York: Bowker, 1982. 129–53.

9. Lemkau, H.L., Jr. "Ellen Gartenfeld, 1938–1984 (Obituary)." *Bulletin of the Medical Library Association.* 73 (1) January 1985. 92.

10. Rees, A.M., ed. "CHIS; Consumer Health Information Service." Sanford, NC: Microfilming Corporation of America, 1983. Supplement. Ann Arbor, MI: University Microfilms International, 1985. Revised Edition. University Microfilms International, 1989.

11. Rees, A.M. and Hoffman, C. *The Consumer Health Information Source Book.* 3rd ed. Phoenix: Oryx Press, 1990.

12. American Council on Science and Health. "1986–1988 ACSH Survey on Nutritional Accuracy in American Magazines. Special report." New York, 1989.

13. Schuman, P.G. "Library Networks: A Means, Not an End." *Library Journal.* 112(2) February 1, 1987. 33–37.

14. Lumin, L.F. and Stein, R. "CHID: A Unique Health Information and Education Database." *Bulletin of the Medical Library Association.* 75(2) April 1987. 95–100.

15. University of Miami, Jackson Medical Center. "Directory of Clinical Services." Miami, 1989.

16. Williams, T.L., Lemkau, H.L., Jr., and Burrows, S. "The Economics of Academic Health Sciences Libraries: Cost Recovery in the Era of Big Science." *Bulletin of the Medical Library Association.* 76(4) October 1988. 317–22.

17. Moore, T.J. "The Cholesterol Myth." *Atlantic Monthly.* 264(3) September 1989. 37–70, passim.

18. "Doubts about the Cholesterol Crusade (editorial)." *The New York Times.* September 14, 1989.

19. "The Oath of Hippocrates." *Encyclopedia Brittanica.* 15th ed. vol. 11. Chicago, 1977.

20. University of Miami, School of Medicine, Louis Calder Memorial Library. "The Ellen Gartenfeld Health Information Network" (Brochure). Miami, 1985.

CHAPTER 7
Community Access to Health Information: The Role of the New York Academy of Medicine

Claudia A. Perry and
Brett A. Kirkpatrick

THE NEW YORK ACADEMY OF MEDICINE AND THE GENERAL PUBLIC

When will my nose stop growing? How does a graduate of a foreign medical school go about finding a residency in the United States? Is Dr. Smith board certified? What information is available for treating earthquake victims and managing the public health problems following such a natural disaster? What diagnosis is indicated by this code in the DSM-III? How can I find out all there is to know about Chronic Epstein-Barr Virus? These are but a few examples of the types of health-related questions encountered at the New York Academy of Medicine Library from the general community.

The diversity of New York and its many visitors is reflected in the variety of users seeking the resources of the Academy, the only major medical research library open to the public in the New York City area. Requests are received by telephone, through the mail, and on-site, and originate not only with local residents but from throughout North and South America and overseas. Both the variety and the steady volume of requests make it a constantly interesting, but nonetheless challenging task to effectively meet the health information needs of the community without neglecting the requirements of primary clientele. The Library's commitment to serve the public has implications for staffing, collection development, hours and levels of service, equipment and budgeting, all of which become even more problematic in times of scarcity. While the Academy is to some degree a unique organization, many of its exper-

Adapted in part from Kirkpatrick, B.A. "Medical Libraries and the Public: Friends, Foes and Frustrations," *Bulletin of the New York Academy of Medicine* 63 (10) December 1987: 968–76; and Perry, C.A. "Patron Medical Queries: A Selected List of Information Sources," *Library Journal* 113 (18) November 1, 1988: 45–50.

iences may nonetheless be generalizable to other medical research libraries that have opened or have considered opening their doors to the world outside.

PUBLIC ACCESS TO HEALTH INFORMATION IN NEW YORK CITY

The Academy Library is a privately supported research collection which exists primarily to serve the needs of its fellows, staff, and subscribers, as well as the professional medical library community, through its role as the Greater Northeastern Regional Medical Library. Despite this emphasis, the Academy Library has nonetheless been open to the public since 1877. Agreements with New York Public Library (NYPL) concluded in 1898 and 1949 created a synergistic partnership between the two organizations. The Public Library discontinued collecting in medical subject areas and the Academy reduced its efforts in acquiring certain allied subject areas, with the understanding that the Academy Library would continue to serve the general public. In effect, this made the Academy the *de facto* public library for medicine in New York City, although the institution has never received any direct public support for performing that function. Nearly 80 percent of the estimated 23,500 reference inquiries received in 1989 can be attributed to the general public. Of these, approximately 60 percent were received by telephone, 39 percent on-site, and less than one percent through the mail. While representing the smallest proportion of inquiries, letters also reflect the most diverse geographic distribution of requesters: New York, New Jersey, Pennsylvania, Puerto Rico, Florida, and Texas, as well as India, Italy, Poland, West Germany, and the U.S.S.R. Most callers and visitors, however, come from the greater New York metropolitan area.

In spite of the fact that New York City boasts one of the nation's largest concentrations of medical libraries in a major metropolitan area, city residents do not have ready access to these collections. There are seven medical school libraries in the five boroughs, none of which has an unrestricted access policy, although a number are providing access for a fee. Many of the approximately 61 hospital and 28 other medical libraries in the area also must place limits on use from nonaffiliated users, or contain very specialized collections or collections of a limited size. Restrictions on use are predictable considering that most medical libraries in New York are affiliated with private institutions and have missions that stress institutional professional support.

This is not to say that citizens cannot find medical information in sites other than the Academy Library. Despite the verbal agreements between the Academy and the New York Public Library, most branch libraries in the city own selected basic medical reference works which may be suitable for assisting a fair proportion of reader requests for health information. While the research libraries of NYPL do not collect in the field of medicine, consumer health materials are collected by the branch libraries, and such collections at larger branches are likely to be more comprehensive than the Academy collection. Moreover, public librarians can provide written referrals to library members of METRO, the

New York Metropolitan Reference and Research Library Agency, when specific items known to be held at private libraries are unavailable at either NYPL or the Academy. The public is also welcome at such specialized libraries as the Center for Medical Consumers, a particularly useful source for information on alternatives to traditional medical practice, or the Brill Library of the New York Psychoanalytic Society. Nonetheless, there is no one single major medical library open to all in the New York City area. Given the degree of interest in health information and the number of potential library users in this city, it is not surprising that a fair proportion of individuals are directed or find their way to the New York Academy of Medicine.

TYPES OF USERS

While a full-scale survey of on-site library use has not been conducted recently, analysis of request patterns from online searches, telephone statistics, user surveys of the Library's CD-ROM Medline system, and past client surveys give a sense of the Library's client population over the last several years. Students—college, high school, medical, and graduate school—form one of the largest single categories of on-site users. Writers, academics, free-lance researchers, and corporate representatives from such fields as law, public relations, advertising, publishing, and insurance call or visit the Library in connection with work-related research. Except for fellows, who receive all services on a priority basis, health professionals are relatively less common direct users of the Academy Library than might be anticipated for a medical library. This is most likely due to the fact that many physicians or nurses have other affiliations through which their health information needs are met. Members of the general public using the services of the Library primarily for personal reasons form the remaining and most diverse segment of the Library's client base.

TYPES OF QUESTIONS

Routine Requests

A large proportion of inquiries from the general public consists of requests for relatively straightforward information to be found in a small number of directories and other reference sources. Requests for information on the background and credentials of physicians and hospitals are among the types of questions received at the Academy Library most often, particularly over the telephone. Requesters want to know the available information in relevant directories—educational background, years of experience, appointments, affiliations, and board certification of physicians—and are sometimes disappointed that the Library does not provide an independent evaluation of specific physicians or hospitals. The Library does not provide referrals to specialists. Instead, requesters are directed to visit the Library or to call local medical societies or hospitals for suggestions. Hospital-based referral services are flourishing in response to the perceived needs of the public for physician or specialist rec-ommendations. Academy librarians provide callers with a choice of avail-able services but advise that these groups generally supply the names of affiliated physicians, and that they may wish to evaluate a recommended physician's credentials independently.

Other frequent requests indicate that members of the public are unaware that the addresses of medical journals are listed in standard periodical directories, that medical books are listed in *Books in Print*,[1] or that the phone numbers of health-oriented associations are very likely available in the *Encyclopedia of Associations*.[2] Health consumers often assume that public libraries do not own medical dictionaries because questions on medical terminology are not common. Unfortunately, a substantial proportion of requests fall into these relatively predictable categories, which should be handled at the local public library level using standard sources. The fact that so many individuals call the Academy, sometimes long-distance, and often hold for as long as 15 minutes, suggests that librarians—both in public and in specialized settings—may need to do a better job of conducting preliminary reference interviews and publicizing the services available in their own neighborhood. Plans to drastically reduce telephone reference at the Academy in the near future in order to better assist clients in other ways make it imperative that alternative sources for answering these routine questions be better ex-plored.

One type of request for which the Academy can be of only limited assistance is for requests for informational pamphlets and handouts. Since the Library does not collect pamphlets for distribution, callers are typi-cally referred to an appropriate agency or organization, or invited to visit the Library in person to conduct their own research on a topic. Such a referral role could also be filled by local public librarians.

Problem Questions

A second category of questions is rather more difficult to deal with, and can be problematic even in the most comprehensive library. These are requests for information about a specific disease or condition with which the requester or a friend or family member is afflicted; interpreta-tions of technical information in lay terminology; diagnosis by someone on the Library staff; information concerning dosage, adverse effects, and contraindications of drugs; information about medical procedures and their appropriate use; information concerning new or experimental proce-dures or treatments recently announced in the media; information de-scribing prognosis; and all the possible information available concerning a general topic such as cancer, hypertension, or lung diseases. Requests for statistical information are particularly challenging, in part because the data are seldom available in precisely the form sought.

Even though the information requested may be available within the Library, these types of questions may cause difficulties for both Library staff and the lay client. With very few exceptions, members of the public who are not health-care professionals have common expectations when they search for health information in a medical library. Generally, they expect to find simple, straightforward answers to what are often very complex questions. They anticipate finding easily understandable printed material describing in specific terms their own unique concerns or problems. They are looking for facts rather than probabilities and possibilities, and perhaps most of all, they want to find information quickly and painlessly, without undue time spent in searching.

In the aggregate, health information consumers share similar characteristics, although their educational and cognitive skills may vary considerably. Many come to the Library with only a limited knowledge of the basics of biology and chemistry. Frequently they have grasped or retained only a portion of what they have been told by a health professional, resulting in misunderstanding and confusion. Previous beliefs and misinformation may interfere with new learning. Most health information consumers do not know the medical literature or the tools to use it effectively but, more importantly, many are not familiar with library research techniques and do not know where to begin. Few, if any, have the ability to think in terms of, or derive meaning from, statistical probabilities, ranges of normal values, or similar representations of information. And very few individuals seem to grasp the concept that a wide range of factors combine to produce unique health situations for unique individuals possessing the same general problem.

USE OF THE LIBRARY BY THE CORPORATE SECTOR

While corporate representatives may be more experienced in using a research library than the typical layperson, skills in legal or business research are not necessarily or readily transferrable to the medical library setting. Individuals delegated to conduct research on behalf of an employer are frequently working under time constraints ("the attorney needs this for trial *immediately*"), and their lack of familiarity with the medical literature may make it more difficult to meet a deadline than they had anticipated. Such researchers may have received information that is limited or incomplete, and their understanding of the research project may be minimal, leading to an insistence on finding an exact phrase rather than a passage with equivalent meaning. This tendency may be reinforced by their awareness of the ease of searching full-text documents for just such an exact phrase in their regular work setting via an online service such as LEXIS or NEXIS.

Various types of corporate research reflect specific categories of questions. Individuals engaged in research for a malpractice case may need to know standards of care or knowledge of adverse effects at a particular point in time, often many years ago. Publishing firms must frequently track down elusive or incorrect citations. Representatives of advertising firms may want clear pictures of particular parts of the body, instruments, or medical situations, while others regularly request videotape or slides of medical procedures or human organs.

AUDIOVISUAL MATERIALS AND ILLUSTRATIONS

Requests for audiovisual materials are particularly difficult to resolve. The Academy Library does not collect audiovisual materials, although slides or photographs of illustrations found in books in the collection may be produced in-house for a fee. The client in such cases holds responsibility for obtaining copyright clearance, if necessary, except in those instances where the Academy holds the copyright to a particular work. While the Library can refer the client to directories such as the *National Library of Medicine Audiovisuals Catalog*,[3] which does list producers and distributors, materials cannot be borrowed on interlibrary loan (ILL) for nonaffiliated requesters. It appears that many libraries will not borrow audiovisual materials on ILL for a number of reasons, including liability and lack of equipment for borrowers to view the materials on-site. Most medical libraries that do collect audiovisuals, at least in New York City, are not open to the public. This makes referrals extremely difficult. Medical libraries that maintain audiovisual collections and that permit on-site access for the public will need to face the issue of access to these materials. Are they to be made available to nonaffiliated users on the same basis as primary clientele? For medical libraries either with or without such collections, the matter of access to audiovisual sources for nonaffiliated users remains problematic.

Even though the Academy Library can reproduce photographs and illustrations for a fee, there is a widespread misunderstanding of the nature of the Library's collection of illustrative material. The Academy's *Illustration Catalog,* organized by subject, provides citations to illustrations in books and journals, but is not an index to a stand-alone picture file.[4] Moreover, many illustrations referenced in this source are historical in nature. Individuals requiring photographs of current material at the Academy must scan appropriate books or journals in search of a picture that meets their needs, a time-consuming and far from systematic process. Although the Academy's *Portrait Catalog* does list the Library's holdings of some 14,000 portraits and photographs, by far the bulk of the work consists of more than 229,000 citations to portraits in various printed sources in the Library's collection.[5] Despite expectations to the contrary, clients cannot simply flip through Library files and select their illustrations on a self-serve basis, which is a source of frustration to many.

LIBRARY SUBSCRIBERS

In response to the demand for priority levels of service from the corporate sector, the Academy Library maintains a Bibliographic Services Unit specifically for this client group. Businesses with a continuing need for immediate, in-depth service can subscribe to the Library on an annual basis, thereby gaining circulation privileges and the opportunity to request citation verification, photocopying, in-depth research, and online computer searches on a rush basis for additional fees. As indicated above, similar services have recently been created at a number of medical school libraries in New York City. Unfortunately, such in-depth assistance is extremely labor-intensive, and staffing levels simply do not permit this level of service for every visitor to the Library. While subscription is one answer to the problems faced by clients needing access to medical information, it is not an appropriate option for every individual using the Library for research. Cost is certainly a deterrent, but in addition, for many the need for medical information is infrequent. Although the concept of a medical information consumer usually calls forth the image of a patient or family member, representatives of the business sector are no less a part of the community surrounding the medical library, nor are their needs less acute. Medical libraries opening their doors to the general public, particularly in urban areas, are likely to encounter an increasing number of business clients as a substantial subset of their nonaffiliated users. Nonetheless, while there are differences, there are also many similarities among users of the medical library who are not health professionals.

FRUSTRATIONS OF LAY USERS

The characteristics and expectations of lay users of medical research libraries—whether their purpose is work-related, school-related, or personal—set the stage for considerable frustration on all sides. A prime irritation relates to the amount of time required to track down relevant information and the degree of independence needed to do so. Library users typically underestimate the time required for research in any library, but particularly so in a closed stack setting. At the Academy, for example, it is virtually impossible to stop at the Library during a lunch hour, scan the indexes, check Library holdings, request journals or books from the stacks, and obtain photocopies of relevant articles or chapters, all in 60 minutes or less. This would challenge the most seasoned library veteran. The task is even more daunting for a first time visitor, who requires guidance at nearly every step. Yet a one-hour turn-around is what many expect.

Apart from the practical difficulties of mastering procedures in a library of some 680,000 cataloged works and over 4,100 current subscriptions housed in 14 floors of closed stacks, orientations to the online public access catalog (OPAC) or CD-ROM version of Medline may be particularly challenging to lay clients who are unfamiliar with computers. Visitors who come unprepared with even such basics as paper, pencil, or reading glasses envision the Library as a far more user-friendly place than it turns out to be. Intimidated by the technology, unfamiliar procedures and terminology, some library users expect to be led by the hand or assume that librarians will do their work for them. The discovery that this is not possible may lead to hostility and resentment, however unwarranted.

Even when relevant information has been identified and obtained, intellectual barriers may create additional tension. Some lay clients become frustrated because they cannot understand the literature, or because they can understand parts of it but not the portions they are most interested in. Information they do identify cannot be interpreted by them in such a way as to apply to a particular situation, and answers, such as they may be, are rarely conclusive. For many it can be equally distressing to find that librarians will not, or cannot, make judgement calls or interpret the information for them.

On the library side, frustration stems from the fact that medical libraries often do not acquire the kind of materials that health information consumers can use most effectively. A more important factor, however, is that medical libraries rarely possess staffing adequate to provide the level of bibliographic instruction needed to assist users in finding the materials and resources that are available. Staff may face a stressful balancing act between meeting their responsibilities to primary clientele and their wish to be as helpful as possible to nonaffiliated users. Such assistance, usually on an individual basis, often takes a great deal of time. Limits on levels of service based on user category are frequently unavoidable.

It is also not uncommon for the public to perceive the library staff as medical experts unwilling to share their medical expertise, rather than as information experts who are sharing their expertise to the fullest. Correcting such faulty perceptions can be a difficult task, with library staff subjected to a wide variety of arm-twisting behaviors, including the occasional offer of bribes. Even when lay users accept and understand the role of the librarian, staff may experience considerable frustration trying to convince people that their questions are simply too complex to be answered simply. Finding a source that clearly lays out the various alternatives surrounding a complicated medical question may be the optimal approach, but how can one identify such a source?

STRATEGIES FOR ASSISTANCE

Given the difficulties experienced by many lay clients in understanding the medical literature, particularly that collected at the research level, there are a number of possible approaches to ameliorate the situation. For example, the nursing literature and sources geared to primary care practitioners may be more easily grasped by the lay reader than materials written for the specialist, and are also more likely to examine psychosocial issues which may be of particular interest to patients or family members. Review articles and general textbooks can provide the client with sufficient background information so that they can begin to understand more specialized sources, and may offer alternative views on treatment or prognosis which can then be pursued further.

Presenting a reader with an appropriate entry from the *Merck Manual* may be as good a starting point as any.[6] It signals to the reader that the librarian is trying to be helpful, and frees the librarian to consider subsequent strategies. Even if the operating principle upon which reference service is based is that the client is responsible for his or her own research, in some cases it may be more practical for the librarian to quickly identify likely titles from the OPAC or card catalog, find a relevant passage in a reference work, or perform a ready reference search to get the client started. This is particularly valid if it appears that guiding the client through the process will demand more of the librarian's time than doing it for the client. This is also the case when it is judged that the client has never visited the library before, is unlikely to do so again, has a fairly limited request, and appears to have difficulty in using the library. Clearly this approach would not be suitable for students or those with extensive or continuing research needs.

MEDLINE ON CD-ROM

One of the most useful aids presently available at the Academy Library for helping the public is a CD-ROM version of Medline, the database equivalent of *Index Medicus*. DIALOG OnDisc Medline makes available the last five years of the complete Medline database in a user-friendly, menu-driven format. Availability of this system has substantially expanded the Library's ability to assist lay readers in getting started with their research, particularly for questions dealing with rare conditions or very current issues, or those questions involving the coordination of several concepts. Users can quickly restrict retrieval by language, review article, or additional delimiters. The presence of abstracts and the ability to search by keyword save users potentially hours of time scanning books and indexes and then requesting possibly relevant journals, for they often can determine from the abstract whether or not an article is likely to be helpful. In a closed stack setting, this can reduce frustration levels substantially in that readers do not have to wait long periods for materials to be retrieved only to discover that they are not relevant or not easily understood. In addition, the availability of such a self-service search system reduces concerns over barriers to access based on financial constraints. Individuals unable to afford subscriber status or a mediated search from a librarian can nonetheless obtain current references without undue difficulty. This can do much to reduce the user frustrations described above.

Staff do need to spend time orienting users to the system, instructing in the use of MeSH headings, assisting with strategy, and changing discs. Currently, slightly more than 20 percent of all on-site reference interactions concern CD-ROM instruction and disc changing. The time commitment may be particularly great for those who have never before used computers. As mentioned previously, this may be an instance where a search by the librarian for the requester might be a more practical use of staff time than instruction in the system's use, particularly if only limited information is required. In other settings, it may be feasible to use stacked multi-disc CD-ROM readers (a slightly more expensive option than a single-disc reader) or to make discs directly available to clients for self-service disc changing. However, changing the discs for users provides staff with a degree of control over monopolization of the system by any one client, and facilitates discussion concerning search strategy and progress.

CONSUMER MATERIALS AND COLLECTION DEVELOPMENT ISSUES

As an alternative or adjunct to a subscription to a CD-ROM version of Medline, medical librarians may wish to consider development of a collection of materials specifically geared to the lay reader. Despite recent improvements in the quality and quantity of materials written specifically for the health consumer, there are very real limits on the ability of the medical library to collect such materials. The pressure of escalating costs for medical and scientific books and serials makes it a continuing challenge for medical libraries to keep pace with purchases for the professional-level materials needed by their primary clientele. The purchase of health-related materials written specifically at the lay level may be difficult to justify unless that aspect of community service is a strong part of the overall institutional mission or can be supported by external funding.

Acquisitions budgets in medical libraries are relatively small when compared with the budgets of university or public library systems. In 1987/1988 the highest acquisitions budget for a medical school library was $1,040,720, and most were far less.[7] In contrast, the lowest materials budget of the 107 libraries reporting such statistics in the Association of Research Libraries annual statistical survey was $1,621,181 for the same period.[8] Historically, prices for medical books and journals also tend to be higher than those of other disciplines, with the exception of chemistry and physics.

In addition to budgetary constraints, there is the matter of selection. The experience in the Academy Library suggests that health information found in the collection is accorded a high degree of credibility by virtue of its very existence in the context of a collection developed for use by health professionals. Consequently, it becomes extremely important to select materials that are medically and scientifically sound.

This self-imposed mandate conflicts directly with the Library's avowed goal to collect materials that represent all facets of medical opinion. The first formal statement of the Academy's Library appeared in 1908 and stated that representatives of all shades of opinion were to be included insofar as possible so that readers might have access to authoritative opinions which they oppose as well as those which they approve.

Significant questions must be posed: What is authoritative? What is accurate, well-documented, and scientifically sound? What is not? What is misleading, faddish, or outright wrong? To find answers to those questions for consumer health information materials, medical librarians apply the same sort of criteria for selection that they would apply to materials produced for consumption by health professionals: Who wrote or produced the work? What is his or her institutional affiliation's scientific and medical reputation? How well is the work documented? Are conclusions and recommendations based upon the latest research results? Do they reflect the prevailing opinion of organized medicine? Are other opinions and alternatives represented? Does the work contain a bibliography listing other sources of information? Is it well-written and easily understood? If research results are reported, is the research methodology sound? If recommendations are made, are risks assessed and explained, probable outcomes discussed, and exceptions to the norm noted?

If all opinions are to be represented in the library, can the health care consumer be expected to discriminate between the authoritative materials and those that are specious? Or should libraries ignore such concerns and follow a policy of *caveat emptor*? There are a host of philosophical issues here which can be argued from many points of view, but which are beyond the scope of the present chapter.

Moreover, even with the availability of high quality consumer health materials and an unlimited acquisitions budget, there is an undeniable delay between the publication of research results in the medical literature and the incorporation of such recent developments in publications geared to a lay audience. Sources written for health professionals are usually updated more often than consumer titles, and are more likely to include information on rare or unusual diseases. The subjects of consumer medical titles, not surprisingly, reflect to a large degree the prevalence of disorders in the general population. Those seeking information on less common medical conditions may be able to turn only to the professional literature.

Fortunately, a greater emphasis on patient education by primary care physicians and the growing sophistication of the general public in health matters means that members of the public increasingly ask for standard sources by name. News reports on the latest studies published in journals such as the *New England Journal of Medicine,* often result in a flurry of requests for the original article. Patients will ask for the *Physician's Desk Reference (PDR)* after seeing it used by their doctor. These requests present an opportunity for librarians to mention the availability of additional or alternative materials on the same topic. As members of the lay public expand the number of sources that they regularly consult, they become better able to use and understand the professional literature. Over time, this greater familiarity with medical terminology and sources should help to reduce considerably many of the user frustrations described earlier in this chapter.

INTERLIBRARY LOAN AND REFERRALS

Another category of problems concerns circulation and interlibrary loan issues. Upon finding a useful book, many users would like to borrow the title for home use. While most materials in medical libraries are available to students or the general public on an interlibrary loan basis, policies usually prohibit immediate loan to the individual. Unfortunately, immediate loan is typically what is desired. Even in those instances where the reader is willing to wait for interlibrary loan, it can be difficult in some instances for the medical librarian to identify the most appropriate library where such a loan request can be initiated. Although such assistance is arguably outside the responsibilities of the medical library, it is nonetheless a question that is likely to arise. In other cases, particularly with students, requesters have been directed to visit the Library precisely because they were unable to wait for materials through interlibrary loan.

Even given the best efforts to assist the lay public from available resources, in many cases people seeking health information from a medical library must be referred to other agencies, libraries, or institutions that can provide the kind and level of information that will prove most useful. While this is undoubtedly a major service in need of being provided, it also carries its own set of problems. There are literally hundreds of agencies—local, regional, national, and international—which provide some sort of health information services. Staying abreast of the programs and services of such agencies could easily occupy a full-time staff member, a luxury few medical libraries can afford. Even when what appears to be an appropriate agency for referral has been identified, one can never know for sure that the desired information is subsequently obtained by the requester. Sometimes one has the uneasy feeling that people with legitimate information needs are bouncing around from referral to referral without ever receiving a satisfactory solution.

TELEPHONE REFERENCE

These problems are particularly acute in the provision of reference service over the telephone. When a member of the public has made the effort to visit the library, staff are in a much better position to provide assistance. There are increased opportunities for extended interaction, for iterative clarification of the problem, and for direct feedback on whether or not information has been helpful.

Moreover, practical and policy issues limit the extent of information provision over the telephone. For fear of misinterpretation and liability, Academy staff do not read definitions or descriptions of diseases, provide drug information, or identify the diagnosis indicated by a particular diagnostic code over the telephone. Other questions are too complicated to handle in five minutes or less. This time limit for telephone reference calls on the public line is in part imposed because of the extremely large volume of calls, which if unchecked would severely limit the ability of staff to deal with their other responsibilities. These restrictions at times prompt callers to ask, "What *do* you provide over the telephone?" The answer, unfortunately, is not much. Staff will refer callers to other agencies, answer questions concerning ownership of materials, provide details on hours and services, and invite the caller to visit the Library. Most of these functions, however, do not require the expertise of medical librarians, and could be provided elsewhere. As has already been mentioned, recognition of the limits of the usefulness of telephone reference has prompted the decision to largely eliminate this service in 1990, so that staff can concentrate efforts in situations where they can be more helpful.

Clearly, the volume of response to public access contributes to some of the hard choices that may arise, particularly in times of scarcity. If they are to survive, medical libraries cannot do everything that might be desirable in the best of all possible worlds. It may be that some popular services must be curtailed or eliminated in order to maintain other programs, or add new services of greater utility. The important thing is that options and choices be carefully considered, with a view to potential repercussions and tradeoffs. At the same time, development of additional reference tools could make it easier for a larger proportion of health information needs to be met at the public or university library, in hospital patient information centers, or even in the physician's office.

A CONSUMER HEALTH INFORMATION WISH LIST

Medical librarians for some time have relied heavily on the databases produced by the National Library of Medicine. Access to medical information without Medline, Catline, Serline, and other Medlars databases is now nearly unthinkable. It is not unreasonable to anticipate the day when electronic access to medical information for health consumers is similarly taken for granted. On-site visitors to the National Library of Medicine can already use a number of Medlars databases through public access terminals, and additional adaptations might further increase the usefulness of these databases for a broader audience. Dirline, for example, an online directory of health and other organizations, could be expanded to include local or statewide organizations, perhaps by subcontract to regional medical libraries. A MeSH tag, added to records in Medline and Catline, could flag records appropriate for lay readers. This could be used to form the core of an additional bibliographic database geared specifically to health consumers, similar to the manner in which a subset of Medline records is augmented by records from the American Hospital Association to form the Health Planning and Administration file. Such a database could be used for collection development purposes and as a useful adjunct to indexes of the general periodical literature. The Combined Health Information Database (CHID), produced by the National Diabetes Information Clearinghouse and vended through BRS Information Technologies, is a source that currently provides bibliographic and selected full-text access on a number of health-related topics. Grouping a variety of databases like these together using CD-ROM technology could bring consumer health materials within reach of a wide audience. While developing and maintaining consumer-oriented databases would be expensive, it would undoubtedly be a cost-effective national resource when one considers the resulting reduction of effort at the local level, and especially the potential for improving consumer access to appropriate information.

Bibliographic access and referral to relevant organizations are important, but like other library users, members of the public seeking medical information increasingly want information, not simply references. The commercial sector is producing a number of full-text electronic databases, both online and in CD-ROM format, and new full-text databases are announced regularly. Some of these electronic sources are simply the online versions of previously existing print sources, such as Martindale's *Extra Pharmacopeia, Merck Manual, Scientific American Medicine,* or the *New England Journal of Medicine.* Others have been created specifically for electronic access.

The full-text, menu-driven PDQ (Physician Data Query) database, produced by the National Cancer Institute, includes a patient information component (PDQI), which could serve as a prototype for future electronic textbooks geared to the layperson. Similarly, a component of the Integrated Academic Information Management System (IAIMS) model being developed at Columbia University Health Sciences Library includes an electronic textbook with various levels of user access. The levels of access are appropriate for individuals—ranging from patients through specialists—with varying levels of medical background.

The popularity of Medline on CD-ROM at the Academy Library suggests that databases using a CD-ROM format—with keyword access, user-friendly menus, and browsing capabilities—have much to offer the nonspecialist, who often has difficulty finding preferred terminology or expressing what it is that is needed. It is frequently that first piece of relevant information that leads the user to what is actually required; for others, a brief printout is sufficient. Users could search electronic textbooks on CD-ROM by keyword and print out relevant sections, just as they presently do successfully with Medline. The textbooks could include bibliographic references for those needing further information. Regularly updated, full-text, consumer-oriented databases, in a convenient and user-friendly format such as CD-ROM, whether created by the National Library of Medicine, academic medical centers, or the commercial sector, could be a major resource for libraries and consumer groups serving the health information needs of the general public in the not too distant future. While the effort involved in developing such electronic textbooks is indeed substantial, it is unlikely that the demand for consumer health information will wane any time in the near future, and the wide dissemination of such products would certainly increase the return on the initial investment.

Convenient electronic sources geared to the health information consumer may take some time to develop, but rapid progress in medical informatics and an encouraging increase in the attention accorded to the medical information needs of the general public suggest that the development of such products is extremely likely. Already, a microcomputer-based software series produced by Clinical Reference Systems, Ltd. makes available a number of patient education materials designed for use in the physician's office (e.g., Patient Education—Pediatrics) which can be searched and printed on demand.[9] The recent release of Health Reference Center by Information Access Corporation goes a long way toward providing the consumer with comprehensive access to some 110 consumer-oriented magazines together with full text for many of the titles and consumer summaries of articles in a number of professional journals.

While one hopes that widespread availability of similar sources will simplify the challenges of providing health information to consumers, even the most ideal information source will not eliminate the need for librarians and traditional print sources for the foreseeable future. Comprehensive, user-friendly sources may, however, make it easier for the lay public to meet basic information needs at the local level, so that medical librarians can spend the needed time to assist clients with more challenging requests.

CONCLUSION

As the preceding discussion suggests, public access to the medical library can be a mixed blessing. For many medical librarians, assisting medical consumers can be a prime source of job satisfaction, and for users the availability of needed information may be of immeasurable value. Nevertheless, problems with user expectations, intellectual access, and adequate staffing levels can create problems. Clients who fully understand what levels of service and information are available at the medical library, and at what cost, are less likely to be frustrated by unrealistic demands. Educating users concerning what they may reasonably expect to find at the medical library is an important task. Ideally, it is one that should be carried out both by medical librarians and by those who refer clients to the medical library.

To some degree, problems with staffing and intellectual access can be reduced if members of the public first exhaust the resources of their local public or university library. The importance of the role of the local library in meeting basic needs of the general public for medical information cannot be overstressed. At the Academy Library, a substantial portion of the reference questions that are perceived as medical are routine ready reference requests that can be answered from standard directory resources. Answers to other frequently asked questions can be found in a relatively small number of basic medical works. If routine needs could be met at the neighborhood library, then medical librarians would be better able to concentrate on more difficult and unusual requests and spend more time with individual users. Clients might still have difficulty understanding materials available at the medical library, but they could build on the more basic information already obtained in their primary setting.

Regardless of whether users can be persuaded to visit their local libraries before coming to the medical library, certain measures may reduce difficulties once they do arrive. Careful selection of a well-organized and conveniently accessed ready reference collection for users can be invaluable for answering a large proportion of regularly encountered inquiries. Such an approach can also reduce the amount of time needed to assist lay clients in the medical library. This is an important goal if adequate staffing is a problem. Clearly written library guides and signs can help make it easier for first-time users to find their way and understand unfamiliar policies and procedures. Coordination of resources and services to the lay public may best be achieved by designating one individual as the user services librarian. Nevertheless, reference assistance should be available from all librarians who normally staff this service point. The user services librarian can also play a central role in maintaining a good working relationship with other local libraries and librarians concerned with consumer access to medical information.

Awareness of the potential problems involved with public access to the medical library, along with careful consideration of relevant issues and concerns, are important determinants of the success of such a venture. While intellectual access to the medical literature is sometimes a problem for the lay client, a number of encouraging developments seem likely to improve the situation. The quality and quantity of consumer-oriented medical titles are increasing, and it appears that the lay public is becoming more knowledgeable about medical information. CD-ROM systems and other new methods of information delivery promise to bring medical information to clients more quickly and easily. Even so, for most individuals use of a specialized medical library is likely to be infrequent, and staff assistance will continue to be essential. Committed and well-trained staff, combined with adequate staffing levels, are likely to be the critical elements in the success of medical libraries in the delivery of medical information to the health consumer. Despite the problems, medical reference will continue to grow and expand as consumers become increasingly sophisticated in their need for health information. In the end, it will be the combination of good reference service and a knowledgeable consumer that will result in a successful resolution to this challenge.

REFERENCES

1. *Books in Print.* New York: Bowker, 1948– . Annual.

2. *Encyclopedia of Associations.* 23rd ed. Detroit: Gale, 1989.

3. *National Library of Medicine Audiovisuals Catalog.* Bethesda, MD: National Library of Medicine, 1977– . Quarterly, annual cumulation.

4. New York Academy of Medicine Library. *Illustration Catalog,* 3rd ed. Boston: G.K. Hall, 1976.

5. New York Academy of Medicine Library. *Portrait Catalog.* 5 vols. Boston: G.K. Hall, 1959– . Supplement 1, 1959-1965; Supplement 2, 1966-1970; Supplement 3, 1971-1975.

6. Berkow, Robert, ed. *The Merck Manual of Diagnosis and Therapy.* 15th ed. Rahway, NJ: Merck, 1987.

7. *Annual Statistics of Medical School Libraries in the United States and Canada, 1987–88,* 11th ed. Houston: Association of Academic Health Sciences Library Directors, 1989, p. 42.

8. *ARL Statistics, 1987–88.* Washington, DC: Association of Research Libraries, 1989, p. 46.

9. Dubynsky, O. "Patient Education—Pediatrics (software review)." *JAMA* 258 December 11, 1987. 3319–3320.

CHAPTER 8
Health Information Services for Pennsylvania Residents Program—College of Physicians of Philadelphia

Andrea Kenyon

INTRODUCTION

Health has become an American preoccupation. Health is used here in the broadest sense to include all factors affecting one's physical and mental well-being. Just think about it. You exercise at a health club, you eat a healthy diet, you pay for health insurance, you visit a physician at a health clinic. Oprah and Donahue talk about it. *Cosmo* and *Good Housekeeping* write about it. TV news reporters quote from *JAMA* and *Lancet*. Newspapers have health features or sections. The Surgeon General sends you pamphlets in the mail explaining it. Health awareness has become our nation's prime preoccupation.

There are thousands of books, pamphlets, and other materials designed for the health consumer. Unfortunately, there is no convenient, systematic way for the public to become aware of consumer health publications; nor is there an organized way for health information providers to identify, acquire, and distribute quality health information designed for the consumer.

Those of us interested in providing health information are trying to assemble a giant jigsaw puzzle. Each of us is quietly working on one section of the total puzzle. The pieces are coming together very slowly, but they are beginning to fit. In the last 10 years, a number of cooperative programs have been developed to pool a wide combination of expertise for the purpose of providing more effective health information services to the community.

This chapter describes the activities at the College of Physicians of Philadelphia. Since the fall of 1985, the College of Physicians has provided health information services to state-supported institutions in Pennsylvania through its Health Information Services for Pennsylvania Residents Program.

CONSUMER HEALTH INFORMATION IN PENNSYLVANIA, 1979–1985

The need for access to consumer health information in Pennsylvania became apparent during the adoption of a statewide Interlibrary Loan Code. After meeting with district library centers, the State Library's consultant determined that access to health information was among the top five concerns of public library officials. A recommendation was made by the Interlibrary Loan Code Development Group in February 1979 encouraging district library centers and local public libraries to explore ways to cooperate with area health science libraries to share resources. During the following two years LSCA grants were awarded to consumer health information programs located in the central and western parts of Pennsylvania. In 1980, an LSCA grant was awarded to the Centre and Clearfield County Library Systems and the Philipsburg State General Hospital to fund a project designed to provide consumer health information to the residents of Centre and Clearfield counties. This was followed in 1981 by an LSCA grant to the York County Library System for the support of a cooperative health information network between the York Hospital Library and the public libraries in York and Adams counties. During the same year, the Health Education Center in Pittsburgh was awarded funds by the National Library of Medicine to provide assistance to health professionals in southwestern Pennsylvania in the selection, acquisition, and effective use of health education materials. In 1982, the Laurel Highlands Health Sciences Library Consortium established a Tel-Med program with funds received from an LSCA grant.[1]

Meanwhile in eastern Pennsylvania, a number of small, independent projects were developed. It soon became apparent that a program was needed that would unite the area's diverse health information providers into one coordinated effort. The Consumer Health Information Network (CHINET) program, proposed and developed by Anthony Aguirre, Director of the Library College of Physicians and Eleanor Goodchild, Director of the University of Pennsylvania Biomedical Library, established a consumer health information network composed of public libraries, health sciences libraries, health-care professionals, consumers, and health agencies in Bucks, Chester, Montgomery, Delaware, and Philadelphia counties.

The project existed from October 1983 to September 1985 with funding from a Title III Library Services and Construction Act Grant (LSCA) from the State Library of Pennsylvania. During the two years of the program, the co-directors of the project, project coordinator, and Advisory Committee accomplished the following activities:[2]

- Assessed, by means of a survey, needs for consumer health information services, existing collections and programs, and policies for access to these.
- Selected institutions to be surveyed for participation in the network and developed a survey instrument.

- Created a database of existing consumer health information materials in the Greater Philadelphia area and methods for obtaining them.
- Developed a workshop for public librarians on the provision of basic biomedical reference and consumer health information.
- Formulated a long-term plan for expansion of the program, addressing future funding, core collections in local libraries, database maintenance, and extended reference services.
- Established a referral network among public libraries, medical libraries, and health agencies for the conveyance of biomedical reference service to the public.

It is important to acknowledge that CHINET and similar health information programs legitimized the dissemination of health information to the public. CHINET laid a firm foundation for the continuation of cooperative activities in consumer health between Pennsylvania public and health science libraries. Many of the earlier relationships formed between public libraries and health science libraries continue today. At the conclusion of CHINET, the College of Physicians decided to expand the Library's consumer health information services and offer them to all librarians at Pennsylvania state-supported institutions. CHINET's reference and educational objectives were expanded and revised, becoming important components of the new program. Before discussing the present program, it may be helpful to provide a brief explanation of the College of Physicians of Philadelphia.

CONSUMER HEALTH INFORMATION AT THE COLLEGE OF PHYSICIANS OF PHILADELPHIA

The College of Physicians of Philadelphia was formed by 24 of Philadelphia's most prominent physicians on January 2, 1787. Their purpose was to establish an organization to promote the exchange of medical information, discuss and debate health care issues, and preserve and uphold the highest ethical standards of the profession. The name "College," derived from the Latin word "collegium," was chosen to describe their coming together as a society of professional colleagues. The College offers membership to physicians in all branches of medicine and other professionals holding doctorates in the biological sciences, nursing, and medical history. The College counts among its membership 1,822 fellows and 208 associate fellows representing 61 medical specialties and scientific and scholarly disciplines from 151 hospitals and academic medical centers throughout the world. Part of the College's mission is to mobilize the diverse capabilities of this talented group for the benefit of the larger community.

Promotion of public health was one of the founders' purposes and continues to play an important role in the activities of the College of Physicians. Throughout its history the College's Committee on Public Health and Preventive Medicine has fostered innovative ideas for health education and public health reform. The College has recently reaffirmed its commitment to public health concerns, developing a plan which will restructure and refocus client services in the Library, redirecting additional resources to support the Public Services Department's provision of health information services to the community.

The various components of the College include the Mutter Museum, founded in 1858 upon the collections of Dr. Thomas Dent Mutter. It is one of the few medical museums in the world. Pathological specimens, medical memorabiliia, and artifacts broaden understanding of the human body and of medical practice past and present. The F.C. Wood Institute for the History of Medicine was founded in 1976 to examine contemporary medical issues in historical perspective.

The Library dates back to 1788, when College Fellow John Morgan donated 16 books from his private collection to the Library. Today the collection has grown to over 322,346 bound books and journals. Its historical collections encompass one of the largest collections of medical history resources in the United States. Aside from providing library services to its fellows, the Library serves as a resource library for the Greater Northeastern Regional Medical Library Program. This is part of a national network of health science libraries, and is funded under contract to the National Library of Medicine. The Library offers a wide range of information services, including reference, computerized literature searching, and photocopy services for a fee to the medical community, law firms, pharmaceutical companies, and other organizations interested in obtaining biomedical information. The Library's extensive collections of scientific and medical journals and monographs, its experience in providing medical information services to the community, together with the College's interest in public health concerns, ideally position it to provide a program of consumer health information services to librarians at Pennsylvania's state supported institutions.

Funding of Consumer Health Information Program

The Pennsylvania legislature has included funds in the state budget to support the provision of medical and consumer health information to residents of the Commonwealth of Pennsylvania. Beginning in 1984, funds were granted to the College of Physicians in support of its service to the community as it approached its bicentennial anniversary. The College receives an annual appropriation of $100,000 which the Library uses to support the Health Information Services for Pennsylvania Residents Program for librarians at Pennsylvania-funded libraries and institutions. Since the Department of Education is responsible for the coordination and promotion of library services to all Commonwealth residents, the College submits an annual budget and performance report to the State Library. The Library Development Division of the State Library administers the monies and monitors the agreement between the College and the Commonwealth as part of its work with grants and subsidies. The College maintains a close relationship with the State Library and submits a year-end report to the state librarian.

The general breakdown of the budget is as follows:

Salaries	33%
Supplies, Postage, Communications, Printing	12%
Travel	6%
Online Searching	2%
Interlibrary Loan	13%
Collection Development	34%
Monographs, professional	5%
Consumer health materials	10%
Reference collection	25%
Journals	60%

Program Purpose and Objectives

The Library's Health Information Services for Pennsylvania Residents Program has the following goals:

- To make health information support services and resources readily available to librarians at state-supported institutions.
- To educate librarians on how to provide medical and consumer health information.
- To encourage cooperation in the collection, management, and provision of health information to Pennsylvania residents.
- To promote the public library as an important source of health information.

Our contract requires that the College of Physicians of Philadelphia Library, for the purpose of providing medical and consumer health information for the libraries and residents of the Commonwealth, shall: Provide the following listed services to all Commonwealth public libraries; community colleges; state hospital libraries; the State System of Higher Education libraries; and the State Library of Pennsylvania:

- Develop resource collections required to serve the needs of the users of the above-mentioned constituencies.
- Provide reference service to the general public by referral from public libraries.
- Supply reference service to libraries (telephone, written requests, location information, citation verification, etc.).
- Offer photocopies of current medical and scientific journal articles at no charge to the above-mentioned libraries.
- Maintain interlibrary loan service of original circulation materials at no charge to the above-mentioned libraries.
- Mount at least two continuing education workshops and develop public information materials that can be used by libraries to promote the consumer health information service.

Target Population

The College's Health Information Services for Pennsylvania Residents Program serves librarians at the following state-supported institutions:

- 669 Public libraries
- 17 Community college libraries
- 10 Correctional institution libraries
- 17 State System of Higher Education libraries
- 42 State hospital libraries
- State Library of Pennsylvania

Commonwealth libraries must respond to a diversified clientele's health information needs. The 1980 U.S. census showed that Pennsylvania had a population of slightly less than 12 million people. The Commonwealth has the nineteenth most urban population of all the states; it is 69 percent urbanized but also has the nation's largest rural population, including 55,535 farms.[3]

Pennsylvania libraries are called upon to supply health information to their users. Often these libraries have insufficient resources to answer successfully every request made for health information. While a number of these libraries rely on informal network contacts (some of which were established during the earlier CHINET program), a large number of state supported libraries seek assistance from the College. The College's services broaden the scope of district and local library resources, offering librarians the means to satisfy a broader spectrum of their patron's health information requests.

Public libraries are the ideal place to promote and disseminate health information since they are the focal point for people seeking all kinds of information and have a long tradition of responsiveness to the needs of their communities. Information sharing must be encouraged between public libraries and the many local, state, and federal health organizations that produce health-oriented books, pamphlets, and audiovisuals.

Public libraries in Pennsylvania are organized with respect to four levels of service: local libraries; library systems (which are optional); district library centers (designated by the state librarian); and regional resource centers (specifically named by law).[4] Local community libraries maintain a basic collection of current materials of an educational, informational, and recreational nature. The quantity and quality of the materials vary with the size of the community and the amount of money available for library service. The collection and services are patron-driven. The library supplies the items and services most requested by members of the community. When other materials are needed, the local library seeks assistance at higher levels through the system or district library center. The library systems are groups of libraries that unite to increase financial support or to coordinate activities that improve the level of service to all users within the system. District library centers are located in the major marketing areas of the Commonwealth. Each district center serves as a local library to its community and as a resource to area libraries within its district. Requests unable to be satisfied at this level can be sent to a regional resource center or, if health-related, to the Library of the College of Physicians of Philadelphia.

Collections

The College's collections serve as a nationwide source of biomedical information supporting research, medical education, patient care, and health policy development. These collections are primarily research-oriented and contain many specialized monographs and symposia. Approximately 2,100 journals are currently received, including over 650 foreign periodicals, representing a wide range of medical subject areas. The historical collections contain over 120,000 books and journals published before 1966. More than 400 are incunabula and 12,000 are pre-1801 imprints. Secondary historical source materials are purchased to complement these materials. Subject area strengths include history of medicine, obstetrics and gynecology, ophthalmology, pediatrics, dermatology, and radiology. Due to the wealth of academic medical libraries and hospitals in the Philadelphia area, the College avoids duplication of their efforts by not purchasing materials in the areas of dentistry, veterinary medicine, nursing, and health administration.

The Library's overall collection development policy is presently undergoing significant changes. A new emphasis is now placed on acquiring materials that support the Library's services to Commonwealth of Pennsylvania libraries. A conscious effort is made to select medical textbooks and other clinical materials that provide answers to questions from librarians at state supported institutions. The journal collection is also becoming more clinically oriented, with the number of foreign and research-oriented journals being reduced in the next two years. Approximately 15 consumer health journals have also been added to the current subscriptions.

The College places great importance on its reference collection since it is used to support many of the programs and services of the College. The reference collection contains many resources that are too expensive or would be underutilized in a public library, such as physician and medical association directories, foreign dictionaries and medical directories, and biomedical indexes.

Prior to the introduction of the Library's Health Information Services for Pennsylvania Residents Program, the College collected very little medical literature specifically written for the consumer. This area of the College's collections has been strengthened to enable the reference staff to deliver quality reference support and to recommend appropriate publications to libraries in Pennsylvania. A large portion of the consumer health collection, 150 reference titles, does not circulate, providing the staff with access to an enormous wealth of information whenever it is needed. This is not a problem since the collections at the College, unlike those of other medical libraries, circulate very little. Despite the fact that post-1900 monographs and periodicals are available for circulation (with a few exceptions), most requests are for photocopies of articles rather than for loan of the original.

The consumer health reference materials are used primarily to answer questions submitted by librarians at state supported institutions. Most of these materials are written for the layperson and provide disease-specific information. Major subject areas covered include:

- Health concerns of women
- Health concerns of men
- Health concerns of the elderly
- Pediatrics
- Cancer
- Mental health
- Surgery
- Nutrition
- Heart disease
- Drug information
- Chronic diseases

Books in the consumer reference collection are sources that provide good reference and referral information. We choose handbooks, directories, bibliographies, and other monographs that can provide succinct answers. Highly favored are those monographs with short chapters and extensive indexes, diagrams, and bibliographies. Information from these books is photocopied, providing the layperson with a concise answer to his/her question.

The general consumer health collection, located in the stacks, includes approximately 250 cataloged pamphlets and a small number of lay materials not appropriate for the reference collection. These materials are available to Pennsylvania residents through interlibrary loan from their public library. The College's consumer health collection excludes materials generally available in most public libraries, such as fad diet books, physical fitness materials, and materials discussing lifestyle changes in relationship to health. Publications written by personal narrators or crusaders, health cookbooks, and most wellness materials are also considered more appropriate for purchase by public libraries. Books that require reading in their entirety, or do not provide indexes or tables of contents, are also avoided.

Our pamphlet file is used regularly for reference services and collection development. Since our walk-in patronage is small, we keep the pamphlet file in the reference office so that it is readily available to the reference staff. The pamphlet file serves as an elaborate reference referral file and includes computer literature searches, health posters, and pamphlets and newspaper articles useful in answering health questions. The pamphlets are arranged utilizing National Library of Medicine Subject Headings. The reference staff constantly weeds, updates, and expands the pamphlet file. This is a very time-consuming but rewarding task, since pamphlet materials are indispensable when responding to consumer health questions. Multiple copies of free pamphlets are ordered and displayed in the reading room and distributed at exhibits and workshops. Locating quality consumer health information materials is a very labor intensive task. The College's library staff spends a large amount of time scanning newspapers and library and medical journals, looking through publishers' booklists, ordering materials from the government and health organizations, checking booklists, and conducting computer searches of the health literature. A dBase file has been developed to measure pamphlet, monograph, and journal usage. Daily interlibrary loan and photocopy request data are entered and tabulated to identify titles frequently requested by state supported institutions. Reference inquiries are also carefully monitored to aid in collection development. These data are used to ensure that the College's collections remain responsive to the needs of our users.

SERVICES TO PENNSYLVANIA STATE-SUPPORTED INSTITUTIONS

Reference Services

Direct Services to Pennsylvania Residents

The health information services provided directly to the consumer are reading room access and limited telephone reference. The Library restricts the use of the College's reading room and its collections. Access to the College's reading room is available to Pennsylvania residents seeking health information by referral from any Pennsylvania public library.

The reading room contains a large reference collection, including medical textbooks, dictionaries, directories, statistical resources, numerous health indexes, and the consumer health collection for easy access by the reference staff and walk-in visitors. If this material is insufficient, patrons must consult the card catalog in order to identify relevant items in our collection, since the Library has closed stacks and no browsing is permitted. This sometimes presents difficulties to public library patrons accustomed to scanning unobtrusively the shelves for materials to meet their information needs. The "unfriendliness" of our card catalogs increases the obstacles that are unintentionally placed in the layperson's path. There are four different card catalogs: a pre-1950 catalog; a post-1950 author/title catalog; a post-1950 subject catalog; and a journal catalog arranged by title.

Since most of our collection is geared towards the health professional, a considerable amount of sleuthing is required to discover material written at a level the layperson will find helpful. These barriers have increased the importance of the reference interview and the need for patrons to relinquish some of their privacy and describe their health concern to one of our staff members. The implementation of an online catalog will aid readers in identifying materials of interest in our collections. Users will then be able to scan a unified catalog for access to a majority of the College's collections. Laypersons planning to visit the Library are encouraged to notify the reference staff in advance so that preliminary work can be done on their question. Staff must work closely with each patron, orienting them with our reading room procedures and determining which resources will address their information needs.

The College's Library is unique in that almost all of our reference work is conducted by telephone, mail, and telefacsimile. On the average, 117 people visit the reading room per month. Patrons include fellows of the College, paralegals, lawyers, students, physicians, historians, and laypersons seeking health information. Reference service provided by telephone to the public is very limited. Consumers may obtain brief definitions, physician credentials, and organization addresses. Neither drug information nor recommendations of physicians or health-care facilities are provided over the telephone.

Consumers often call requesting subject information which they assume can be relayed to them over the telephone. Consumers have very high expectations regarding the response time necessary to answer what are often complex questions. Although the question may be simple, the answer can be elusive. Most consumers want simple answers, fact not theory, certainty rather than hypothesis. Consumers are surprised and frustrated when they are told that the answer to their question is too complex to be dealt with over the telephone and that the library staff cannot interpret medical information. They also find it difficult to accept that the available material does not address their specific situations.

Laypersons requesting more than a dictionary definition are informed about the free services provided to librarians at Pennsylvania state supported institutions and encouraged to avail themselves of these services through their local public library. This information is reinforced by giving the caller our name and telling them to have the public librarian call us if the library staff is not familiar with our services. Callers are encouraged to contact us if they feel their health information needs are not being met. In this connection, consumers should consider their public library as their primary information resource. The College Library wishes to be considered the "librarian's library," a valuable biomedical resource for the information specialist seeking elusive health information for his or her patron.

Reference Services to Librarians

Reference services provided to librarians at state supported institutions include requests for subject information, citation verification, statistics, and document delivery locations for ILL purposes. Table 8-1 below provides data on the number of reference requests received from Commonwealth librarians per year.

TABLE 8-1: Reference Services Statistics

	1985	*1986*	*1987*	*1988*
Total Number of Questions	451	472	514	584

Most requests are for subject information. Subject requests submitted by public librarians fall into the following categories:

- Specific aspects of a chronic condition, such as Alzheimer's, diabetes, arthritis
- Surgical procedures, such as balloon angioplasty
- Nutrition, including diet therapy
- Adverse effects of drugs and information concerning new drugs
- Current, experimental, or alternative therapies
- Disease prognosis
- Anything announced by a television reporter as appearing in a recent issue of *JAMA* or *Lancet.*

Some of our more unusual question topics have included:

- People who set themselves on fire
- How to donate a human body to science
- Sex predetermination
- Adverse effects of deep meditation
- History of wheelchairs
- Cannibalism causing "laughing disease"

Most of the subject requests we receive from state supported institutions are for patrons who are unfamiliar with the world of biomedicine. Every attempt is made to identify materials designed for the general public. The consumer health collection, the ever-growing pamphlet file, and computerized databases are consulted. These resources are usually adequate for the more "popular diseases" or if someone wants a general overview of a topic. But often the questions we receive are more specific. Such questions have already been screened by a public librarian who has utilized local and district resources in an attempt to answer the question. In these instances, our staff must locate more in-depth resources for patrons wanting more than a brief definition or an explanation found in a medical encyclopedia.

Consumer health materials are not sufficient to answer approximately 40 percent of the questions we receive from state supported institutions. When we cannot find appropriate material in our popular consumer literature, we then turn to the professional collection. We look for concisely written, easily understood materials from the medical and nursing literature. We often perform a Medline search and photocopy several articles from our collection which are relatively easy to understand. Questions requiring recourse to the professional literature usually fall into the following categories:

- Syndromes such as Dandy Walker Syndrome, Horner's Syndrome
- Surgical procedures such as Shouldice hernia technique, pig valves for use in open heart surgery, suspended animation surgery
- Advances in medicine and/or alternative therapies, such as chelation therapy, recent advances in the treatment of glaucoma, Tourette's Syndrome
- Uncommon diseases and conditions, such as discoid tumors, progeria, microcephaly, and Morton's neuroma

We always try to send some type of written material back to the requesting library. A bibliography of additional resources is often included in the event the patron requires more information. The names and addresses of agencies providing services in the requested subject area are also enclosed. A cover letter addressed to the requesting librarian accompanies each completed request, encouraging the consumer to consult a health professional should they have any questions regarding the enclosed information. The librarian is reminded to contact the College if follow-up information is required.

Libraries, particularly in the public library system, have different approaches and levels of service with regard to providing health information. Originally, local libraries were required to send requests for library support services through their district library. This was found to be cumbersome by some libraries, slowing down service to patrons. The College then decided to answer requests from any state supported institution librarian. Many district centers continue to encourage libraries to follow a hierarchical procedure while others do not. We encourage district centers to establish policies and procedures regarding what library level will directly access the College's services and communicate these policies to their area libraries.

It is interesting to note that procedures for public libraries requesting reference information vary from those of medical libraries. Public libraries often submit subject requests on interlibrary loan forms. This was a foreign procedure to the College reference staff. The College decided to discourage this practice since requests were sometimes delayed in our Document Delivery Department. Consequently, the reference staff developed a special reference request form which the College distributed throughout the state.

Workshops

The reference staff conducts a half-day workshop for librarians who are interested in providing health information to their community. The "Consumer Health Information in Public Libraries Workshop" discusses criteria for the selection of materials for building and maintaining a consumer health collection. Emphasis is placed upon the importance of the reference interview and useful health information materials. Legal and ethical issues involved in providing health information along with guidelines for answering medical questions are also discussed.

A special effort is made in the workshops to reinforce the importance of weeding the health collection. This is an activity which some public libraries are reluctant to pursue, since they do not have the funding to replace many of the outdated items. Exploration of community referral sources and library cooperation are encouraged. We also stress the importance of establishing guidelines and policies that will prevent librarians from overstepping their role when providing health information.

These workshops have been very well received. The librarians particularly appreciate the opportunity to examine and discuss the health information materials available. The smaller libraries find our hand-outs describing free and low cost health information from health organizations and state and federal agencies very useful. Public librarians are free to voice their problems and concerns about providing health information. After attending our course, most public librarians feel more comfortable answering health information questions. They have also had a chance to exchange ideas with us and we are no longer a remote entity. They discover that we share similar concerns in our efforts to respond to consumers' health information needs.

Approximately four workshops are presented each year with an average of 30 people in attendance. Presenting workshops across the state for various library districts has given us the opportunity to promote our services and to gain insight into the types of health collections public librarians utilize to assist their patrons. We also gain an understanding of how we can better serve Commonwealth public librarians.

Interlibrary Loan and Photocopy Services

Photocopied articles or loans of original materials in the College of Physicians of Philadelphia's collections are available free of charge to Pennsylvania state supported institution libraries. Requests may be sent by mail, OCLC, Docline, Palinet electronic mail, Ontyme II electronic mail, or telefacsimile. Due to staffing limitations we do not accept telephone or in-person requests. Mailed requests for ILL or photocopies must be submitted on ALA interlibrary loan forms or the ILL/photocopy request form designed specifically by the College for librarians at Commonwealth libraries. Requests for items not in the College's collections will be returned to the requestor unless they ask for a referral to another library and agree to assume the costs required by the document supplier. If we do not own an item, the College's reference staff will provide free document delivery locations, enabling Commonwealth libraries to send their requests directly to the lending library. Table 8-2 below provides data regarding ILL services.

TABLE 8-2: Document Delivery Statistics

	1985	1986	1987	1988
Filled	1594	1962	1394	2151
Unfilled	302	249	133	425
Total Requests	1896	2211	1527	2576

Consultations

Consultations are available in connection with collection development and maintenance. We encourage state supported institution libraries to develop health collections that are current, of high quality, accurate, relevant, authoritative, and assist consumers in making an intelligent decision regarding their health care.

Publications

Our newsletter, *Consumer Health Resources,* is published quarterly and highlights the free services that we provide to Commonwealth Libraries. It also identifies sources of consumer health information and offers advice on health reference and referral services. This publication is sent to the 850 libraries and interested individuals on our mailing list. *Consumer Health Updates* list resources on a specific health topic. *Updates* are made available through Palinet's electronic mail system and distributed by mail upon request. Topics covered in the past included colorectal cancer, drunken and drugged driver awareness, Parkinson's disease, and Lyme disease. Each state supported institution library has been sent a copy of our brochure *Health Information for Librarians at Pennsylvania State Supported Institutions,* which describes the services available and how to access them. *A Suggested List of Medical Reference Sources* for librarians furnishing health information to consumers is reviewed and updated on a regular basis, distributed at workshops, and is available upon request.

Promotional Activities

Promotion is vital to the success of any health information program. In the last two years we have intensified our efforts to increase our visibility to state supported institution libraries. Distance and diversity of user needs are de-emphasized through marketing and public relations. We constantly remind our primary users, the librarians at Pennsylvania state supported institutions, that we are available to support them in their health information activities.

The emergence of telefacsimile as a means for library-to-library communication has encouraged state supported institution libraries to utilize our services from remote locations. Geographical distance no longer impedes services since requests and answers can be sent across the state in a matter of minutes.

A group mailbox on Palinet's CALL (Computer Access Linking Libraries) service has been established for the approximately 109 Pennsylvania state supported institution libraries that are users of the electronic mail and bulletin board system. *Consumer Health Updates* are sent electronically to district centers and then downloaded and distributed to affiliated libraries.

An effective strategy of Pennsylvania's statewide library legislative program is an annual Library Legislative Day. Librarians, trustees, friends, and other library supporters from all over the state meet in Harrisburg for a day-long session. They are brought up to date on library legislation, visit with legislators, and formally show legislators their appreciation with an afternoon reception. Staff members from the College attend this event to keep legislators informed of our program and stress the importance of the program's continuance.

Staff

The entire Library staff contributes in some way to the provision of services to Commonwealth librarians. The associate librarian for public services coordinates the program's activities, ensuring that its goals and objectives are met. The reference/circulation staff consists of the associate librarian for public services, a reference librarian, and two full-time technicians. The reference staff is responsible for the reference, publishing, educational, promotional, and collection development aspects of this program. In addition to these responsibilities, the reference staff manages Library circulation, and provides computer literature searches and reference services to the fellows of the College, the legal and pharmaceutical communities, hospitals, and other institutions interested in obtaining health information.

The reference technicians have been trained to conduct reference interviews and provide answers to brief reference questions. They screen reference calls and assist reading room patrons, referring difficult questions to a reference librarian. The utilization of technicians at the reference/circulation desk has enabled the professional staff to direct their energies toward planning, problem-solving, and providing in-depth reference service to the librarians at state supported institutions. The enthusiasm of the reference technicians regarding this program is apparent in their willingness to assume additional responsibilities for production of the newsletter, management of the pamphlet file, and other projects outside the normal range of their duties.

Interlibrary loans are processed by the Document Delivery Department of the Library. This is a large operation since the Library serves as a resource library for the Greater Northeastern Regional Medical Library Program. This is part of a national network of health science libraries, and is funded under contract by the National Library of Medicine. All document delivery requests are routed to the document delivery coordinator who distributes the work load to five document delivery clerks. The College receives approximately 150 document delivery requests per day, 10 of which are state requests.

CONCLUSION

The College's Health Information Services for Pennsylvania Residents Program has evolved from a regional program into an invaluable resource that librarians at state supported institutions have come to rely upon for health information support services. We hope to continue providing a program that encourages librarians in Pennsylvania to expand their knowledge of health information resources, to develop sound health collections, and to guide the public in its quest for quality health information. The College's emphasis on educational and promotional activities has increased the visibility and the use of the program's services. Librarians at these institutions know they can turn to the College for assistance with their patrons' health information needs.

Commonwealth librarians are not the only ones benefiting from this program. The staff at the College has gained a sense of satisfaction knowing their work is helping Pennsylvania residents to make informed decisions about their health. The pieces of the consumer health information jigsaw puzzle are indeed coming together as demonstrated by the success of this cooperative program, but much work still lies ahead. Efforts must be made to inform the public that they can obtain health information at their public library. Those of us involved in providing consumer health information have the obligation of sharing our ideas regarding health information resources and services.

REFERENCES

1. Consumer Health Information Network. Proposal for LSCA Title III Grant, June 1983.

2. Consumer Health Information Network. Final LSCA Program Report, October 1984–September 1985.

3. *Pennsylvania Government Manual.* Harrisburg: Department of General Services, 1987.

4. State Library of Pennsylvania. *A Handbook for Public Library Trustees.* 3rd ed. Harrisburg: State Library of Pennsylvania, 1987.

CHAPTER 9
HealthAnswers:
Targeting Resources to the
Hospital's Market

Rya Ben-Shir

INTRODUCTION

HealthAnswers, MacNeal Hospital's consumer health information service, was introduced to its 12 target market communities in September 1984. This information service illustrates a mutually beneficial partnership between 12 public libraries and one hospital library. HealthAnswers is one of the ways that the Health Science Resource Center (HSRC) actively supports MacNeal Hospital's strategic goals of strengthening community linkages and increasing market share.

The Hospital

MacNeal Hospital is a 427-bed, not-for-profit, community teaching hospital in Berwyn, a near western suburb of Chicago. It was started in 1921, with much civic pride, by a local physician. Due in part to similar civic pride repeatedly expressed throughout metropolitan Chicago, this market is among the most overbedded in the country.

In 1983, MacNeal moved from its aging buildings to a new state-of-the-art replacement facility. With all the space in the new building allocated, no area for a consumer health information service had been designated. The Hospital Library (Health Science Resource Center), had recently been moved to a building across the street from the Hospital, near the medical residency offices.

The Community

MacNeal's target market communities include a number of near western suburbs of Chicago, totaling 680,000 consumers, including a high concentration of elderly. In the midst of a very competitive marketplace, MacNeal decided in 1983 to go back to its consumers to evaluate levels of satisfaction and unmet needs. It commissioned an extensive market survey, interviewing 769 adults, with a margin of error of plus or minus 3 percent.

The targeted market communities MacNeal surveyed were and still are where the Hospital seeks to increase its market share and penetration. One of the many goals of the survey was to understand how the community obtained health information. One of the conclusions reached was related to the quality and accessibility of the information available to the local residents. Expressing an unmet need, many of those interviewed (51%) stated that "quality information was hard to find when they really needed it."[1] At the time, "residents did not appear to be particularly resourceful in locating information for the purpose of making thoughtful health-care decisions. Once they asked their physicians (28%) and friends (53%), they were not altogether sure where to turn. Residents did perceive a hospital as a possible third informational alternative."[2] Additionally, they would rely on these same sources for information about hospitals and other health care services. One of the study's recommendations was that the "challenge to hospital's communications efforts may be not only to increase the flow of information to area residents in formats they will respond to, but also to educate them on where to look for information and how to evaluate it effectively. Area physicians and hospital staff would be useful conduits of that educational information . . . Using them would enable the hospital to network through them to patients and their families."[3]

The Health Science Resource Center (HSRC)

The Health Science Resource Center is staffed by two full-time Master's level medical librarians and one full-time library technician. Library staffing is supplemented by volunteers, who are instrumental in the delivery of the HealthAnswers service. Virtually all major library functions are automated.

As with the majority of hospital libraries in the United States and Canada, the HSRC was not open to the public, being geared strictly toward the needs of the medical and nursing staff and employees. The Library was relocated in 1981 to a new facility outside the Hospital in the Professional Services Building.

Strategic Moves

During the presentation of the extensive target market survey, the vice president of marketing announced a number of strategies to address the unmet needs of the community, including the setting up of a consumer information center. Library staff doubted that these plans included any involvement of the Health Science Resource Center. Taking into consideration the layoffs and downsizing of hospitals nationally during the first years of DRGs (Diagnostic Related Groups) motivated the HSRC to be proactive in planning and establishing its own consumer health information service before the Marketing Division could establish one.

This action was taken for a number of reasons. Who better than librarians could develop a comprehensive special collection of nontechnical sources of medical information? Who better than librarians could conduct a thorough and compassionate reference interview? Who better than librarians could organize a collection specifically geared to rapid turn-around?

At a time when hospitals nationally were laying off staff due to comprehensive changes in reimbursement, it was felt that the Library had to be in the forefront of a strategic effort to strengthen its place in the marketplace.

The approach adopted had, however, to satisfy a number of criteria:

1. Meet the information needs of the community
2. Enhance the image of the Hospital as a caring institution
3. Maintain the current "staff only" status of the HSRC
4. Offer the service in a manner that would be acceptable to the medical staff
5. Provide service in an authoritative, professional, and caring manner that would not put the Hospital at risk of a lawsuit
6. Accomplish all the above using a minimum of money, space, and with no additional personnel

Realizing that most of the population (our consumers) are healthy most of the time, and believing that they seek out their public libraries when they have specific information needs, the first step of the needs assessment process was to contact the head librarians and reference staff of each of the public libraries located in our targeted communities. As we were increasingly contacted by consumers for medical information, we were not surprised when virtually all public libraries expressed a need for medical information to be made readily available for their clientele, and preferably without cost. In the wake of California's Proposition 13, public libraries in metropolitan Chicago were trying to do even more, with even less. Even though they were faced with a growing consumer's movement in healthcare, the public libraries could not afford to develop collections to respond to the plethora of new health questions. What they did own, often amounted to anecdotal stories about survival with a disease or out-of-date medical tomes.

THE MACNEAL HEALTHANSWERS MODEL

As our corporate goals included increased visibility in the community, MacNeal Hospital's HSRC adopted the model of a wholesale/retail relationship with the 12 public libraries in our target market areas. To this end, the 12 public library directors and reference staffs were invited to a workshop about the HealthAnswers service. As these librarians would be our service representatives to the public, the Hospital rolled out the red carpet to welcome them. The orientation included a tour of the Hospital facility; the Health Science Resource Center; the HealthAnswers' collection; and a discussion of the policies, procedures, and concerns regarding the service. We also discussed the three-month trial period of HealthAnswers service just completed with one of the public libraries.

Each public library receiving the service was asked to display Mac-Neal Hospital's HealthAnswers color-coordinated posters and bookmarks in highly visible areas. All promotional materials were provided free to all participating libraries. They were also asked to credit MacNeal Hospital with the provision of the service. They were not asked to make any endorsement of the Hospital.

All promotional materials, such as bookmarks, posters, and Health-Answers stationery, were provided free of charge to all participating public libraries. The Marketing Division agreed to allow the HSRC to provide the consumer health information service and it in turn designed and paid for the promotional materials. It also developed a series of classes and workshops on health topics that is very dependent on the HealthAnswers collection. Follow-up with each of the libraries and their staffs has continued and has included site visits to each public library with fresh supplies of book marks and posters and repeat workshops for new staff.

MacNeal would provide the public libraries and their clientele a comprehensive, consumer health information service, free of charge. The service would be accessible entirely by telephone, either by the library staff or by the clients themselves. A written and researched response was guaranteed to be in the mail to the client's home address within two business days, and when this was not possible, the client would be alerted of the delay and the reasons for it.

ROLES AND RESPONSIBILITIES

Unlike any other service that a hospital library might offer, HealthAnswers is one that required a great deal of thought and consideration before it could be started. As good quality, accurate, and understandable information dealing with health and disease is very hard to acquire when it is needed, a library may find itself barraged by desperate, upset people. It will also have to cope with the lonely, demanding, unreasonable, and psychotic patrons who avail themselves of free community services. Public librarians are very familiar with such users. As these same clients are also potential patients of the Hospital, they must be accorded patience, understanding, and time. This is not an easy task. Added to this is the specter of malpractice. Since a client may blame the consumer health information service for information that may have led him or her to a poor outcome, the consumer health information librarian must never interpret any information and must always document every interaction and all information sent to clients.

At MacNeal Hospital's HealthAnswers service, we believe our role should be to:

1. Facilitate better understanding of consumers' medical conditions. For consumers we can provide an independent verification of what their physician has told them. Most consumers have many more

questions than they think to ask when in a physician's office. Often when a patient is informed of a diagnosis, the rest of the family is not present, but still has many questions about what to expect. When consumers understand a disease's process and their options, they will be more satisfied and feel in greater control of the situation.

2. Educate and aid in the referral process. We will often introduce the concept of what "board certification" means, and when a "board certified specialist" makes sense. Where appropriate, we refer the client to our physician referral service. A consumer health information service can provide a hospital with something that people in sales call a "warm sell." Often a consumer will call and indicate a high level of dissatisfaction with a physician. Although consumers cannot evaluate a physician's knowledge or technical ability, they can judge his/her interpersonal skills and ability to answer their questions or simply to be available on the telephone to answer questions. This is the ideal opportunity to offer them referral services to the Hospital's physicians. The physician referral service number is printed on the HealthAnswers bookmark along with the HealthAnswers and Community Education telephone numbers.

3. Help problem consumers get the information that they need. Some clients are simply difficult. They are demanding, never satisfied, and their physicians do not relish dealing with them. These clients still need information. Despite the poor quality of their interpersonal skills, they are often very intelligent and frustrated with the health-care system.

COLLECTION DEVELOPMENT

Quite surprising to us was how much good quality, authoritative material was available free or at low cost. Post cards to request three copies of any consumer/patient related materials for our new consumer information service were sent to hundreds of selected associations listed in the Health and Medical Organizations section of the *Encyclopedia of Associations*. Multiple copies of each Krames and Scriptographic pamphlet were purchased. Local book stores and consumer health information services were visited and books were examined and purchased. We subscribed to the following journals (whenever possible back to the first issue) and these were clipped and filed by health topic:

- *Consumer Reports*
- *Consumer Reports Health Letter*
- *FDA Consumer*
- *Harvard Medical School Health Letter*
- *Health Facts*
- *Health Letter*
- *Healthline*
- *Health Resources*

- *Hippocrates* (now *In-Health*)
- *Johns Hopkins University Health Letter*
- *Mayo Clinic Health Letter*
- *New York Times*
- *Newsweek*
- *Nutrition News*
- *Time*
- *Tufts University Health and Nutrition Newsletter*

Appropriate articles from the nursing and medical literature were included when evaluated as suitable for inclusion.

As one of the logistical goals of the collections was that the reference staff would be able to look in one place and be able to answer virtually any question, it was decided that all books, articles, pamphlets (and the occasional audiovisual) dealing with a single topic be housed together in one integrated file, with all files in alphabetical order. An authority file of subject headings was developed to avoid duplicate files being developed (for example, high blood pressure and hypertension). When resources were found to be inadequate to answer a question, computer searches of the popular press as well as the nursing and medical literature were conducted and articles were obtained to develop files on new topics or to supplement existing resources.

Currently, it is estimated that there are approximately 2,500 to 3,000 subject files housed in five file cabinets. Approximately 250 new articles, pamphlets, and books are added each month to update the collection.

To meet the requirement of keeping the physical setting of the Health Science Resource Center off limits to the public, the service was developed to be accessible only by telephone request, with a guarantee that a researched response would be in the mail within two business days. By being available by telephone to the clients themselves or to public libraries, and being accessible to the housebound, the disabled, the elderly, or the sick, we have removed many of the obstacles involved in finding the time and parking to seek desperately needed information.

EXAMPLE OF TYPICAL USAGE

As HealthAnswers is accessible by telephone, we addressed the public librarian's concern that HSRC might displace them with their patrons by offering two possibilities for the all important reference interview. Either the public librarian could conduct the reference interview or the librarian could simply refer the consumer to HealthAnswers directly. There was no attempt to circumvent the reference librarian. Our HealthAnswers poster states: "Questions about health? Now there's HealthAnswers: a service of your public library and MacNeal Hospital. Ask your Librarian for complete details!" It was felt that if the promotional materials promoted the public librarian, it was more likely that they would in turn promote HealthAnswers. We also offered a workshop and handouts that listed the data elements needed to answer questions. These elements were the client's name, telephone number, mailing address, how they were referred to the service, the name of the condition or disease, and what they wanted to know (treatment, alternatives, diet, etc.). Initially, we received a number of librarians calling for their patrons, but today more than 90 percent of all calls come in directly from the consumer. During business hours (7:30 a.m. to 5:00 p.m.) their calls come in on the HealthAnswers line (708-795-2222) and they speak to a librarian. A thorough reference interview is done. After hours and on weekends, the call is recorded by an answering machine. All callers are contacted for the reference interview. The Health Science Resource Center is never mentioned by name. The reason for this is that although the Hospital wishes to attract potential patients, the HSRC does not want to attract walk-in visitors. It is important that the client know that the Hospital, rather than the Library, is the provider of the service.

The questions are researched, first by consulting the most appropriate files and HealthAnswers reference books. If an answer has not been found, then the nursing and medical collection will be accessed. For drug and diet related questions, the hospital pharmacists or clinical dieticians would be contacted and they can speak to the consumer, if necessary. If it seems that the client does not have a personal physician or is dissatisfied with their physician or hospital, we offer to transfer the call to the physician referral service after the reference interview is completed.

All appropriate pages that directly answer the question are photocopied. Whenever possible, original pamphlets are included rather than copied. All titles, authors or sponsoring agencies, and dates are highlighted as well as where the related section begins. Each item is stamped with a disclaimer: "These materials are intended to educate you about subjects pertinent to your health, not as a substitute for consultation with a personal physician." The entire interaction is completely documented in the HealthAnswers log book, including the data elements discussed above, and an itemized list of every item included in the information package. This documentation is to protect the hospital in the unlikely event of a client lawsuit. A cover letter to the client is typed on HealthAnswers stationery mentioning the requester's name; title of the reference question, as we understood it; and identification of any support groups or other information that is not contained in the documents supplied. The whole package is put into a MacNeal Hospital folder. The latest community health education calendar of courses is included in the package. It is mailed generally within 24 to 48 hours of receiving the telephone call.

PROBLEMS NOT ANTICIPATED

We expected a grateful and polite clientele, and by and large the vast majority of callers to the HealthAnswers service make our service extremely gratifying. However, there were problems that we never expected. These can be characterized as follows:

1. The Terrible Diagnosis
2. Problem, Repeat Callers

3. Confused and Rambling Callers
4. Callers Contemplating a Lawsuit Against Their Physician or the Hospital
5. Practical Jokers

The Terrible Diagnosis

Another name for the Terrible Diagnosis is the "Worst Case Scenario." Every librarian's nightmare has to be the caller who does not appear to be aware of the seriousness of the diagnosis and its implications. This can be the result of patients not registering everything told them by the physician, or the physician not taking the necessary time to fully explain or using language that was too technical. We get a few such calls every year and they are very troubling for us. Whether the caller seems to be aware of the disease outcome or not we handle the question the same way.

Our policy in this connection is that the caller has a right to know and by calling us has indicated a willingness and readiness to know. Shielding or protecting the caller from the information, regardless of how painful, is in fact becoming a part of the problem of conspiring to keep laypersons in the dark. The constructive stance is to become a part of the solution and to give the client the information to help take control of his or her life.

The crucial part of the equation is that the consumer called Health-Answers with a specific question. HealthAnswers is not forcing anything on an unwilling person. The client is taking an active role, perhaps to verify or reinforce what he or she has already heard, or to seek alternatives.

An example of such a call was when a young woman called wanting to know about the prognosis, treatment, and outcome of chronic myelogenous leukemia. She said that she had recently been diagnosed, but did not seem to know much about it. At MacNeal our policy is always to find the best nontechnical source. The PDQ database was determined to be the best source and the information retrieved indicated that the prognosis was poor. The PDQ printout was sent to her and was accompanied by the HealthAnswers cover sheet on which we recommended that she discuss the attached information with her physician. About a year later she called us again to see if there were any new research findings. She mentioned how much we had helped her and that no one had been open with her up to that point. With the HealthAnswers materials in hand, she was able to discuss her specific situation with her physician as well as put her own affairs in order.

Problem, Repeat Callers

Such clients will call frequently, detailing minute aspects of a disease. Any reference interview results in many more totally unrelated, but very specific questions. This caller will also call on behalf of others. Since we are dealing with an information gatekeeper, it is not possible to do a satisfactory reference interview or follow-up to find out whether the information sent was helpful. Often, this type of caller also tends to be an extremely demanding and abusive client. Although HealthAnswers is a public service offered gratis by MacNeal Hospital, this does not mean that our staff can be treated abrasively or that any client has the right to demand special treatment. Without a doubt, this is the downside of offering a free service. Thankfully, these difficult clients are the very rare exception.

It is recommended that problem clients be anticipated and that an appropriate response be planned. Consultation with the departments of Marketing or Guest Relations will be helpful when establishing policies and procedures for this type of problem.

Confused and Rambling Callers

The unclear and rambling client will call for a telephone diagnosis with " . . . it hurts here when I do this. . . ." For obvious reasons, we are not permitted to help the client self diagnose and instead offer a referral to our physician referral service. The HealthAnswers staff informs them that they have contacted MacNeal Hospital's Medical Library and that they are speaking with a librarian. If the client persists, we tell the client that legally we cannot guess what their problem is because we would in effect be practicing medicine without a license. We offer to help them after they have been seen by a physician and have a specific diagnosis.

Such questions are frustrating, but still need to be handled compassionately. Every client has the right to be treated with respect, whether or not they can express their needs articulately. Hospitals and libraries can be very intimidating for some people.

Callers Contemplating a Lawsuit

This type of call represents a malpractice suit in the making. As MacNeal Hospital is in Cook County, the area with more malpractice suits per capita than any other in the country, this was one problem that was anticipated. It is our mandate that HealthAnswers is not equipped or prepared to help clients or their lawyers sue their doctors or hospitals. When callers request that we search the technical literature to find evidence that something very specific should not have happened as a result of surgery or therapy, we inform them that the HealthAnswers collection is a nontechnical and lay collection. We inform them that HealthAnswers is not a suitable resource for their needs and refer them to an academic medical center library.

Practical Jokers

When we least expect it, someone will call with a strange question. Although we may suspect that the question is really a joke or wager, we treat it seriously. If after some effort no answer can be found, we try to call the client's telephone number. We document the question and our inability to find an answer in our HealthAnswers log book and write the client to inform them that we could not find an answer.

We make every effort to treat all our clients and their questions with dignity, even in the event that they might be difficult or demanding. Most callers are very grateful for the information provided. If anyone on staff feels themselves becoming jaundiced to the needs of HealthAnswers' clients, we provide them the opportunity to remove themselves from the service. This nonresponsive attitude would quickly become apparent to the clients, who would resent it and the institution. For many clients, HealthAnswers may be their first contact with MacNeal.

Problems Expected, But Never Encountered

The one obstacle that all hospital librarians anticipate when initiating a consumer health information service is opposition from physicians. This has never happened at MacNeal Hospital. I believe that our medical staff is no different from any other at a community hospital in that we have our share of physicians who disdain the current health consumer movement. We did three things, and refrained from a fourth, which enabled us to offer the service with no opposition on the part of the medical staff.

1. We (as information professionals) set high but realistic standards about what would and would not be included in the HealthAnswers collection. Information that would be included would come from government agencies (National Cancer Institute); specialty organizations (American College of Surgeons); disease-oriented organizations (Multiple Sclerosis Society); periodicals from authoritative sources geared to the consumer (*Harvard Medical School Health Letter*); and books written by physicians, nurses, dieticians, social workers, or authoritative sources (*Boston Children's Hospital: New Child Health Encyclopedia*).

2. We were open about the service we were developing, always making it clear that the Hospital was going to offer this service, whether through the Marketing Division, or the Health Science Resource Center. We explained that it was considered necessary in light of the current competitive environment and that HealthAnswers would link callers to the physician referral service, (and their practices). We encouraged physicians (and nursing units) to select appropriate items from our files to purchase for their practices. We also urged them to consult our HealthAnswers file collection when developing educational classes and presentations to community groups. As our files are constantly being updated, they are confident that HealthAnswers is the best place to "shop" for consumer health information for purchase for their offices or to hand out at classes. Once physicians have used the collection or service, they refer their patients, families, and other physicians to the resource.

3. We inform the primary care physician when a call is received from one of their patients currently in the Hospital. The patient/physician relationship is of paramount importance, and alerting the physician of the request for more information lets the doctor know that the patient or family has some unresolved questions. We tell the physician when the package of information will be delivered and invite them to review it if they wish, provided it does not delay the delivery. Only once has a physician reviewed a package, and in that instance it had been developed at the physician's behest. Receiving calls for patients in-house happens very rarely. Due to the emphasis on outpatient care, when a patient is admitted he or she is often very ill or a decision has already been made about treatment. Research has shown "that patients prefer that the physician take the major role as decision maker, especially in severe illness."[4]

The one action that we did not take at any point was to ask for permission or approval from physicians or nurses. To ask for approval of materials is to inject unending interference and complication into an already complex service. If high standards are established and maintained for the collection, no approval process is necessary.

COSTS AND USAGE

Since HealthAnswers utilizes the same staff and occupies the same space as the Health Science Resource Center, actual costs were very low. To start up, we purchased four file cabinets ($2,000) and 1,000 file folders and a file organizing system ($450). The initial book, periodical, and pamphlet file cost was approximately $5,000. Other requirements included the installation of an additional telephone line ($200); an answering machine for off hours ($100); design and printing of posters, 50,000 bookmarks, and 25 pads of coversheets ($3,000). The staff hours to contact all the public libraries to do a needs analysis; visit other consumer health information services; develop and organize the collection; create policies and procedures; and conduct a trial of the service totalled eight months of one full-time professional librarian or 1,280 hours. With the exception of the design and printing of promotional materials, all the costs were absorbed by the Health Science Resource Center. No additional staff or funds were budgeted or used with the single exception of the file cabinets and folders. The literature for Health-Answers was very inexpensive and easy to accommodate when compared with medical textbooks and periodicals.

In relation to the costs involved in delivering the service, the expenditures include: either photocopies of pages of articles, pamphlets, or books (average of 15 pages per package) or original pamphlets; HealthAnswers stationery for the coversheet; HealthAnswers bookmark; MacNeal Hospital binder; mailing envelope; and postage (average $.60 per package). The average time per call, including reference interview, researching the question, processing the materials, and documenting the interaction and materials sent, is 30 minutes. The photocopying and refiling of materials is done by volunteers and takes an average of eight minutes per package. Additional costs include a disclaimer stamp ($25) and HealthAnswers log books ($15 per year).

In 1985, the first complete year, HealthAnswers responded to 368 calls; in 1986, 478; in 1987, 565; and in 1988, 707. Each call represents about three questions (not always related). With the exception of four articles in MacNeal's public relations publication, and four mentions in MacNeal's Community Health Education advertisements in the local press, all promotion has been through the public libraries. The response to each of the articles or advertisements was to double or triple typical monthly volume, with requests coming also from outside of MacNeal's targeted markets. Without a doubt, this is a service that meets a great need, but we are now at a point where the service cannot be promoted unless more staff are added. Currently, there is no way to document that HealthAnswers has contributed to any growth in Hospital admissions or market share.

SURVEY OF HEALTHANSWERS CLIENTS

In August 1988, we surveyed 100 previous HealthAnswers clients to ascertain their level of satisfaction with the service and whether the service had any effect on their perceptions of MacNeal Hospital. To avoid any bias in the administration of the pretested survey, we employed a recent library school graduate who had no previous relationship with MacNeal or any consumer health information service. The methodology used was to contact every fourth client as documented in the HealthAnswers log books as of September 1984, the starting date of our service. Approximately 400 clients were called to eventually survey 100 adults.

Of those surveyed, 40 percent came from our primary target market communities, where we have good market penetration; 51 percent from the secondary targeted areas, where MacNeal would like to increase its market share; and 9 percent from outside our market areas. As all the telephone calls were placed during business hours to home telephone numbers, it is not surprising that 96 percent of those surveyed were female. (In general, 35 percent of HealthAnswers callers are male.)

As HealthAnswers is primarily marketed through public libraries, 35 percent stated that they were referred to our service from their public libraries; 25 percent read an article or noticed the telephone number in MacNeal's publication *Health Call*; 19 percent were referred by a friend or family member; 10 percent mentioned that the service was included in advertisements listing MacNeal's Community Health Seminars; 9 percent were unaware of the service and simply called the Hospital wanting health information; while 2 percent were referred by their physician.

We asked respondents where else they had gone in the past for nontechnical medical information, asking them to list as many resources as were appropriate. Given our major referral source, it is not surprising that 30 percent stated that they looked to their public libraries for answers to their health questions; 20 percent mentioned books, magazines, and newspapers; 17 percent mentioned physicians; 11 percent stated that they did not know where to get this kind of information; 7 percent resourcefully contacted other hospitals or associations; and the remaining 15 percent asked friends or family.

After identifying the topic of their question, 93 percent said that HealthAnswers had provided a satisfactory answer. The same number agreed with the statement, "The information sent was just right. I understood most everything and my questions were answered." It is of interest that despite the efforts to provide nontechnical information, 7 percent still found the materials "too difficult to understand." Eighty-seven percent appreciated that HealthAnswers was accessible by telephone and mail and 88 percent said that the information arrived fast enough to meet their needs. It is significant that 13 percent said that they would like the face-to-face contact and that they would have liked to be able to come in themselves to follow up on their questions.

We asked the respondents whether they had used the Hospital or any of its services prior to, and after, utilizing HealthAnswers. The answers seem inconclusive, as some clients had first contacted the service almost four years earlier, while other respondents had called only two months earlier. For 45 percent of survey respondents, HealthAnswers was their first and only contact with MacNeal Hospital.

When asked which hospital they considered to be "their hospital" or to which hospital would they go for treatment, 36 percent named Mac-Neal. Twenty-nine percent named one of MacNeal's five primary competitors; 19 percent named other hospitals considered to be too far geographically to be in competition; and the remaining 16 percent stated that they did not know which hospital they would use.

Fifty-one percent did not know that medical librarians had provided the HealthAnswers service and 65 percent stated that they did not know that hospitals had libraries. One hundred percent of respondents said that they would refer a friend or family member to MacNeal's HealthAnswers service.

We ended the survey with an open ended question: "Does the fact that MacNeal offers the HealthAnswers service affect or change the way you think about MacNeal Hospital?" Most of the comments were extremely positive in regards to HealthAnswers and MacNeal. One of the comments that best exemplifies this is: "The HealthAnswers staff know a lot about getting the information quickly. They are always very polite. It makes you feel comfortable if HealthAnswers staff is so competent, then the rest of MacNeal's staff must be also."

SUMMARY

There is no doubt that MacNeal's HealthAnswers has fulfilled its mandate of improving community linkages and the way consumers in its targeted market area view the Hospital. For many consumers, HealthAnswers will be the first contact with the Hospital and it may continue to be the only one. Today's consumer is very sophisticated in many ways. Despite a dazzling array of health-care offerings, from the pages of comments we solicited, it seems that two factors are still very important:

geography (the closest hospital) and where their doctor is affiliated. They know which hospital they will call for health information, but it may not be where they spend their health-care dollars, no matter how much they may appreciate the information service. However, a service like HealthAnswers can make a difference in the case of a consumer who is dissatisfied with his/her current situation or one who does not "have" a doctor or hospital. Considering that in 1983 our community told us that they ask their friends and family (51 percent) to recommend hospitals, the spillover effect of HealthAnswers might be substantial, but unmeasureable.

Those surveyed reiterated what the literature states: consumers want to understand what their options are and will go beyond their physician if necessary to seek out information. Since it takes time to "erode" market share and to have an impact, we believe that the jury is still out as to whether a consumer health information service can have a positive impact on a hospital's market share.

REFERENCES

1. *MacNeal Hospital Market Area Study, October 1983.* New York: Research & Forecasts, Inc., 1983. 11.

2. Ibid., 12.

3. Ibid., 218.

4. Ende, Jack. et al. "Measuring Patients' Desire for Autonomy: Decision Making and Information Seeking Preferences Among Medical Patients." *Journal of General Internal Medicine.* January/February. 23.

BIBLIOGRAPHY

Droste, T. "Education Centers Are Subtle Marketing Tools." *Hospitals.* 63 September 20, 1989. 76.

Ende, J. et al. "Measuring Patients' Desire for Autonomy: Decision Making and Information Seeking Preferences Among Medical Patients." *Journal of General Internal Medicine.* 4 January/February 1989. 23–30.

Hibbard, J.H. "Consumerism in Health Care: Prevalence and Predictors." *Medical Care.* 25 1987. 1019–1032.

Inguanzo, J.M. and Harju, M. "How Do Consumers Receive Local Health Care Information?" *Hospitals.* 59 April 1, 1985. 74–76.

MacNeal Hospital Market Area Study, October 1983. New York: Research & Forecasts, Inc., 1983. 250pp.

"Market Focus: Chicago." *Modern Healthcare.* 18 August 12, 1988. 54–56, 58, 61–63.

Rynne, S. "Women's Health Programs: A Loss or a Real Leader?" *Hospitals.* 63 September 20, 1989. 112.

Shapiro, R.S. et al. "A Survey of Sued and Nonsued Physicians and Suing Patients." *Archives of Internal Medicine.* 149 (1989). 2190–2193.

CHAPTER 10
The Consumer Health Information Library at Overlook Hospital

Kathleen A. Moeller

COMMUNITY SERVED

Overlook Hospital is a 620-bed, community, nonprofit hospital founded in 1906 and is affiliated with Columbia University. Overlook is a major teaching hospital with residency programs in five medical specialities. Summit is an affluent suburb in the greater metropolitan New York area. Since Summit is only 30 miles from midtown Manhattan, it is an easy commute and many New York City executives and their families live in Summit. The standard of living is quite high, and the populace is well-educated and politically active. There is much volunteerism, as evidenced by a large Red Cross office in town, a historical society, a SAGE office, and a store for senior citizens. Over 110,000 hours of volunteer service are given to the Hospital each year. Local organizations such as Scouts, Junior League, and Jaycees are very active. The demographic profile of Overlook Hospital indicates sophisticated health concerns and information needs.

Health Information and Health Education at Overlook Hospital

The Consumer Health Information Library was first planned in 1979. At that time considerable change was taking place. The growing national trend towards self-responsibility for medical care and increasing costs combined to make consumers aware that they could have a real impact on their own health. With this connection, the demand for medical information grew.

At Overlook, this trend was first acknowledged by the establishment of a Community Health Education Department. This Department offered a number of educational courses for the public, including parenting, childbirth, respiratory diseases, and diabetes. One-day or one-evening seminars were also sponsored with such speakers as Dr. Benjamin Spock on childrearing. The attraction of more people to the Hospital had an impact on the Library.

As people became aware that there was a library in the Hospital, they came to the Library asking for information. The number of calls for information from the general public, patients, and patient families also increased. Like most hospital libraries at that time, Overlook's Library was officially restricted to use by Hospital staff. However, the Library staff would attempt to provide information for the public if possible. This attempt proved to be most frustrating, because the collection was developed to support the needs of health-care professionals, and was written in highly technical language.

Early in 1979, a new building program was announced. The new building would have no beds, and was to be named the Center for Community Health (CCH). It was intended to house outpatient testing, admissions, a family practice center, a dental center, outpatient surgery, and most exciting, an entire floor devoted to education. The education floor included offices for Medical Education, Community Health Education, and Nursing Education. It also housed a nursing arts classroom, a conference center with conference rooms in various sizes, an audiovisual production unit with a studio, and a new, greatly expanded Library.

Fortunately, the Hospital gave the department heads involved a great deal of decision-making power with the building's architects. At one of the architectural planning meetings, the Community Health Education director asked that a small area of the new Library be devoted to housing materials requested by people attending hospital-run classes. The director stated, "They always ask for more to read! I have a small collection, but have nowhere to put it, and no way to keep track of it." This information, together with the increasing number of questions the Library was getting from the public, clearly indicated that further planning was needed.

Determination of Need

A Library Development Task Force was formed and charged with determining the scope of consumer health information services needed at Overlook. Task Force members included representatives from school and public libraries, hospital administration, consumer groups, medical staff, nursing instructors, a local bookstore owner, and Overlook Hospital Library staff.

The Task Force conducted a community-wide survey during the month of October 1980. Full results of the survey were published in the *Bulletin of the Medical Library Association.* Two thousand questionnaires were distributed through four channels: local pharmacies, public libraries, junior and senior high school health classes, and elementary schools. The elementary school children were instructed to take the questionnaire home to their parents. Five hundred forty-three (27 percent) questionnaires were returned. In summary, results of the survey uncovered a large information gap. Seventy-two percent of the respondents stated that they had needed information on health or disease during the past year and 38 percent could not find it, indicating a serious problem for consumers.

A further analysis showed that 47 percent of public library users reported their health information needs unfulfilled, and 45 percent of students could not find what they wanted. Yet when asked where they generally sought medical information, 55 percent, as might be expected, listed their physician as the first choice, and the public library as the next source.

With seven out of 10 consumers needing health information and four out of 10 not finding it, the need for a local consumer health collection was apparent. The overwhelming majority of comments were most favorable about Overlook's plans to open such a library. Requests for specific services included a referral service to physicians, extended weekend and evening library hours, access to Overlook's consumer health collection for the surrounding community public libraries, telephone reference service manned by professional medical librarians, videotapes, and repeatedly, information that is easily understood by laypeople.

After the survey was completed, the Task Force worked on its final project, the development of a philosophy statement. The wording of the philosophy was important and is still in effect: "Access to reliable, up-to-date health information is the right of every individual in our society, and is an integral part of health care delivery and education."

Implementation

By the beginning of 1981, the planning process was complete and the building was under construction. The building itself was directly adjacent and connected to the main Hospital. The Library had 6,000 square feet with 1,500 square feet for offices, 1,500 square feet for the consumer health section, and 3,000 square feet for the professional collection. Because there was to be only one Library staff to serve both libraries, one large circulation/information desk was designed. Moveable modular wall panels were chosen. The shelves, index tables, card catalogs, and desks in the public areas hang on the wall panels and are also movable. The only stationary walls are around the Library offices, and these have half-height walls with windows above. Thus, the Library staff can see the entire Library from the offices.

In choosing furniture, a variety of study styles was considered. In both the consumer section and the professional sections of the Library, there are tables for those who need to spread out, carrels in the main reading and in more private areas, and lounge-type chairs.

Financing for the entire building was supplied by the Hospital through a major fund-raising effort, and by a Series C bond issue. A total of $21,900 was budgeted for the Consumer Library. This included $6,000 for consumer health books, and $9,000 for consumer health journal subscriptions. Other expenses were $4,000 for moving costs, $6,500 for a theft detection system and supplies, $2,500 for audiovisual equipment and software, $1,600 for a circulation charging system and supplies, and $400 for office supplies. This amount was spent in addition to the Library's annual budget.

The Library staff was expanded and reorganized. Three new staff members were hired. The new staff consisted of three professionals (director, assistant director, medical librarian), and three clerical staff. Library hours were extended to 9:00 p.m., Monday through Thursday. Saturday hours were retained as usual, 9:00 a.m. to 5:00 p.m.

The move to the new Library actually took place in February 1982. Two months were spent in ordering, cataloging, and processing consumer health materials. During that time, a reviewing panel was established. A file of physicians and nurses willing to review materials under consideration for the Consumer Library was assembled. Every item would be reviewed for medical accuracy, authority, and suitability for consumers.

In April 1982, the Consumer Health Information Library officially opened. A major publicity campaign was mounted and local and regional newspapers published several articles about the new Library. An open house was held for residents of the 14 communities in the Hospital's primary service area. Another open house and workshop for school and public librarians was held. A brochure was developed and included in a publicity packet prepared and distributed to libraries, pharmacies, and doctors' offices in the area.

CURRENT PROGRAM

The consumer health information program has changed considerably since its inception as a result of several factors. The original certificate-of-need for the new building, including the Library and salaries for a full-time staff of six, was written and approved in the late 1970s. By the beginning of the 1980s, however, health-care costs became much more regulated, and prospective payment plans began. New Jersey was one of the first states to adopt the DRG system. Overlook Hospital had to mandate cost containment measures including staff downsizing throughout the early 1980s. Accordingly, the most important factor affecting the Consumer Health Library as a recurring cost containment measure was a drastic cutback in staff.

In both 1983 and 1984 one professional position was deleted. In 1985, one-half of a clerical position was deleted. The current staff consists of one professional medical librarian, one paraprofessional, and two clericals, one part-time and one full-time. The loss of professional and support staff has had a predictable effect. With fewer staff hours available, Library hours were curtailed and evening hours eliminated, although Saturday hours were maintained.

Due to lack of staff, publicity efforts had to be revised. Today, to maintain visibility in the community, three one-day publicity efforts are undertaken each year. For example, in 1988 a National Nutrition Day program was held in the Library. Working with the American Dietetic Association, school classes from kindergarten to junior high school ages were invited to come to the Library and learn what to eat. Dieticians met with the children to answer their nutrition questions and to present them with "healthy" snacks. The Library has its nutrition collection on display and bibliographies and pamphlets were distributed. Library staff time for this type of one-day program is minimal in relation to the amount of publicity generated.

In another effort to streamline time-consuming procedures, the reviewing process was eliminated. By 1984, the Library staff had sufficient experience in consumer health collection development to feel comfortable in selecting materials without advice. The review process had proved to be extremely time-consuming in that once an item was ordered it had to be recorded as received, and then sent to a health professional for review. The turn-around time was very slow, averaging one to two months. This required much follow-up and nagging by the Library staff. If the item was rejected, it often could no longer be returned. Reviewing was found to be a good idea in theory, and necessary initially, but difficult to maintain on a practical basis.

Fortunately, at the time of the staff cutbacks, the Hospital recognized and supported the need to automate. The Library was one of the first departments to request microcomputers and administrative approval was given to purchase three IBM machines. Today, the Library has four microcomputers, and the most labor-intensive and time-consuming systems have been gradually automated. As in most hospital libraries, integrated library systems were simply too expensive, and automation was done with several different software programs. Besides database searching and word processing, systems that have been automated include circulation, serials control, and acquisitions management. Due to the microcomputing capabilities, no direct-to-patron services have been curtailed despite the staff cutbacks.

COLLECTIONS

Other factors affecting the current program stem from lessons learned through experience. When the Consumer Library was first opened, subscriptions to 60 consumer journals were purchased. However, these proved to be an unimportant part of the collection. The Library staff soon observed that, unlike professional medical journals, the consumer journals were simply not used. People visiting the Library indicated a desire to have something to take home, similar to having a prescription from a visit to the doctor's office. Since the journals do not circulate, they were not used. Most people come into the Library with a specific question about a specific medical problem and do not wish to browse through health magazines. Therefore, the current consumer journal collection has been cut to 25 titles. The most popular title by far is *Shape,* with an attractive girl on the cover of each issue. The second most popular title is *Consumer Reports.*

Another factor affecting the current program was learned through experience and was unexpected. This was the discovery of consumer health pamphlets. Shortly after opening, it became apparent that the consumer pamphlets were disappearing at an amazing rate. People seemed to be extremely happy to have a small anonymous piece of information that did not have to be checked out or returned. The consumer pamphlets on embarrassing topics, such as hemorrhoids or sexual diseases, disappeared even when there were no actual reference questions presented. Patrons are free to go into the Library and pick up a pamphlet and no one has to be aware of it. With this knowledge gained, more pamphlet display shelving and racks were added.

One Library volunteer, who works two days a week, was placed in charge of the consumer pamphlet collection. A 200-square-foot area in the back of the Library was partitioned off with shelving and the volunteer set up a consumer pamphlet storehouse where pamplet stock is maintained. In the storehouse, consumer pamphlets are filed alphabetically by title. In the Consumer Library itself, one copy of each title is kept in a vertical file, with over 1,500 files labeled with National Library of Medicine medical subject headings. A written list of vendors, addresses, sources, prices, and pamphlets ordered is soon to be computerized with the acquisitions management software. The Library has virtually no budget for consumer health pamphlets, but they are obtained at little or no cost. When only one copy can be obtained free, it is placed in the vertical file. There is no fee charged for pamphlets, and these are supplied free to all patrons. The vertical file is a valuable resource and is used often. Substantial consumer pamphlets, those with 25 or more pages, or those with a unique subject, are cataloged and kept in the book collection.

Another lesson learned, much to the staff's dismay, is that there are some areas of medicine that are just not covered very well by popular health literature. For example, there is very little written on radiology. Also, because consumer health books are trade books, they do not stay in print long. It is most discouraging to find a good bibliography on a particular topic and discover that most of the material is out of print. There are very few classics in the consumer health field.

Being in a hospital setting has proven to be ideal, because the professional collection can be used as a back-up. For 25 to 30 percent of the questions, the Consumer Library is not adequate. This is probably because the Library is hospital-based and people come in with illness specific requests. One example is a request for information on eosinophilic enteritis, which is a rare form of gastroenteritis. As can be expected with such a specific disease-related topic, very little could be found in the Consumer Library.

The present collection, now eight years old, houses 2,000 books, hundreds of pamphlet titles, 75 audiovisual programs, 25 journal subscriptions, and 1,500 vertical files.

REFERENCE POLICIES

Providing consumer health information forces an examination of the ethics of service. Two issues need to be considered. First is a recognition of the characteristics of sick people and their families. They can be angry, disbelieving, sad, and distraught. They have lost control of their most important possession, their own or a loved one's body, and may be overly demanding in an effort to regain some form of control. Many people are close to a state of shock. They will say, "I know my doctor told me all about this, but I was just too shocked to hear. Now I need to find out more."

The problem patron who talks incessantly, or is verbally abusive, appears from time to time. At Overlook, two resources are used to handle problem patrons. First is public library literature on the topic. Public librarians have been faced with problem patrons for years, and there is a great deal of literature on how to cope. The other resource available at the Hospital is the counselling departments. These include the Social Work Department, the chaplaincy, the substance abuse programs, and the Psychiatric Department. If there is an upset patron, we can ask, "Would you like to have someone to talk to?," and then call a social worker or other professional.

The second ethical issue to be considered is related to our own humanness. It is very tempting to be overly kind and censor information. For example, presenting prognosis information is difficult. In keeping with our philosophy that if a person is asking for information they are entitled to have it, the staff at Overlook tries very hard not to restrict information. If a person is asking for information, it is assumed that they really do want it. At the same time, it is important to honor our own ethics. If we feel uncomfortable, we can try to give the patron a choice. We may say, "There is information here regarding the outcome of the disease. Would you like me to continue or would you prefer to have a copy and discuss it with your doctor?" Almost invariably, the patron already knows the information we are afraid to give.

One example of honoring our own ethics is when a public library called Overlook's Library with a request from a young mother for pictures of burns so that she could teach her children not to play with matches. The Library staff felt too uncomfortable sending out such gruesome photos for that purpose. The staff member involved called the public library back and stated her feelings and suggested that the mother was welcome to come into the Library and preview the pictures herself.

REFERENCE STATISTICS

In 1982 and 1983, reference statistics showed that consumers asked an average of 70 questions a month. In later years, reference statistics were not kept due to staff time restrictions.

However, in March 1989, Overlook's Library was named as the Consumer Health Information Center for two counties in New Jersey. Part of the obligation for funding as a Center involved reporting statistics on a monthly basis. A detailed form was developed. The statistics reported below in Table 10-1 represent the first six months of operation as a Center, April–September 1989. Statistics include all consumer requests, including those generated by libraries or referred from other sources.

TABLE 10-1: Reference Statistics

1989	Apr	May	June	July	Aug	Sept	Total	Percent
No. of Queries:	52	88	107	84	65	74	470	
In Person	12	38	74	32	9	29	194	41%
By Phone	40	50	33	52	56	45	276	59%
From Libraries	17	20	28	10	19	11	105	22%
From Patron Direct	35	68	79	74	46	63	365	78%
Answered	46	85	103	79	60	71	444	94%
Completely								
Referred	6	3	4	5	5	3	26	6%
Average Time Spent	9.9	9.2	9.5	9.4	9.7	9.3	9.5	
(Minutes)								
Document Delivery:								
Pamphlets	28	58	41	37	31	39	234	
Journal Articles	19	24	21	24	12	24	124	
Books	11	23	57	16	13	17	137	
AV's			2				2	
Computer Searches	6	4	6	4	6	5	31	

An analysis of the statistics reveals several important points. First is in regard to the in-person vs. phone inquiries ratio. It should be noted that parking at the Hospital is somewhat difficult to find and expensive. If a patron asks, the Library will provide a parking pass to park free. However, this is not a well-known fact and the parking cost may keep people away and explains the large number of requests by phone.

Second, the number of inquiries from libraries is lower than might be expected. However, Overlook's Library is intended for supplemental reference. There are three area reference libraries in the two countries served, and they all have large reference collections. Although public and school librarians can go directly to Overlook for medical information, their normal channels for other types of information are the area reference libraries. Approximately one-third of the library inquiries received at Overlook come from the area reference libraries themselves.

With regard to outcome data, questions are referred for two reasons. First is that the specific material requested is unavailable at Overlook. This may be a request for a particular book or journal article. These questions are referred to a larger medical library, the University of Medicine and Dentistry of New Jersey. The second referral reason is that information requested cannot be located. This is a rare occasion and has only happened twice.

From the statistics, it can easily be seen that answering reference questions for the consumer is much more time-consuming (9.5 minutes average) than answering professional questions (3.8 minutes average). The health-care professional usually has a particular patient in mind and knows exactly what to ask. The consumer may have sketchy knowledge to begin with, and have little or no idea what resources are available to consult. Developing reference interviewing skills is particularly important when providing consumer health information.

FURTHER FUNDING AND EXPANSION

As previously mentioned, in March 1989, the Library was designated as the Consumer Health Information Center for two counties in New Jersey. The funding agency, Linx, is a Regional Library Cooperative established by the State Library. There are six geographical regions in New Jersey, and each region has its own independent Regional Library Cooperative. The Cooperatives receive state funds to provide multi-type library networking and library services throughout the state.

Overlook's Library received a contract with Linx to provide supplemental health-care information services to the libraries and residents of Union and Middlesex counties. Funding of $9,624 covered the period from March 1, 1989 through December 31, 1989. The budget included $6,524 for a part-time library assistant. This was needed to provide evening and Sunday coverage requested by the public libraries.

Other items included in the contract were $1,600 for reference materials, resources, and database searching. Operating costs were set at $1,500. Services provided by Overlook include reference back-up and document delivery of materials in the Consumer Library. Interlibrary loans and database searching are not part of the funded services. These are provided by other large medical reference libraries and the OCLC network. Database searching is done at Overlook only if needed to answer a consumer reference question. The contract with Linx has been renewed for 1990, and all medical database searching will now be Overlook's responsibility. This will be much less confusing to public and school libraries. Other services offered by Overlook are training classes and consumer health updates for public librarians.

USE STUDY

With the addition of a computerized circulation system in 1987, use patterns of the consumer collection could be tracked by library patron category. Categories were designated as follows: attending physicians, resident physicians and interns, consumers, nursing staff (including all RNs, LPNs, and aides), allied health workers (employees who are not doctors or nurses but are involved in direct patient care), and other employees. The other employees category included administrators, secretaries, and other staff not involved in direct patient care.

TABLE 10-2: Use Study

Patron Categories	1987	1988	1989 (through Sept)
Attendings	4%	3%	5%
Residents	1%	4%	1%
Consumers	38%	39%	36%
Nursing	16%	14%	14%
Allied Health	29%	29%	24%
Other Employees	12%	11%	20%

Results of the use study proved to be most interesting. The Library staff had noticed early on that the Consumer Library was used a great deal by the Hospital staff for their own personal health information needs. The statistics proved this observation to be true. Although the Consumer Library patrons took out the most material, the Hospital staff accounted for more than half of the total circulation. Adding consumer health services allows the Hospital Library to become a "full-service" library, with materials for everyone to read.

As can be seen in Table 10–3, the total number of circulated items has steadily increased. This can be attributed to publicity efforts, an increasing collection size, and word-of-mouth good will in the surrounding communities.

TABLE 10-3: Circulation Statistics

	1987	*1988*	*1989 (Projected)*
Books	996	1079	1298
AV's	61	64	75
Total	1057	1143	1373

CONCLUSION

Adding consumer health information services is one of the best survival strategies for hospital libraries. It is not an expensive undertaking. At Overlook, only $4,000 a year is spent on consumer health materials. Consumer books are trade books with prices like $10.95 or $15.95 that do not compare with the hundreds of dollars needed to purchase professional medical books. For this small amount of money, nearly 100 people a month not associated with the Hospital are drawn in to use the Library. This is the best return-on-investment of any area of the Hospital, or any public relations event, and the administration is aware of this fact. The Library staff encourages satisfied patrons to write letters of praise, and they do. Since the Consumer Library opened, Overlook's Library has not had a budget cut. With the goodwill and expectations of service in both the community and other libraries, Overlook has a commitment to keeping the Library strong.

Providing consumer health services greatly enhances the Library staff's job satisfaction. People really do have a difficult time finding medical information. They are overwhelmingly grateful for the help we provide.

CHAPTER 11
Swedish Medical Center Health Information Service

Sandra K. Parker

INTRODUCTION

The Health Information Service at Swedish Medical Center has been in existence since 1983. During that time, it has evolved into a program that does not entirely correspond with the originators' model. Many changes have occurred as the result of adaptation rather than intentional alteration. Even though reference is made to the Health Information Service in this chapter as a program, it is only done for the purpose of description. In its current form it is a fully integrated library service.

Swedish Medical Center (SMC) is a not-for-profit, 328-bed community hospital located in Englewood, Colorado. Englewood, with a population of 30,000, is one of several suburban communities bordering South Denver. Swedish Medical Center provides a full-service emergency department and trauma center serving the South Denver metropolitan area. The Hospital shares its campus with two leading rehabilitation centers: Craig Hospital and Spalding Rehabilitation Hospital South. The three hospitals work cooperatively, providing a continuum of care for people with a spinal cord injury, head injury, stroke, neurological disorder, or complex orthopedic problem. In addition, the Colorado Neurological Institute, the Rocky Mountain Multiple Sclerosis Society, the Colorado Epilepsy Foundation, the National Stroke Association, and the Center for Spine Rehabilitation are located on the campus complementing the comprehensive neurological services offered by Swedish Medical Center.

The SMC Library serves health professionals and staff members of the three hospitals and the other organizations mentioned above. This new Library, completed three years ago, is larger and more accessible than that of its former location. The Library is currently located on the first floor of SMC near the main patient elevators and adjacent to the physicians' lounge. A staff of four, including two professional librarians, is assisted by three volunteers and a part-time shelving and photocopy clerk.

ORIGINS OF THE HEALTH INFORMATION SERVICE

The Health Information Service at SMC began informally early in 1982 when the director of the nearby Englewood Public Library requested a meeting with the librarian at Swedish. She was concerned about the growing number of medical inquiries from the public which could not be satisfied from the resources of the public library. This conversation initiated discussions concerning a joint effort to meet the needs of the community and the Hospital patients. Several additional meetings followed until a Letter of Administrative Agreement was drafted and signed (Appendix I). In the meantime, the librarian at Swedish contacted the patient educator in order to involve her in subsequent program planning.

The initial investment of time and resources was remarkably modest. In late 1982, the Swedish librarian, in a memo to the patient educator, committed 21 linear feet of shelf space, $1,000 for materials, two hours of volunteer time, and two hours per week of professional time. She suggested that they "plan to implement a limited patient education library service." At that time, the limitations were perceived to be its budget and staff.

In an effort to overcome these limitations, the medical librarian and patient educator submitted in early 1983 a formal project request to the Hospital administration. The request documented the lack of useful and accurate health information resources to meet patient and community needs and requested support to develop a health information service in cooperation with the Englewood Public Library. The objectives as stated in the proposal were:

1. To monitor and respond to the consumer health information needs of the community.
2. To establish a collaborative relationship with the Englewood Public Library to give the public greater accessibility to health information.
3. To promote and support the overall mission and values of Swedish Medical Center.
4. To provide information resources on campus for inpatients and families.
5. To provide a means of networking between area industry, business, schools, and libraries.

At that time, the Hospital Library located on the fourth floor at the rear of the Hospital was quite small and crowded and difficult to find. Seating and study space were severely limited. However, the initial proposal did not suggest a new facility nor did it recommend expansion of the current space. Instead, it proposed to refer all outpatient and community requests to the public library. The SMC Library staff would fill inpatient requests with the cooperation of the nursing staff. They would also serve a "back-up" function for the public library when requests requiring additional research were received. They proposed to assist the public librarians in collection development and to participate in staff training.

FUNDING

The proposal asked for a grand total of $6,000. The requested budget included collection development ($2,600), promotion ($1,600), and contract labor ($1,800). The proposal was approved and the funds were made available for the 1984 fiscal year. The "patient library" has since become a line item in the medical library budget and is currently funded at a level of $3,000 annually. These funds are now used exclusively for collection development. Promotional costs have been integrated into the overall Hospital marketing budget. The contract labor expenses, so crucial during the initial development process, were not extended past the first year.

GETTING STARTED

The public library already owned a substantial collection of books on preventive health topics—holistic medicine, nutrition, child care—but it was not equipped to answer detailed questions on specific diseases. The Hospital Library staff provided a list of basic medical and nursing texts and recommended a number of medical and nursing journals and a subscription to *Abridged Index Medicus*. During the first year of the program, SMC Library staff offered two training sessions for the public librarians. These were informal meetings covering the introduction of medical reference sources and how to use them.

The Hospital Library needed to significantly expand the collection of resources for patient use. Since the public library collection was geared toward holism and prevention, the decision was made to concentrate on developing a comprehensive collection of disease-specific titles. However, no conscious effort was made to prevent duplication of books. The acquisitions process was facilitated by two excellent local bookstores committed to stocking consumer health books. The two librarians (hospital and public) agreed to provide each other with a catalog card for each book added to the collection. The card selected was a duplicate shelf list card so that each library would at least have subject access to the other's book collection.

The public library added journal subscriptions such as the *Journal of the American Medical Association,* the *American Journal of Nursing,* and the *New England Journal of Medicine;* while the Hospital Library added consumer health newsletters and, when it became available, the *Consumer Health and Nutrition Index.*[1]

An extensive pamphlet collection was planned at the Swedish Library for patients. A local librarian was hired with project funds to work for one day per week to develop a good basic collection. The *Consumer Health Information Source Book*[2] provided sources for pamphlets, but contacting the various organizations and pre-paying for materials involved extensive paperwork. Today, this process is facilitated by a word-processing and label-producing program.

Initially, the staff was concerned that the physicians might object to the service or take exception to the content of some of the materials. A book selection form contained in the first edition of *Developing Consumer Health Information Services* was adopted for use in the evaluation of each title.[3] However, the individual review of every title consumed too much time and sometimes the books were out for weeks for evaluation. Therefore, a decision was made to seek evaluations only for controversial titles, such as *No More Hysterectomies.* This procedure resulted in the creation of a small and highly select group of expert evaluators consisting of physician friends and program supporters who were not necessarily representative of the entire medical staff. Eventually, almost all content evaluation by physicians was suspended for the sake of expediency. At present, only books authored by credentialed health professionals and meeting defined criteria (such as the presence of a useful index and publication by a reputable publishing house) are selected. This set of criteria has worked well. Printed reviews from *Medical Self-Care, Hippocrates,* (now *In-Health*) and *Library Journal* are also valuable for selection purposes. Only one book has been withdrawn from the collection based on user criticism. The request came from a dietician who had uncovered some inaccurate information in the content. Today, the Health Information collection consists of 550 books, 1,550 pamphlets, and 10 magazine and six newsletter subscriptions.

ACCESSING THE SERVICE

In the first year of the program, the patient educator developed an in-house institutional policy with associated procedures to be circulated to all departments describing the service and how it could be accessed (Appendix II). The policy called for nursing staff to fill out the "Patient Information Library Request" form and to deliver the request to the Library. Phone calls were to be accepted only under RUSH circumstances. However, telephone requests soon preempted the forms and now almost all of the in-house information requests are taken by telephone. The Library staff either delivers the requested information to the nurses' station or a volunteer from the unit collects it.

Community patrons are encouraged to access the service initially through the Englewood Public Library. The Hospital Library staff refers callers to the public library and explains the cooperative nature of the service. The expanded medical reference materials at the Englewood Public Library aid the reference librarians in satisfying more complex medical questions than was previously feasible. The public librarians contact SMC Library whenever more in-depth research is needed or when specialized resources are required. The Hospital Library staff can usually locate the requested information and send it to the public library within 24 hours. This procedure works well as public library patrons often prefer to return to the public library a day or two later to obtain the information rather than venture into an unfamiliar hospital. Materials are sent between the two libraries by a daily library courier. This service is made available through the Colorado State Library System and most metropolitan area libraries—public, academic, and special—participate.

Occasionally a caller may insist that he or she has exhausted the public library resources. These assertions are not questioned since the objective is to facilitate access to health information in any way possible. In such a case, an offer is made to accommodate the caller by mailing the information or by extending an invitation to visit the Library to obtain the appropriate information in person.

All walk-in users are accommodated since a referral in such circumstances might be needlessly discouraging. Full reference service and self-service photocopying are provided at no charge. A complementary computer search may be necessary to locate the needed information.

TYPES OF INQUIRIES

The nature of inquiries received from the patients and the public cover a very broad spectrum, yet certain patterns emerge. Many questions originating at SMC concern multiple sclerosis, head injury, and neurological and spinal disorders and reflect the specialized services of the Hospital. Infertility and gynecologic concerns are also common inquiries and again reflect the typical Swedish patient population. Many cancer-related questions can be attributed to a dynamic oncology clinical specialist who works closely with the Library staff.

The public library inquiry can be anything from "How long does a sunburn last?" to day-care for the aged. There is the obvious interest in medications and their side effects. The *Directory of Medical Specialists* and medical dictionaries are consulted extensively. Both libraries see a continuing interest in medical procedures and diagnostic tests. Regional concerns are also reflected in questions on altitude sickness, Rocky Mountain Spotted Fever, wilderness survival, and poisonous snakes and spiders.

CIRCULATION

Approximately 55 books per month circulate from the Health Information Collection. Information requests from patients and the community rarely exceed 15 per week and usually average around 10. In general, more patient family members than patients utilize the Medical Library in person. Many community patrons have either been patients at Swedish or plan to be patients in the future. The extent to which the collection is used by the employees at the three hospitals has been surprising. Many of the users are not health professionals, but are personnel from the business office, medical records, dietary, housekeeping, social services, materials management, administration, and the fitness center. For the most part, these are new patrons who had not previously used the Library. The health information service has helped to dispel the exclusive image of the "doctor's library."

PUBLICITY

The Health Information Service was introduced to the Swedish staff and the public library community at concurrent open houses. Brochures, bookmarks, and promotional signs were designed with the assistance of the Hospital's Public Relations Department. A flyer announcing the event was mailed to 17,000 homes in the South Denver suburban area. Attendance at the Swedish open house was somewhat disappointing, probably due to inadequate publicity. However, the attendance at the public library was much larger as a result of a mass mailing, with the local press present. A few weeks later, representatives from the public library and the Hospital Library were asked to appear on a local Denver television program to discuss the Health Information Service.

At Swedish, the new service was also announced through in-house publications and meetings of department heads. The head nurses and nurse educators were particularly targeted. The patients are currently advised of the service via closed-circuit television. An early effort to reach the patient and family through printed brochures in the patient rooms was not successful. Attractive in-house brochures were designed to be displayed on the nightstands by the patient beds. They described the service for friends and family as well as to patients, and gave the Library location and telephone number. The housekeeping staff was asked to distribute the brochures on a daily basis, placing one in each room as it was cleaned for a new occupant. The director and the chief supervisor of Environmental Services agreed to the plan and the brochures were delivered to their department. However, that was the last time they were seen by anyone. The nursing staff were also unaware of the brochures. No calls were received from patients as a result of the brochure. Though the mystery was never solved, the Library staff learned not to depend on an uninvolved third party to accomplish an objective.

The patient educator and the librarian spent many lunch hours delivering brochures to the Hospital's satellite emergency care centers and local pharmacies. A letter introducing the program and brochures were mailed to each medical staff physician. Those who expressed an interest in publicizing the service in their offices were offered a free acrylic brochure display with a supply of brochures. Several physicians called to accept the offer. A few months later, a bibliography was compiled of the books and journals in the health information collection and mailed to physicians' offices.

RELATIONSHIP TO PATIENT EDUCATION AND NURSING

Shortly after the Health Information Service was introduced, the patient educator, who contributed extensively to the planning process, resigned from her position. Since her resignation occurred during a critical budget period at the Hospital, a decision was made not to replace her. For the past six years there has been no coordinated housewide patient education policy. However, a new employee in the Nursing Education Department has recently undertaken a diabetes education project. Also, the oncology nurse clinician received funds in 1989 to acquire educational resources for cancer patients, and the cardiac nurse clinician is investigating the acquisition of patient and family resources developed by *Heartmates*. These three nursing educators, the director of the Audiovisual Department, and the library director are planning to pool budget resources and investigate outside funding for the development of a videocassette library for patients. This project promises to lead to a renewal of interest in the education of patients among the nursing staff and to opportunities for further cooperative projects. It is difficult for librarians who have little patient contact to be accurate in identifying the needs of the patients. Nurses can be most valuable allies in selection and program planning and are also an important channel for facilitating patient awareness and access to health information services.

NETWORKING

The relationship with Englewood Public Library has changed over the five years since the project began. Meetings between the two library staffs have become very occasional during the past few years. Catalog cards are no longer exchanged due to automated catalogs at both libraries. Unfortunately, the two libraries participate in different electronic networks which has hindered collection access. However, a network link is about to be established which should alleviate that problem.

The Swedish Library has become the *first* point of access for more community patrons than originally anticipated. Frequently, a community member will telephone or come in without a referral since the location is more accessible than before and visitor parking is now much easier. Requestors are also referred from other public libraries in the metro area, by the hospital staff or volunteers, by former requestors, and by physicians. The Englewood public librarians still contact the medical library to request backup reference or to obtain information on behalf of a patron, and they also send people directly to the Swedish Library if it is appropriate. Publicity for the program is now entirely independent. However, the mutual cooperative spirit continues.

An outgrowth of the Swedish Health Information Service has been the development of an informal network with the Health Reach Library, located at Saint Joseph Hospital in Denver and described in Chapter 12 of this book. Though the services operate quite differently, the librarians selected and purchased modular display equipment, sharing both the cost and the equipment, and have exhibited jointly at local meetings. While no official networking relationship exists between the two institutions, enormous benefit is realized from shared objectives and experiences.

IMPACT OF AUTOMATION

During the first two years of the program, the consumer health books were cataloged on OCLC. In 1986, the SMC Library joined a small consortium of hospital libraries contracting with the University of Colorado Health Sciences Center's Denison Library for centralized cataloging and began sharing the CLSI automated circulation and catalog system. The St. Joseph Hospital Health Reach Library is also a member of the consortium. CLSI displays a book record in the database and identifies the libraries in the group that own that title. This online public catalog has brought in occasional patrons from the medical school library and the Health Reach Library. It is current policy to circulate materials in the health information collection to the public.

Denison Library and the other five libraries in the consortium, including the Swedish Library, are now in the process of changing from CLSI to the CARL (Colorado Alliance of Research Libraries) automated system. This change involves more than just a new vendor. There are currently 15 member libraries using CARL. Many other libraries access the system through network links. Most of these libraries are public and academic. Public telephone lines provide dial-in access for people from their homes and offices. As a member of CARL, SMC Library's holdings will be available for viewing on terminals in most of the libraries and in many homes both within Colorado and outside the state. This change may impact collection and circulation policies.

EVALUATION

The first formal evaluation effort is presently underway. Within six weeks after a patron has used the health information service, a survey is mailed to the home with a letter of explanation. A self-addressed, postage-paid envelope is enclosed. The return rate has been around 50 percent so far, though the sample is still small. There is concern that the "halo" effect may be at work since all of the returned surveys have been positive. The assumption is that the program is a success. However, the reality is that the vital question still remains unanswered—does the service benefit the institution and how can that be measured?

FUTURE

In retrospect, initial fears from the early days of the program, such as that of inadvertently revealing the fatality of an illness to a requestor, seem minor now. The patron almost invariably knows, or at least suspects, the seriousness of the situation before coming to the Library. Another initial concern—that the physicians will object to the service—has also proven to be unfounded. Many patrons are referred by their physicians. Other concerns, such as shortage of staff, time, and resources and the uncertain benefit accruing to the institution, can also affect the decision to offer consumer health information services. However, experience has shown that it can be offered with a relatively small investment of resources. Providing health information has brought to the Library many new users and friends in the community and within the institution itself. It also provides a significant degree of personal satisfaction in so far as it enables the Library staff to use professional skills to help people access the information needed to make personal health decisions with respect to their health care.

Realistically, it is possible that library-based consumer information health services may not be needed in the future. Sophisticated technology and media will someday make comprehensive health information readily available to former patrons in their homes by means of electronic technology. Perhaps those who have committed professional energy in this area will have a role to play in extending the service outside the walls of their institutions. It is gratifying to imagine that these programs may ultimately contribute to the development of a worldwide consumer data bank of complete, accurate, and comprehensible medical information available to all people.

REFERENCES

1. Rees, Alan M., ed. *Consumer Health & Nutrition Index.* Phoenix: Oryx Press, 1985– .

2. Rees, Alan M. and Hoffman, Catherine. *Consumer Health Information Source Book.* 3rd ed. Phoenix: Oryx, 1990.

3. Rees, Alan M., ed. *Developing Consumer Health Information Services.* New York: R.R. Bowker, 1982.

APPENDIX I:
Letter of Administrative Agreement

Englewood Public Library
Swedish Medical Center Library

Because both libraries share a commitment to serve the health information needs of the community, we agree to share responsibility for serving these needs in the following manner.

Requests from the community to Swedish Medical Center Library will be referred to the Englewood Public Library.

The Englewood Public Library will attempt to satisfy health information requests with a basic collection of medical reference books.

Swedish Medical Center Library will provide the Englewood Public Library, upon request, with selection and reference consultation to ensure a quality medical reference collection and service.

Health information requests which cannot be satisfied by the Englewood Public Library will be referred to the Swedish Medical Center Library.

Englewood Public Library will encourage patrons to call the Swedish Medical Center Library to describe the nature of the request and to arrange for use of the library.

Englewood Public Library and Swedish Medical Center Library agree to provide for each other basic reference and interlibrary loan service.

Both parties will attempt to document contacts and referrals and will meet twice a year to discuss this agreement.

This agreement is effective immediately and will continue until one party wishes to negotiate a change.

_____   _____
Director of Libraries   Director, Library Services
Englewood Public Library   Swedish Medical Center Library

APPENDIX II:
Swedish Medical Center Policy Procedure

SUBJECT: USE OF PATIENT HEALTH INFORMATION LIBRARY
"HEALTHLINK: YOUR HEALTH INFORMATION SERVICE"

PURPOSE: To describe how inpatients of Swedish Medical Center may receive medically related information from the Swedish Health Information Library

POLICY STATEMENT:

1. Consumer health information is available for utilization and education by Swedish Medical Center inpatients and their families through the Health Information Library located at Swedish.
2. Swedish Medical Center out-patients or other consumers are encouraged to use the Health Information Service at the Englewood Public Library, 3400 S. Elati, Englewood, Colorado, for any information needs or requests.

PROCEDURE:

1. Medically related and appropriate information may be requested for inpatients from the Health Information Library by:
   a. Patients and/or their families
   b. Physicians
   c. SMC professional staff

2. To obtain information from "HEALTHLINK: HEALTH INFORMATION LIBRARY," staff should fill out the Library Information Request Form.

3. Request Form is to be addressographed and delivered to the library by staff, volunteer or, if time allows, inter-departmental mail. If information is needed immediately, a call may be made to the library and a staff member may go to pick it up when notified that material is ready.

4. Request is in three parts. One part is to be retained by the library, one part to be retained by the unit, and one part given to the patient.

5. Unit copy to be retained as a reminder that the patient has library materials needing to be returned, and to aid in documentation of information given for educational purposes.

6. If materials are to be returned to the library after use, and prior to discharge, the appropriate box will be checked on the request form.

7. Nursing staff will remind inpatients upon discharge of their need to return any remaining checked out material to the nurse's station or library.

8. Materials may be returned to the library via the inter-hospital mail system, or delivered there by staff.

CHAPTER 12
Saint Joseph Hospital Health Reach Library

Margaret Bandy

Saint Joseph Hospital is a private, nonprofit, 565-bed regional medical center located in Denver, Colorado. It was founded in 1873 by the Sisters of Charity of Leavenworth and is still owned and operated by the Sisters. Services range from primary care to tertiary care, and the Hospital has Level III maternity and newborn designation. Patient education is an integral part of patient care at Saint Joseph Hospital; in 1984 the Hospital received an Outstanding Achievement Award from the American Hospital Association for patient education activities.

BACKGROUND

In 1983, the patient education coordinator and the medical librarian met to discuss problems regarding patient education in the Hospital. Although there were classes for diabetic and heart patients, closed-circuit television, and one-on-one teaching on the units, some patients' needs were not being met. Problems existed in connection with the lack of time by nurses for such activities and illnesses for which no teaching packages had been developed. The staff of the Health Sciences Library had also encountered frustration in trying to serve the needs of patients and family members who had come to the Library seeking information. Although there was no policy against serving them, there was little in the collection that was useful to most laypersons. The Health Sciences Library's capacity to serve patients was further limited by its small size, and by the large number of house staff who used it. During early discussions, the goal of establishing a separate library, located near the Health Sciences Library, that could respond to the information needs of the patients was formulated. Later, the idea was expanded to allow access by the Denver community. Because of the state of health care financing, it was also decided to try to fund the start-up costs through donations, and to staff the Library with volunteers.

THE PLANNING PROCESS

The planning process lasted nearly two years and involved research, seeking political support, the preparation of a convincing proposal to present to Hospital administration, and, following approval, received, the work involved in getting the Library ready to open. The various revisions of the proposal were reviewed by the Library's administrator, and additional information incorporated into each revision. Midway in the process, a most welcome donation of $5,000 was received from the Denver Clinic (now called Accord Medical Centers).

The key elements of the "Proposal to Establish a Health Information Library at Saint Joseph Hospital" were the rationale for establishing such a service, the results of a formal needs assessment, an environmental competitive analysis performed to place the proposal in the context of the current health-care scene, the presentation of alternative solutions to disseminating information to patients and families, the recommended solution, and the issues for implementation. Implementation issues included location, staffing, funding, and selection policy for collection development.

Rationale

In order to bring the decision-makers to an understanding of the state-of-the-art in patient education, the proposal pointed out the support of patient education by the American Hospital Association, an established authority acknowledged by the Hospital administration. The AHA Policy and Statement of the Hospital's Responsibility for Patient Education states that "patient education/information services be provided as an integral part of care to assist patients in making informed decisions about their use of health-care services, managing their illnesses and implementing follow-up care." The proposal also noted that because of decreasing length of stay, the Hospital should consider alternative modalities for providing such education/information in an efficient and cost-effective manner.

The proposal suggested that the patient library in an acute care hospital was becoming a well-recognized mode of providing education to patients about their specific illnesses, treatment methods, and healthy lifestyles, and some experts were supporting the creation of resource centers for the purpose.[1,2] In this connection, a patient library allows patients to select and read materials at their own reading level, encourages them to become more self-directed in their learning and self-care, and provides an alternative to the standard one-to-one teaching currently employed by hospital staff. Many patients actively seek information about health, illnesses, and health-care options and need to be exposed to such information in an environment responsive to their questions and concerns. Materials provided in a hospital-based patient library would be authoritative, unlike that which the patient might find in a local public library or bookstore. The proposal argued that this Hospital's experience with a "mini-library" for maternity patients had shown that patients are interested in and do utilize such a facility; 350 to 500 free pamphlets and photocopied materials were daily taken from the maternity library by patients and their families.

The rationale also pointed out that most physicians want their patients to be well-informed, and would like them to have access to accurate and appropriate information. One of the planning activities involved drafting a memo of support that was sent to a number of physicians for their signature (Appendix I). A sufficient number of influential physicians responded positively. In addition, the medical librarian and the patient education coordinator (a Planning Committee of two) attended several Medical Staff Committee meetings to present the idea and document medical staff support for the Library.

Finally, the proposal cited research within the health field that showed inadequate explanation of the various aspects of their diagnosis and treatment to be rated consistently by patients as the most stressful aspect of hospitalization.[3] Other research revealed that patients tend to be more dissatisfied by the lack of information they receive than by any other aspect of their care.[4] The proposal suggested that a patient library could improve patient satisfaction, enhance staff-patient relations, and serve as a tangible manifestation of the Hospital's concern for the total well-being of the patient.

Needs Assessment

Informal observation by library and nursing education staff indicated that patients, family members, outpatients with acute or chronic illnesses, and members of the community at large periodically contacted Saint Joseph Hospital for health-related information and literature. To more accurately determine the information needs, the Planning Committee decided to survey inpatients. The Hospital's planning office assisted in the development of the patient survey. On May 1, 1984, approximately 100 surveys were distributed and retrieved by auxiliary volunteers (Appendix II). The survey included most segments of the patient population. A summary of results revealed the following:

- 91 percent would definitely or probably be interested in reading about their own illness, operation, or physical condition.
- 90 percent would definitely or probably be interested in materials about good physical or mental health in general.
- 78 percent thought that their family members would be interested in such materials.
- 87 percent would definitely or probably visit a patient library if one were available.
- 50 percent would like copies of articles or pamphlets they could keep.
- 25 percent would like materials that could be checked out and returned.
- 25 percent would like either to check-out or keep items.

The survey also revealed some reasons why a patient might not visit the Library. One patient pointed out that the tendency is for patients to remain on their floor and not wander about, while another commented that they were from out of state and hoped not to spend much time here. Typical comments were:

- "sounds like an excellent program"
- "a healthy mind leads to a healthy body; knowledge is crucial"
- "this would be a great patient service"
- "any pamphlets or materials on this disease would help me and my family maybe understand"
- "I think it would be a big breakthrough for many people. Most people could cope better with their medical problems knowing . . . and their family would be more knowledgeable."

A part of the survey also involved a compilation of the reasons for hospitalization and organizing them into National Library of Medicine classification areas.

Environmental Competitive Analysis

Following a review of one of the early versions of the proposal, the Library's administrator requested that a small environmental competitive analysis be performed. This involved looking at the competition to see what was being done, and reviewing established programs to analyze their success. At that time, the Swedish Medical Center/Englewood Public Library HealthLink Project had begun, but there were no acute care hospitals in Denver that had separate consumer health libraries for their patients. Other activities in Denver at that time were the plans of Children's Hospital to develop a health information collection for parents, and the formation by the Colorado Council of Medical Librarians of a Patient and Community Health Information Interest Group to promote resource sharing.

In order to identify existing programs in acute care hospitals throughout the country, contact was made with the Hospital Library Section of the Medical Library Association. In 1983 the Section had undertaken a survey of patient and consumer health library programs; 60–70 of the respondents had been identified as having viable programs. Although the survey had not yet been tabulated, the chairman of the Section's Patient Education Committee, Katherine Lindner, shared copies of 15 completed survey forms. These together with five programs that had been described in the literature formed the basis of a survey to ascertain the success of the programs. Of the 20, 17 served not only patients, but also the community on a walk-in, call-in, or interlibrary loan basis. All felt that their programs were successful.

Alternative Solutions

The patient survey and the survey of existing programs provided evidence to the Hospital administration that patients thought a health information library would be worthwhile, and that other institutions had established successful patient library programs. These facts were incorporated into the final proposal. However, the medical librarian and the patient education coordinator knew that a convincing proposal should include other possible solutions to the problem of information dissemination to patients, family members, and the community. The four options were defined as follows:

Option #1: Patient Education Materials in the Health Sciences Library

Advantages: The Health Sciences Library has established procedures for handling print materials; staff is knowledgeable about the subject matter; there would be limited budget impact initially.
Disadvantages: The Health Sciences Library cannot accommodate lay users because of lack of seating space; conversation by house staff that would not be appropriate for patients and visitors to hear; lack of shelving space; and lack of staff time for responding to information requests, and for ordering and processing materials.

Option #2: Dissemination of Materials on the Nursing Unit

Advantages: Materials convenient for nursing staff; nurses are familiar with patients and their needs.
Disadvantages: Dissemination of materials is contingent upon the time and interest of the nurses; available space is suitable for only a small amount of materials.

Option #3: Refer All Requests for Information to the Denver Public Library

Advantages: No resources or staff time expended by Saint Joseph Hospital; convenient for Denver residents.
Disadvantages: Materials have not been screened for accuracy by health-care professionals; not convenient for the Hospital's many non-Denver patients and families.

Option #4: Establish a Separate Library for Patients and Visitors

Advantages: A separate library would maintain the privacy of physicians and other staff members who use the Health Sciences Library; could accommodate more materials and provide seating especially for the patients and families; and could more easily be open to those outside the Hospital.
Disadvantages: This solution requires adequate resolution of several issues, such as location, staffing, funding, and selection of materials.

Implementation Issues

The decisions that the medical librarian and the patient education coordinator made on implementation issues were critical to the success of the proposal because they focused on such political concerns as location (space in the Hospital was at a premium), staffing (approval for additional FTE's would be impossible), funding (budget constraints were already being felt), and selection of materials (administrators and Hospital staff worried about liability and physician approval).

Location: The Planning Committee had investigated several options for location of the Library and recommended a little used classroom one floor below the Health Sciences Library. It was approximately 375 square feet, and although it was a little out of the mainstream of hospital activity, it was close to all elevators.

Staffing: The question of staffing was more difficult. The administration would not approve paid staff for a new, untried program. Although paid staff would have been ideal, the use of volunteers, not necessarily drawn from the Hospital Auxiliary but recruited especially to work in the Library, was explored. Once the proposal was approved, volunteers were recruited by advertising in the Hospital publications and in the Non-Practicing and Part-Time Nurses Association Newsletter. A position description was written that covered the primary responsibilities of the volunteer staff, including assisting patrons by phone and in person, processing materials, maintaining statistics on Library usage, updating materials in pamphlet racks throughout the Hospital, and monitoring subject areas that needed to be added to the Library (Appendix III). Difficult questions or those for which no materials are on hand would be referred to the medical librarian.

A policy regarding the use of volunteers in the Library was drafted for approval by Hospital administration (Appendix IV). When the Library opened in 1985, volunteer staff included two former RNs, one LPN, a former nursing school instructor, an individual with experience in school and public libraries, and two members of the Hospital Auxiliary. Training covered the subject areas and organization of the collection, and the difference between giving information and dispensing medical advice. A "Trigger Tape" film developed by Luella Allen and Martha Manning at the Health Sciences Library of the State University of New York at Buffalo was used. This tape, developed for training public librarians to handle medical reference questions, presents various vignettes that can be used to explore sensitive areas such as dealing with the emotional patron, commenting on specific physicians, or providing medical advice.[5]

Funding: The Denver Clinic contribution was to be used for materials, processing, and promotional activities. The Nursing Education Department also committed $1,000. The intention during the planning process, and as outlined in the proposal, was to locate some surplus Hospital furniture and perhaps in-kind donations for shelving, in the hope of holding down costs. We estimated that an additional $5,800 would be needed, either from donations or from Hospital funds.

Selection Policy: During the planning stages, the development of a selection policy assumed major importance. In addition to clarifying the components of the collection, the policy addressed the concerns of physicians regarding the materials their patients would be reading, and the fears of the support staff regarding malpractice issues. Criteria developed by the InfoHealth Project in Cleveland used seven major variables for evaluating materials. These were adapted for the evaluation form that our expert reviewers would use.[6] A decision was made not to acquire fad books or polemics antipathetic to the medical profession. The goals and objectives did not require that the Library provide this type of consumer health information, and to do so might work against the credibility the planners wanted to establish within the Hospital and community. As one consumer later said: "I came here because I knew you would have accurate information."

Midway through the planning process, the patient education coordinator, who chaired the Patient Education Committee, invited the medical librarian to join the Committee. The Committee is composed of several nurse educator specialists, such as the ostomy nurse, representatives of respiratory therapy, diagnostic imaging, social services, cancer education and counseling, and dietary. The Committee made recommendations for acquisitions and also proposed the idea of inserting a disclaimer into each book. The disclaimer is printed on self-sticking paper and states: "The materials in Saint Joseph Hospital Health Reach Library are intended to provide general information for you. Some material may contain information that is the opinion of the author and not necessarily that of your physician. Please consult your physician on specific medical questions."

Other elements of collection development policy evolved during the planning process. Subjects to be collected in depth would reflect the 10 most common discharge diagnoses of the Hospital. These include normal delivery and other indications for care in pregnancy, vascular disorders (primarily stroke), neoplastic disorders, cardiovascular disorders, gynecologic disorders, mental disorders, and arthropathies and related disorders. Other subject areas would be represented but with less depth. Materials presenting diverse points of view by authoritative authors would be purchased.

Initially, all books were reviewed for accuracy by the Patient Education Committee or a physician. After one year the Library was able to dispense with this slow process, since very few of the medical librarian's selections were rejected. The opinion of experts is still sought on occasion for certain topics, for example, nutrition.

Although the patient survey indicated that material on general physical and mental health was desirable, the need for health promotion material is minimal. The collection includes information on diet, especially cholesterol; physical fitness; stress reduction; and holistic health topics. Tools used in collection development include publishers' and vendors' notices, reviews in *Library Journal,* lists of reviews in the *Consumer Health & Nutrition Index* (Oryx Press), and a Catline SDI on Popular Works shared by the Swedish Medical Center librarian.

The collection currently contains over 600 books and approximately 20 subscriptions to magazines and newsletters. The latter includes general publications, such as the *Mayo Clinic Health Letter* and support group newsletters such as *Let's Face It,* for individuals who are facially disfigured or disabled. There are currently only a few audiotapes but there are plans to expand the audiovisual collection, especially in the subject areas of humor, stress reduction, and mental health topics.

Although not important to the acceptance of the proposal, another decision made during the planning process was to organize the book collection according to National Library of Medicine Classification. Most pamphlets are filed according to NLM Medical Subject Headings (MeSH), although there are some exceptions. For example, the term "miscarriage" is used rather than "Abortion." After approval of the program, two field work students from the University of Denver Library School helped organize the pamphlet collection and the community resource file.

After nearly two years of planning, the Health Reach Library opened in July 1985. The name "Health Reach" was selected because the Hospital had community education programs under that name. The Library is now located in a room of about 200 square feet adjacent to the Health Sciences Library that could be remodeled for use as the Library. Although this is more convenient for Library staff to manage, it is less accessible to patients and the public, and user statistics reflect this fact.

CURRENT SERVICES

The collection is open to all patients, their family members, employees of the Hospital, and people from the community (adults only). Books and periodicals can be checked out or used in the Library; the circulation period is two weeks. Patrons not affiliated with the Hospital fill out a form and are issued a library card, but are not entered into the automated circulation system patron file at this time. Photocopying is provided free of charge for up to 10 pages; the charge after that is 10 cents per page. In addition to books and periodicals, a popular feature of the Library is the pamphlet collection. Multiple copies of pamphlets on common conditions are available on open shelves for patrons to take. Single copies of more expensive pamphlets are filed and can be checked out.

Many of the individuals who use the Library's telephone reference service have been referred by physicians, other libraries, and a local bookstore. Brief answers, such as definitions, are read over the phone; lengthier information is photocopied and mailed to the user. Telephone queries provide the greatest variety of subject matter and often require the most time and effort to answer.

The questions the Library receives from the community do not always fall into neat categories as do the inpatient requests. There may be one request regarding eye diseases once every six months, whereas we disseminate information on stroke to inpatients almost weekly. Over the past four years, the Health Reach Library has received phone requests for information on corneal dysplasia, Tourette Syndrome, "fingerprint" dystrophy, chelation therapy, ocular albinism, vertigo, uterine fibroids, lupus, syringomyelia, porphyria, narcolepsy, and peripheral artery disease.

Many questions deal with infectious diseases. Often consumers will want to know the latest or alternative treatments for a disease. For many of these kinds of questions, the consumer literature would probably be inadequate, and the Health Reach Library would supplement an item from the consumer collection with something from the professional collection. In addition, many patients with chronic illnesses require more specific information than is available in lay materials. A computer search may be performed to assist the Library staff when the collection does not contain appropriate information. The Rare Disease Database on Compuserve and the Combined Health Information Database on BRS are often useful. The medical librarian may also search Medline either online or on compact disc to identify professional materials that can help to answer questions.

The Health Reach Library staff sees these services as essential. If a consumer health library defines itself as a health library for consumers, not merely a collection of consumer or lay-level materials, it must be prepared to offer access to the professional literature in some fashion, such as by allowing users to access the collection, by performing literature searches, or by referring users to other sources of information. The last item sometimes simply means explaining to users how to access the interlibrary loan services of their local public library.

Other services offered on a regular basis include providing lists of patient materials in the Health Reach Library to patient educators conducting classes on such topics as diabetes, stroke, or women's health issues.

Two days each week, the volunteers take a book cart of selections from the Library to several patient units, including mother/baby care, dialysis, and orthopedics. Use of materials is not high, especially since inpatients today are very sick, but the cart serves as a public relations tool, reminding the nursing staff of the availability of the service for patients. Materials will also be delivered to patients' rooms at their request or that of physicians and/or nurses even if it is not a day for cart service.

LIBRARY USAGE STATISTICS

Since the Library opened in July 1985, the volunteers have attempted to keep accurate statistics on Library use. Statistics include new registrants by category, gross statistics on walk-in and other usage, and use of the book collection by subject area. A study performed after the first year showed that usage was almost evenly divided between Hospital employees and three groups—patients, family/friends, and people from the community. Table 12-1 shows the breakdown for all four years.

TABLE 12-1: Health Reach Library New Registrants

	1985-86	*1986-87*	*1987-88*	*1988-89*	*Total*
Patients	54	66	82	69	271
Family/Friends	49	36	33	22	140
Community	46	30	31	22	129
Total	149	132	146	113	540

During the first year, the largest use was by the 30–39 age group (32 percent); while use by women was 82 percent. Those percentages have remained approximately the same each year.

The volunteers also keep monthly statistics to reflect total usage in certain categories, but not by user group. Four of these categories are shown in Table 12-2. As a point of clarification, "Mat. Use" refers to Library materials checked-out, free pamphlets taken, or materials used in the Library. "Searches" means that to find information for a user, the volunteer or, usually, the medical librarian, had to go beyond finding a book or pamphlet in the Health Reach Library collection as in the examples discussed in the section on services.

TABLE 12-2: Health Reach Library Utilization by Selected Categories

	1985-86	*1986-87*	*1987-88*	*1988-89*	*Total*
Walk-In	1333	1309	1132	974	4748
Calls	205	287	293	201	986
Mat. Use	928	1327	1120	930	4305
Searches	17	40	54	49	160

During the past four years, the subjects most used in the book collection have been psychiatry/psychology, women's health, pediatric topics, heart disease, cancer, nervous system disorders, orthopedics, gastrointestinal disorders, and diabetes. Employee usage reflects both personal and professional needs. For example, pastoral care personnel use the materials on grief or on cancer if they are working with cancer patients. Other employees may have a family member with a chronic illness, or may wish to deal with their own stress or diet needs.

To date only informal, anecdotal evaluations have been done. Patrons mention that they have been better able to communicate with their physicians because of reading something in the Library. Several patients who have a chronic illness have said that for the first time they understood something about it. One patron told a volunteer that reading the material gave her courage to consult a physician. Follow-up evaluations are now being planned to more accurately ascertain the usefulness of the service.

PUBLIC RELATIONS

The Health Reach Library has never been part of the Hospital's public relations efforts, so promotion has been a challenge for Library staff. Several open houses have been held primarily to promote the Library to nursing staff. When the library first opened, a local television station producer happened to be in the Hospital and was interested in the service; subsequently the television station ran a short feature story about it. There were also press releases in the local papers during the first year of operation. Direct mailing of information and a Rolodex card to physicians was done to encourage referrals. Other promotional pieces currently in use are a card describing the Library services that are offered, and a bookmark that is put in each book that is checked out. On a continuing basis there are articles and book notes in the various hospital publications, bulletin board displays in the lobby, pamphlet racks in patient waiting areas and solariums that direct people to the Library, and a "bulletin board" announcement on the Hospital's closed-circuit patient television station. During Patient Education Week each November, the Health Reach Library display in the main lobby shows samples of materials that are available to our patients and the community. The Library is also listed in the city telephone directory as part of the main Hospital listing.

NETWORKING

Because the Health Reach Library was originally conceived to meet the information needs of our patients and their families, many of whom are not from the Denver area, no formal cooperative links to public libraries were established. There have been many informal, librarian-to-librarian linkages, and the services have been publicized through the Colorado State Library and the Central Colorado Library System newsletters. The Colorado Council of Medical Librarians maintains a strong cooperative network, and the Health Reach Library has received many referrals through these channels. The earliest and most enduring link is with the Swedish Medical Center Health Information Service.

Informal links exist with many of the patient support groups in the area. One of the most interesting links has been with a large bookstore that is noted for the high level of customer service they provide. The store frequently refers its customers to the Health Reach Library when unable to provide a publication that meets the customer's needs.

In May 1986 the Health Sciences Library signed a formal agreement with the University of Colorado Health Sciences Center Library allowing the installation of a dedicated line terminal to the University Library computer. The holdings of both the Saint Joseph Hospital Health Sciences Library and the Health Reach Library became searchable online to patrons of both libraries, and to the other libraries that joined the shared system, including Swedish Medical Center. As a result of this link, many referrals to the Health Reach Library have been made. In 1990 the University and the libraries sharing the system will move all automated processes to the Colorado Alliance of Research Libraries (CARL). The CARL system includes the collections of nine colleges and universities in Colorado, five community colleges, the Denver Public Library, public libraries in western Colorado, the University of Wyoming, and Arizona State University. CARL is also available for searching on Internet, a collection of networks available to hundreds of institutions across the country.

As part of the CARL system, the Health Reach Library collection will become more accessible to the community via the public and university libraries that use the CARL Public Access Catalog. The Health Reach Library now receives several interlibrary loan requests each month via the OCLC Interlibrary Loan Subsystem and it is anticipated that both the ILL's and walk-in use will increase when the collection is available on CARL. Users of the public access terminals in all of the public, college, and university libraries throughout the state will be able to browse the consumer health collections at both Saint Joseph and Swedish; this will give them subject access to the collections for the first time. When both libraries begin using the circulation functions, they will also be able to determine whether the item is actually available.

Use of the CARL circulation system will give the Health Reach Library more efficient tracking of utilization by user groups and subject. The current plan is not to enter each individual patient or community user into the system; this would be impractical because usage is often a one-time occurrence. However, a generic card will be created for the patient and community user in order to take full advantage of the CARL statistical functions.

THE FUTURE

The Health Reach Library moves into the 1990s facing many challenges. After the first year and a half, some of the volunteers left and the staff now includes three individuals working a total of 36 hours per week. There are particular challenges inherent in relying on volunteers—recruiting, training, and retraining individuals who may not have experience with libraries and/or medical terminology. The Health Reach Library has been extremely fortunate in the caliber of volunteer, especially in their commitment to the concept of consumer health information.

Ongoing funding was to have been provided initially by the Education Department and Nursing Education. Each department agreed to allocate $500 annually for materials, but due to budgeting restrictions this amount has not always been provided. The Library is again seeking grant funding through the Hospital Foundation and will probably always need to rely on such funding in order to maintain a quality collection.

Despite the challenges, the rewards of providing consumer health information are many. As the medical librarian noted in an article in the *Saint Joseph Hospital Primary Care Bulletin,* people seek consumer health information for a variety of reasons, but one emotion nearly all of these information seekers share is fear. Information that can be obtained in a nonthreatening environment, or that can be requested by phone and read in the privacy of the home can often help individuals cope with these fears. In the four years that the Health Reach Library has been providing information, there has not been one complaint from a physician.

The success of the Health Reach Library is best measured not by statistics but by the appreciation of the patients, family members, and community persons who have found answers to their most difficult questions during times of acute stress. Many users have said: "Every hospital should have something like this." The Health Reach Library program demonstrates that these services can be provided on a small scale, with limited funds. The critical factor is a dedicated library staff that sees these services as an essential ingredient in quality patient care, and sees consumer health information as an appropriate role for the hospital library to undertake.

REFERENCES

1. Skillkern, P. "A Planned System of Patient Education." *JAMA.* 238 (1977). 878–79.

2. Hoffman, L. "Patient Education: How We Designed Our Own Program." *Group Practice.* 25 (5) (1976). 21–24.

3. Volcer, B. "Perceived Levels of Stress Events Associated with the Experience of Hospitalization." *Nursing Research.* 23 (1977). 4955–5005.

4. Waitzkin, H. and Stoeckle, J. "The Communication of Information About Illness." *Adv Psychosom Med.* 8 (1972). 180–90.

5. Bain, Christine, ed. *Health Information from the Public Library: A Report of Two Pilot Projects.* Albany: The State Library of New York, 1984.

6. Rees, Alan M. ed. *Developing Consumer Health Information Services.* New York: Bowker, 1982.

APPENDIX I:
Memo Signed by Physician Supporters

I am aware that you are proposing that a patient information library be instituted at Saint Joseph Hospital. I am also aware that all patient education materials will be reviewed by expert medical or hospital staff prior to placement in the library. I support this proposal and believe that a patient information library would be an added benefit to patient care at this hospital.

APPENDIX II:
Survey of Patients

(**Note:** Questions 1–4 had as choices Definitely, Probably, Probably Not, Definitely Not, Don't Know)

Dear Saint Joseph Hospital Guest,

Because of the growing interest of patients in maintaining a healthy lifestyle and in caring for their own well-being, Saint Joseph Hospital is studying the feasibility of establishing a Patient Health Information Library to provide material on medical conditions and health care.

Would you take a few minutes of your time to complete the following survey which would help us determine the benefits to patients of establishing such a library?

Please check the appropriate blank:

1. If reading materials were available in the hospital about your illness, operation, or physical condition, would you be interested?
2. Would you be interested in materials about good physical and mental health in general?
3. Would members of your family be interested in reading such material?
4. If the hospital had a patient library, would you visit it?
5. What subjects would be of greatest interest to you?
6. What types of printed materials would be most useful?
   _____ Books, pamphlets, etc., that could be checked out and
          returned later
   _____ Pamphlets, brochures, or copies of articles that you
          could keep
   _____ Doesn't make any difference
   _____ Other—please explain
7. What times would be most convenient for you to visit a library in the hospital?
   9-11 am _____ 1-3 pm _____ 3-5 pm _____ 7-9 pm _____ Other _____

8. About you . . .
   Reason for hospital stay _____
   Age Group: Under 21 _____ 20-29 _____ 30-39 _____
   40-49 _____ 50-59 _____ 60-69 _____ 70 and over _____
   Sex: Male _____ Female _____

APPENDIX III:
Position Description, Saint Joseph Hospital, Denver, Colorado

Position: Health Information Library Assistant

Job Summary: Under direct supervision of the Medical Librarian, assists in the establishment and daily maintenance of the Health Information Library.

Training: The Health Information Library Assistant will receive special training in addition to the regular hospital orientation and library activity training. This training will include the following:

1. Familiarization with subject areas, as well as with the cataloging and classification schemes used.
2. How to interview patients, etc., in order to identify information needs.
3. Understanding the difference between health information dissemination and medical advice.

Responsibilities:

1. Assist patrons by phone and in person.
2. Order and process materials for the library.
3. Review selected periodicals to identify potential additions to the library.
4. Maintain statistics on library use.
5. Assist in evaluation of library services.
6. Update materials in information racks throughout the hospital.
7. Monitor subject areas that need to be added to the collection.
8. Maintain circulation records.
9. Perform other related duties as assigned.

Skills: Interpersonal skills are essential because of potential contact with patients. These include tact, discretion, sympathy for patients and their family members, good judgement, maturity.

APPENDIX IV:
Policy Regarding the Use of Volunteers in the Health Information Library

General

A staff of volunteers to support the activities of the health information library will be established. The primary role of the volunteer is to provide medical and health information in the library collection to patrons. Under no circumstances is the volunteer library assistant to give medical advice. Medical advice includes the following:

1. Recommending a method or procedure of treatment to follow.
2. Recommending an alternate drug that may produce the same results as the one presently being taken.
3. Assisting the patron in diagnosing him or herself.
4. Interpreting medical information to the patron.

Requirements

An application form and interview with the Medical Librarian will determine the applicant's suitability. Requirements include the following:

1. **Physical.** The volunteer must be able to lift, carry, and shelve books.
2. **Knowledge and skills.** Medical knowledge and/or library experience is preferred.
3. **Personal characteristics.** Tact, discretion, and sympathy for patients and family members; good judgment and maturity.

General Responsibilities

1. **Time commitment.** The volunteer must work at least three (3) consecutive hours per week in the library.
2. **Name tag.** A regulation name tag must be worn while on duty.
3. **Absences.** The volunteer must notify the Medical Librarian in advance of the time due on duty if he/she will be absent. After three (3) unexcused absences the volunteer will be considered for possible dismissal.

Orientation and Training

1. The volunteer will attend the hospital orientation.
2. The volunteer will be trained by the Medical Librarian to staff the library. Areas included in training are described in the position description.

CHAPTER 13
The Planetree Health Resource Center

Tracey Cosgrove

INTRODUCTION

Planetree is a national, nonprofit consumer health organization dedicated to helping people become active participants in their health and medical care. Named for the tree that Hippocrates sat beneath when he taught his first medical students, the Planetree Health Resource Center provides the general public with access to health and medical information.

THE PLANETREE ORGANIZATION

Planetree was founded in 1978 by a layperson, Angelica R. Thieriot, as a result of several hospital experiences that left her frustrated and angry. As a patient, she envisioned a hospital modeled on the Greek tradition of healing that not only supported the physical needs of patients, but also met their emotional, intellectual, and spiritual needs. Mrs. Thieriot's vision attracted a diverse group of physicians, civic, business, cultural, and health-care leaders who became the founding board of directors, dedicated to the creation of innovative models for humanized health care.

The Planetree Health Resource Center model is dedicated to empowering health consumers by providing access to current health and medical information. One of the ways patients are disempowered within the health-care system is that they do not always have clear access to the health and medical information needed to make their own informed health-care decisions. As a patient, a patient's family member, or loved one, the lay health consumer is often left out of the network of information resources available to the health-care team. Patients rarely have direct access to their own medical charts or to the current medical literature available through the hospital medical library. People can go to local public libraries for health information, but public libraries usually have limited collections that may not contain the in-depth range of

The author gratefully acknowledges Candace Ford, M.L.S. and Janna Katz for their assistance with this chapter.

current health information that is needed to make complicated health-care decisions.

The general public can sometimes access the resources of a local medical school library or a hospital medical library. However, these collections are created for health professionals. When they do contain publications in lay language, it is rarely above the sophistication of a pamphlet collection. These collections often fail to address topics beyond the scope of their health-care institution's services and usually do not offer information on increasingly popular complementary or alternative therapy approaches.

Planetree's solution was to create a free-standing library collection that would provide access to a wide range of health and medical information to any member of the community, both layperson and health practitioner. The first Planetree Health Resource Center opened in 1981 in San Francisco. The Center currently serves 12,000 patrons each year, and houses a 2,500-volume medical library, a health bookstore, clipping files of current medical information, an Information and Reference System of voluntary health organizations, support groups and health practitioner listings, and a Health Information Service by mail. The Center hosts a fall and spring health lecture series and publishes a semiannual newsletter and health catalog.

OTHER PLANETREE PROGRAMS

In a pioneering effort to humanize the hospital setting, the Planetree organization opened a Model Hospital Unit in 1985 at Pacific Presbyterian Medical Center in San Francisco. This 13-bed medical-surgical unit combines the best of modern technology with the most ancient concepts of nurturing and supportive care.

In 1989 a second Planetree Health Resource Center opened in San Jose, California, in conjunction with San Jose Medical Center. The new Planetree Health Resource Center occupies a beautifully renovated Victorian house on the San Jose Medical Center grounds. Within the Hospital there is a 25-bed Planetree Unit. In addition, Planetree is developing Health Resource Centers and Planetree Hospital Unit sites in Oregon, New York, and central California. In building towards the future of humanized health care, Planetree is working toward the creation of the Planetree Institute, a "think tank" for the discussion of humanistic health-care policies.

The overall Planetree goal is to bring positive changes to the health-care system that will empower health consumers to fully participate in their own health-care decisions.

THE PLANETREE HEALTH RESOURCE CENTER IN SAN FRANCISCO

Overview

The purpose of the Planetree Health Resource Center is to:

* provide the layperson with open access to a broad spectrum of current health and medical information;
* empower individuals to make informed health-care decisions; and
* encourage individuals to take greater responsibility for their own health.

The Planetree Health Resource Center Library is free and open to the public. The Library contains a wide variety of medical information that reflects the health information needs and interests of the community.

There are no public access restrictions to any of the information in the Health Resource Center collection. On-site information can be accessed by any member of the public or any staff member whether she or he is a layperson or health professional. We have posted a sign at the front of the Library which states that information available in the Library collection does not imply recommendation or endorsement by Planetree.

The collection contains over 2,500 health and medical books. The technical level of material ranges from current medical textbooks to lay health books and professional publications on complementary therapies. Over 100 serials titles are received with an emphasis on consumer health newsletters, magazines, and popular medical journals. A 24-drawer clipping file system containing articles from the current (last two to four years) medical and consumer health literature is constantly updated and maintained. The audiovisual library offers over 75 video- and audiocassette titles on health-related topics.

Patrons can borrow material from the Library collection by obtaining an annual library card ($20 in 1989) or membership. Membership is available with an annual fee ($35 in 1989) and constitutes a tax-deductible contribution to Planetree. Membership privileges include a library card for the Health Resource Center in San Francisco; a 10 percent discount on books and products for sale; a subscription to *Planetalk,* the semiannual Planetree newsletter; discounts on the Planetree Health Lecture Series; and notification of Planetree events and classes.

All audiovisual tapes and most of the book collection, excluding medical textbooks and reference works, can be borrowed. These items circulate from the collection for a two-week period, and can be renewed for an additional two weeks if they have not been reserved for another patron. Journals, magazines, newsletters, and clipping file materials do not circulate from the collection. Patrons are encouraged to photocopy from these materials (10 cents a page in 1989) to take home with them. The Planetree Health Resource Center is open to the public Tuesday through Friday and the first and third Saturdays of the month from 11 a.m. to 5 p.m. On Wednesday, hours are extended from 11 a.m. to 7 p.m.

The Library Environment

The Planetree Health Resource Center offers a comfortable physical environment in a noninstitutional setting. The Center is located on street level in the original Stanford Medical School Library, a historical landmark built in the 1920s. The Library's design incorporates day lighting, nonfluorescent fixtures, and nonglare surfaces. Tables, chairs, bookshelves, countertops, and the journal display rack are constructed in light oak; bright colored directors' chairs are arranged in the reading and audiovisual areas. To help create an attractive environment for patrons and staff, the Center includes green plants, fresh-cut flowers, and Japanese silk screen and English garden art prints. A play space for children is located in one of the reading areas. This "Kids Corner" is a low bookshelf stocked with toys, crayons and paper, anatomical models, and health books written for children. This play space offers children an area of their own to play in, yet allows them to stay close to their guardian.

Collection Development

The range of materials in the Health Resource Center collection includes general medical texts and journals, lay language books and periodicals, books and journals on complementary medical therapies, indices to the consumer health and medical literature, lay health audiocassette and videocassette tapes and compact discs, and selected health information pamphlets and computer software. The collection includes all major areas of medical interest to the general public, ranging from diagnostic tests to Mind/Body visualization techniques. The primary focus of collection development is for current health and medical information written or recorded for the layperson. For all major medical specialities, at least one current edition of a professional medical textbook is collected.

The selection of material for the Library is the responsibility of the medical librarian following the guideliness of the collection development policy. Items considered are assessed by subject content, currency of information, publisher reputation, author credentials, foreign-language relevancy, organization and presentation of contents, and cost. In Planetree's experience, the decision to include an item cannot be based on a single criterion alone. Conversely, every point of assessment listed may not be appropriate for all items. Suggestions for materials to be included in the collection are accepted from staff, patrons, and health professionals. It is understood that by selecting specific materials, Planetree does not endorse any particular method of treatment, specific physician, health practitioner, organization, or health-care facility. Health Resource Center staff and volunteers cannot verify the scientific accuracy of materials included in the collection.

In general, the collection is developed to reflect the pluralistic needs and interests of Health Resource Center patrons from the local community, and requests of the Health Information Service. The depth and range of any particular subject collected is based on consumer interest and need, and the availability and affordability of those materials. Whenever possible, for each medical specialty or major diagnostic category, we collect published materials from the perspectives of conventional medical therapeutics, from complementary therapies, and from investigational therapies. Lay health books are purchased to circulate from the collection. Lay books on popular health topics or those written by popular authors are purchased in multiple copies.

Audiovisual Collection

The Health Resource Center in San Francisco currently maintains circulating audiocassette and videocassette collections. The types of audiovisuals in the collection can be characterized by their different styles of presentation of health information:

- **Instructional:** Actively educational or motivational in presenting information. This category can include patient education tapes and health lectures.
- **Relaxation/Inspirational:** Uses primarily music, color, scenery or images, and guided visualization or personal stories to assist and perhaps transport listeners/viewers.
- **Combination:** Using elements of both categories to present information.

The Planetree Audiovisual Collection consists primarily of relaxation/inspirational tapes and combination tapes. Our experience has shown that the general public is interested in the most current health information available.

The Health Resource Center Library is formally reviewed twice a year to assess the currency and usage of the collection. Informally, the process of updating and refining the collection occurs constantly. Collection development resources are reviewed weekly by the medical librarian and the bookstore manager.

Clipping Files

The most accessed component of the Library collection is the Planetree clipping files. This 24-drawer vertical file system provides easy subject access to a wide variety of current health information. Files are organized alphabetically within broad subject categories. For example, the subject division for Heart/Heart Diseases includes files on Angioplasty, Cardiomyopathy, Heart Attack, Mitral Valve Prolapse, Valvuloplasty, and more. "See references" are used liberally to map medical diagnoses to lay health topics. While the emphasis is to select a main subject heading that is a common lay term, i.e., Heart Attack for Myocardial Infarction, we will sometimes prefer the common medical diagnostic term over the lay term when it is most commonly the one used by patrons to request information. We also use the medical term if it is used widely in the health and medical literature; for example, Chondromalacia Patella over

Jumper's Knee. We also attempt to define subject categories in the most unbiased and least subjective way possible. For example, we use the diagnosis Seizure Disorder over Epilepsy and the topic Street Drugs over Drug Abuse.

Articles for the clipping files are selected from the professional medical journals, consumer health newsletters and magazines, and newspapers that we receive by subscription or donation. We regularly conduct Medline searches for citations of new articles to update the information in our files and to create files on popular or health topics.

Health information pamphlets are included in the clipping files when the pamphlet is exceptional in its presentation of information, offers unique information, covers a rare diagnosis or disorder, or offers an excellent presentation of information in a language other than English. We collect pamphlets with an especially critical eye, excluding any undated materials. We prefer not to keep pamphlets that have not been updated within the last two to four years. We do not acquire health information pamphlets and fliers written by drug companies or producers of health-care products and devices that are intended as subjective promotional material.

Some of the areas where we do collect pamphlets in our clipping files are "safe" sex pamphlets from the San Francisco AIDS Foundation in Chinese and Spanish; health information pamphlets on surgical procedures produced by Krames Communications; and self-care pamphlets produced by the Brain Tumor Research Group from Scripps University in San Diego.

Circulation Control

Planetree's philosophy supports free and open access to all information in the collection. Since we are a health library open to the public, our patrons are sometimes ill themselves or emotionally upset by a loved one's health condition or death. Our expectation is that the loss rate in our Library might be higher than in other specialty libraries because our patrons may be unable to return materials. Overdue notices are sent after two weeks from the due date to encourage the return of items; there are no overdue fines to penalize patrons for late returns. The Health Resource Center does not contain a security system and there are no plans to install one in the future. Like many other bookstores, we keep one copy of our bookstore stock on display, and empty boxes of our audio- and videotape inventory; library copies of these tapes are available to sample on-site in our audiovisual center.

Classification Scheme

Planetree made a decision in 1981 to create a unique classification scheme for the organization of consumer health information. Originally, we considered using the National Library of Medicine (NLM) classification scheme for the medical literature. However, the NLM scheme contained several features we felt were necessary for the organization of the Library: subject specificity for the medical literature; broad organization by diagnostics, therapeutics, body systems, and the fields of medicine; the simplicity of consistent numbers assigned fixed meanings (i.e., 100s for general works); specific classification numbers for individual diagnoses and a broad number range within each subject division to allow for the creation of future numbers for new diagnoses. We elected not to use the NLM scheme for a consumer health information library for several reasons. In many cases the medical subject heading is not the commonly used lay term for the topic; the organization of the scheme did not group related subjects, making this system less conducive to browsing; several major subject divisions for consumer health information were not included in the NLM scheme, for example, Men's Health information is located under Urology; some subject placement in the classification scheme appeared either antiquated or philosophically biased, for example, many complementary therapy techniques are categorized under the subject Therapeutic Cults. Other classification schemes that used medical terminology more appropriate for the lay health consumer, like the Library of Congress, were not considered because they did not provide classification numbers for specific diagnoses and because the subject headings were often false or artificial sounding, using, for example, inverted subject headings.

The Planetree Classification Scheme organizes the books, journals, audiovisuals, clipping files, and Information and Reference System. It consists of an alphanumeric numbering system that is tailored to the field of consumer health information and a subject thesaurus that exclusively represents this body of literature. Special effort is taken to maintain flexibility with classification numbers that allow for the metamorphosis of the scheme to suit the changing trends in consumer health literature. For example, when we created the second generation of our classification scheme this year, we discovered that some subject classifications were obsolete. We removed the topic of Self-Care, which we felt had become redundant, because so many books incorporate a self-care perspective within general health or diagnostic specific books. We determined it was necessary to include new subject headings for diagnoses and topics that were not a part of the medical literature nine years ago, like Codependency and Chronic Fatigue Syndrome.

The Planetree Classification Scheme was developed to organize a health and medical library so that people could find the information they are seeking without the specialized knowledge of a health professional. Philosophically, we believe that the organization of the collection should be as self-service as possible so that people may choose not to interact with Library staff. Additionally, we believe in the value of serendipity. Our experience is that many people find helpful and useful information not by direct approach but by personally browsing through material and discovering the myriad of information sources and options available to them. Specific topics are organized within broad subject divisions that bring together relevant information. Unlike a classification scheme organized alphabetically that places melanoma next to migraine, patrons find melanoma information within the cancer section near useful information on coping with chemotherapy, cancer therapy utilizing Chinese herbal medicine, and support for the families of cancer patients.

Our cataloging emphasizes the organization of library materials by their anticipated usage rather than just their descriptive value. We try to consider the users' point of view, and their purposes for seeking information. For example, a book on yoga and the disabled would be found with the books on physical disability. This allows patrons looking at books for the disabled to find a book on a topic that they may not have originally considered. Additional references within the system alert persons looking for yoga books to the presence of this specialized book in the collection.

Reference Service Guidelines

The reference desk is staffed during all Library hours with volunteers and/or paid staff. A Library orientation tour and the availability of reference assistance is offered to each patron visiting the Library. The reference desk staff is trained to respect the confidentiality and privacy of patrons who do not want to interact with staff.

The Health Resource Center is not staffed by medical professionals, therefore volunteers and staff cannot legally provide clarification or interpretation of the medical literature, advice, or recommendations. Staff encourage callers seeking medical advice to contact their physician or health-care practitioner, visit the Health Resource Center to research their question, or contact an appropriate health agency or support group for assistance. The Health Resource Center will provide callers with phone numbers of health agencies and support groups listed in our Information and Reference System.

A log book is kept at the reference desk to record daily statistics, including the sex, ethnic group, topic interest, and estimated age of visitors. This information is recorded in a confidential manner without directly asking patrons. The log book data provide useful information for collection development and for the assessment of high use periods in the Center.

To provide the best possible reference assistance, staff are encouraged to interview the Library patron to gain the information necessary to be helpful. A successful reference interview not only is helpful to the patron, but can help a reference desk volunteer ascertain whether further professional staff assistance is needed. Some useful interview questions to ask the patron are:

- Is this a specific diagnosis or lay term?
- Is this the correct spelling?
- What part of the body or body system is affected?
- Are there other common names for the topic?
- What is the source of the person's information?
- What amount of information is needed?
- For drug names, is the patron requesting the generic or brand name?

Sometimes, the patron may have been given a diagnosis that is a medical slang term or colloquialism. If the term cannot be found in the reference book collection and the patron has no more information for clarification, we will conduct an online search in Medline for quick reference.

Infrequently, but nevertheless significantly, a patron may come to the Library looking for information about a diagnosis, unaware of the ramifications of the term or its prognostic significance. For example, one young woman came into the library to find out about her mother's newly diagnosed lymphoma. It was shocking for her to discover that lymphoma is a type of cancer. We attempt to handle these difficulties with sensitivity and compassion. We are available to listen to patrons in these situations and to assist them in finding resources for support. In cases where a patron may be confused about their topic or diagnosis, we have found it appropriate to refer the person to their health-care practitioner or to the original source of information about the topic for clarification.

The Health Resource Center may not be the best place to answer all health information requests. It is sometimes more appropriate to refer a person to his or her health practitioner for answers to specific questions related to a particular diagnosis, to local support groups for sharing experiences, or to a national or local health organization dedicated to a specific diagnosis.

We refer patrons to other libraries if the Health Resource Center collection does not contain the specific piece of information, book, or journal article the patron wants to obtain. For more technical medical information, patrons are referred to their nearest medical school library.

Planetree Information and Reference System

In 1981, Planetree created an original Information and Reference System of health resources. The System is designed to provide the public with extensive information regarding national and local services offered by health practitioners and support groups. Housed in mylar-protected sheets in detachable open binders, the system is available for public access in the Health Resource Center. It includes a local Physician's Questionnaire Section, a Health Agencies and Support Services Section, a Complementary Therapy Services Section, and a Consumer Health Network. In 1989, we began construction of an in-house online database for the Information and Reference System. Our goal is to create a standardized Information and Reference System that can be mutually maintained and updated for various sites—from health resource centers and public libraries to hospital units and admitting departments.

Physician's Questionnaire Section

The purpose of the Physician Questionnaire is to provide consumers with qualitative information about a physician, without implying recommendation. The Questionnaire was designed to solicit the kinds of information a patient might want to know about a prospective physician.

The two-sided single page form asks local physicians to provide information on their educational background, board certification, practice associates, office hours and availability, HMO and PPO participation, fees for service, and insurance and billing information. Physicians are asked to provide information about their philosophy about patient care: whether they will refer patients to stress reduction programs, nutritionists, or complementary therapists; whether they will encourage patients to seek a second opinion; whether they will respect a patient's wishes regarding a living will or interest in contraceptive and/or abortion services; and whether they permit patients to view their medical records. There is room on the form for physicians to discuss a diagnostic emphasis or special areas of service in their practices.

The original Physician's Questionnaire was sent to members of the San Francisco Medical Society in 1981. An updated Physician's Questionnaire was distributed in 1989. Completed questionnaires are displayed alphabetically by specialty, including acupuncture (M.D.s trained in acupuncture), cardiology, dentistry, endocrinology, gynecology, internal medicine, oncology, ophthalmology, plastic and reconstructive surgery, and others. The questionnaire is available to all physicians upon request, and the current information is formally updated every three years. Planetree staff do not evaluate a participating physician or make specific recommendations to patrons from the Physician's Questionnaire.

Health Agencies and Support Service Section

The Health Agencies and Support Service Section of the Information and Reference System is the largest division, listing over 2,000 national and local voluntary health organizations, support groups, and health services. This Section is the first to be input to the database because it is constantly accessed to assist telephone reference questions. The database fields include contact information for the group or organization; hours of service; services provided; publications available from; non-English languages spoken; wheelchair accessibility; fees for services; and subject accessibility. Currently, this database covers over 100 health categories and lists over 500 local and national groups.

Complementary Therapies Section

The Complementary Therapies Section of the System includes a wide variety of resource listings for individual practitioners, and local and national professional organizations. Each subject division begins with a one-page description on the philosophy and techniques of the practice designed to familiarize and educate the user to the particular form of therapy. Complementary therapy topic areas cover acupuncture, aromatherapy, bodywork techniques, homeopathy, massage, music therapy, Native American nutrition, yoga, and more. Individual practitioner and organization listings include information about the educational, professional, and philosophical background of the practitioner or group.

The Consumer Health Network

Sometimes the most useful information that can help someone face an illness or a loved one's diagnosis is experiential knowledge not found in books or computer databases. The Planetree Consumer Health Network was created to provide a method for consumers to locate and communicate with others who share their particular diagnosis or health interest. Through this Network, Planetree encourages consumers to gain the benefit of a support group or informal, one-to-one information sharing. To participate in the Network, consumers are asked to complete a Network form indicating the topic(s) that they are interested in discussing and the preferred method of contact (by phone, mail, or computer). Network forms are attainable in the Library. They are also included in all Planetree health information packets and are available by mail or faxed upon request. Participation in the Network is completely voluntary and there is no charge to be listed or to access listings. Forms are dated and respondents are asked annually if they wish to remain in the Network. The completed forms are organized in topic order and available for public reference at the Health Resource Center Library. When appropriate, forms are photocopied and included in the Planetree health information packets or mailed individually in response to reference questions.

Information and Reference System Limitations

The Planetree Information and Reference System is not a referral system; patrons are not referred to specific services or practitioners to the exclusion of others. Specifically with telephone inquiries, staff will answer a patron's request for names, addresses, and telephone numbers of organizations or practitioners when the patron is looking for information by topic, specialty, name, or geographical location. Planetree will not recommend a practitioner to a patron based on a general inquiry, such as "Can you find me a good doctor for gallstone removal?" or "Who is the best Feldenkrais bodyworker in Mill Valley?" Patrons are encouraged to qualitatively evaluate the information listings for themselves and, if appropriate, may be referred to specific medical societies and voluntary health organizations that offer a referral service. Inclusion, or absence, of a listing in the Planetree Information and Reference System does not constitute a recommendation in favor of, or against, a specific practitioner, organization, individual, or physician. There is one exception: if two or more complaints are received against any group, organization, or practitioner, the listing will be removed from our files. While we have attempted with our computerization of the System data to provide the most up-to-date information, we cannot guarantee that all information stated on the forms, especially fees and specific policies, are necessarily accurate or current.

The Planetree Health Information Service

It was not long after the Planetree Health Resource Center opened in 1981 that we began to receive requests for health information from people who were not able to use the Library. Many people cannot come to the Library because of illness, geographic location, or travel restrictions. Responding to this need, we developed a mail-order Health Information Service that sends health information to people at home.

The Planetree Health Information Service prepares individually researched packets of information on requested medical topics or diagnoses. The packet can include a selection of current articles from our consumer health library collection; materials describing both traditional and complementary therapy options; a computer-searched bibliography of the current medical literature on the topic; references for further sources of information; support group listings and national or local voluntary health organizations; and advocacy groups dedicated to providing services or information on the topic. We also utilize the collections of other medical libraries within the Bay Area for material not available on-site.

Since the inception of this service in 1982, requests for information have radically increased in their sophistication and in the technical level of material desired. Common requests were, in the past, for information about nondrug therapies for hypertension or coping with Alzheimer's disease. We still receive requests for these topics, but also for information on less common diagnoses, such as glossopharyngeal neuralgia, tardive dyskinesia, and seizures in newborns.

We receive requests for information from all over the world and currently prepare 80–100 information packets each month. Our priority is to respond to packet requests from people who need information regarding an illness or diagnosis. We will not accept information packet requests to perform research beyond the scope of our services. Typical of these situations are:

- Requests for information about a group of symptoms or for interpretation of medical conditions or diagnostic test results.
- Requests from attorneys for information to be used in legal proceedings.
- Requests for information packets for the purpose of fulfilling a student's research report requirements.

To assist patrons in conducting their own research, we can prepare computerized bibliographies and databank printouts from the National Library of Medicine's Medline database. The most frequently requested computer searches are for the Physician Data Query (PDQ) databank. PDQ is a full-text database produced by the National Cancer Institute and is available through Medline. It provides concise and current information on the prognosis, staging, and treatment options for specific cancer diagnoses.

Research packets are prepared by a paid staff trained in medical library research methods. Each member of the research staff possesses working or educational experience from within the health or medical field.

The Health Information Service is a negligible source of income. Currently, the fees for computer searches and information packets range from $15 to $75 and are charged according to online time, overhead costs, and staff preparation time.

Planetree Patient Health Information Service

Since 1985, the Health Information Service has offered information packets at no charge to patients of the Planetree Unit. At both Planetree Units in San Francisco and San Jose, patients can request an information packet through their nurse or directly from the Planetree Unit Health Information Resource Staff.

Patients often request information about self-care procedures for their specific diagnoses. Requests are also frequently made for information on improving health and lifestyle habits that may impact on chronic health problems such as smoking cessation, weight loss, or stress reduction. Families of Planetree Unit patients may also request information packets. This service has been greatly appreciated because it provides take-home material to help patients and their families understand how to take care of their health.

Planetree Health Bookstore

The Planetree Bookstore provides patrons with the opportunity to purchase many of the books and tapes available in the Resource Center's collection. Planetree encourages consumers to build their own home medical library and the bookstore inventory reflects the diverse health interests and information needs of patrons. Popular titles have focused on health promotion and self-care perspectives of chronic illness, home medical texts, adult children of dysfunctional families, mind-body healing, coping with cancer, and relaxation audiotapes.

The Planetree Hospital Book Cart

As a service to hospital patients and their families, Planetree sponsors a health information book cart at Pacific Presbyterian Medical Center in San Francisco. The cart features a sampling of the Planetree Health Resource Center Library collection, including current and popular titles on particular diagnoses as well as information on coping with illness and surgery, attitudinal healing, selected complementary therapies, and promoting healthy lifestyle habits. Patients and their family members may borrow books and pamphlets for the length of their hospital stay.

Personnel

Planetree is administered by an executive director, an associate director, and a development coordinator governed by the board of directors. The Health Resource Center staff includes a medical librarian, bookstore manager, office manager, volunteer staff, and four part-time high school student clerks. The Planetree Health Information Service consists of 3½ full-time research staff members.

Funding

Early funding for the Planetree Health Resource Center relied heavily upon grants from local foundations interested in supporting health-related projects of benefit to the community. For Planetree's first five years of planning and operations, major fundraising events contributed annually to the Center's operating expenses. Planetree currently receives its funding from private foundations, individual donors, proceeds from fund-raising events, and licensing and consulting fees.

Since its inception, Planetree has been supported by membership contributions. Memberships entitle individuals to circulation privileges from the the Library, a 10 percent discount on purchases from the health bookstore; a subscription to *Planetalk,* a biannual health newsletter; new book updates; a 50 percent discount on admission to the biannual health lecture series; and other special events mailings. In addition, the Planetree Health Resource Center in San Francisco generates some revenue from the sale of books, the Health Information Service, and the Planetree Health Lecture Series. These services do not support the overhead costs of the Resource Center.

Planetree has received grants from local foundations and businesses to fund the development of special projects. Some of these projects include: a Planetree Health Bookstore Catalog; the Planetree Information and Reference System; the Planetree Hospital book cart; and the Model Hospital Project Patient Health Information Packets.

Planetree Consulting Services

Over the last several years, Planetree has been contacted by hospitals, health organizations, community service groups, and individuals for our advice and experience in the development of their consumer health resource center. In response to this need, Planetree has developed a consulting division that provides a range of services and assistance according to the needs of specific community projects.

Through our consulting service, we are able to provide to other health resource centers components of our Health Resource Center collection and the library systems that we have developed for ongoing maintenance. These include: the Planetree Collection Recommendation List; the Planetree Classification Scheme; the Planetree Information and Reference System and Core Collection; the Planetree Clipping File System and

Core Collection; and the Health Resource Center Policy and Operations Manual.

Planetree staff have assisted many organizations considering the development of a consumer health resource center by providing a feasibility study for the project, a development timeline and implementation plan, on-site library training, and ongoing collection update support for the library. Groups we have assisted with the development of their health resource centers include Stanford University Hospital, The Sierra Foundation, and The Lutheran Hospital and Homes Society.

Public Relations

The purpose of Planetree's community outreach is to promote awareness and support of the Health Resource Center and its services. Promotional efforts include public speaking, media promotion, special events, tours, and participation in community events.

The Planetree Health Lecture Series

The Planetree Health Lecture Series was created to provide further opportunity for community access to health information and to promote the resources available in the Library. The Health Resource Center invites speakers, such as health practitioners, licensed professionals and qualified laypersons in a particular topic area, and authors of new health books, to share their experience and knowledge with the general public. Lecture topics and speakers are selected based on topic appropriateness, public interest, and availability. All lectures are held at the Health Resource Center on Thursday evenings from 7 p.m. to 9 p.m. Although there is a limited seating capacity of only 45, we feel that the Resource Center is an important setting; it provides a comfortable environment and draws attention to Resource Center services. Library materials are immediately available to provide information on the lecture topic.

Classes held at the Planetree Health Resource Center in San Francisco have included consumer health issues such as "How to Choose a Health Insurance Plan" and "Choosing and Using Alternative Therapies." Other lectures have addressed specific subject areas or health promotion topics such as "Infertility" and "Nutrition and Immune System Support." Lectures on personal growth issues, self-help techniques, and complementary therapies are often the most popular classes and have included "Music and Healing" and "Adult Children of Alcoholics" Guest lecturers donate their time to Planetree and receive a complimentary membership to the Health Resource Center. A nominal admission fee of $3 for members and $6 for nonmembers is charged to cover promotional costs of the series.

PLANETREE AT SAN JOSE MEDICAL CENTER

San Jose Medical Center in San Jose, California, is the first health-care institution to replicate The Planetree Health Resource Center and The Planetree Hospital Unit Models. The Planetree Health Resource Center in San Jose is a community service affiliated with San Jose Medical Center (SJMC). Open since February 1989, this consumer health library offers the public free access to health and medical information in the comforting ambiance of a renovated 1885 Victorian home. The Library includes health books, medical textbooks, periodicals, clipping files containing articles from the medical and consumer health literature, and audio- and videotapes. Patrons can purchase a library card for $20 a year to borrow books and audiocassettes from the collection, but the emphasis in promoting the Library to the community is that the use of the collection is free to the public.

The collection of over 1,000 titles was selected from a core consumer health library list based on the Planetree Health Resource Center collection in San Francisco. In addition, specific collection development research yielded titles that were pertinent to the multi-cultural health needs of the South Bay community.

Community services provided by the Health Resource Center include an on-site bookstore offering health books and audiotapes for sale, the Planetree Health Information and Reference System, and a health lecture series. While Planetree in San Jose does not operate a by-mail Health Information Service, Medline, Physician Data Query (PDQ), and other database searches are available for a fee. Planetree staff members have circulating privileges to the Hospital Library collection only open to the medical staff. Journal articles can also be retrieved for Planetree patrons through ILL from area medical libraries. On the Planetree Patient Care Unit within the Medical Center, patients can request individualized information packets on health and medical topics.

Funding

The Planetree Health Resource Center in San Jose is funded by San Jose Medical Center, a private, nonprofit 529-bed hospital founded in 1923. The Library's initial budget of $75,000 covers building the initial Library collection and excludes building renovations and staff salaries.

Fund-raising efforts through the San Jose Medical Center (SJMC) Foundation successfully raised substantial community support towards start-up costs for the collection, furnishings, and extensive renovation of the 980 square foot building. There has been much fund-raising support from within the institution itself, including generous contributions from many Medical Center employees and the SJMC Auxiliary.

The Medical Center's Foundation continues to provide initial contacts and grantwriting assistance to outside foundations, agencies, and individuals. Most sources prefer to offer grants for expansion or enhancement of services, rather than for operational costs. For example, one grant was received to develop a multi-cultural health video collection. Hospital vendors proved to be a further source for in-house donation opportunities. The Health Resource Center received a microcomputer and a special arrangement for a photocopy machine from companies that have contracts with the Medical Center.

Another funding source which brought many people to Planetree for the first time was the first "Tree to Tree Run," a 10K race through downtown San Jose parks which finished in front of the Library. Sponsored by San Jose Medical Center, with contributions from several local businesses, the Run will be an annual event to publicize and benefit the Health Resource Center.

In addition to funding, San Jose Medical Center provides support to Planetree through its Public Relations and Marketing departments. Brochures, bookmarks, advertising, and media coverage continue to be coordinated with the Planetree librarian and the strength of the Hospital's contacts throughout the county has helped to publicize its "gift to the community." Strong administrative leadership at San Jose Medical Center and a vision of what the Planetree program means to the community has underscored the successful affiliation between the Medical Center and the Planetree organization.

Challenges

Though the Health Resource Center is institutionally sponsored and supported, the content authority for the Library collection is maintained by the Planetree librarian at the Health Resource Center. The San Jose Medical Center Planetree welcomes collection suggestions from physicians, other health-care professionals, and consumers, but it is the librarian's responsibility to add or delete a title. Being consumer-driven is one element that differentiates Planetree library services from many other medical libraries.

The Health Resource Center is located across the street from the main Hospital campus and that location, as well as the independent name for the Library, has promoted our community identity as a collection that anyone can use without being a patient, employee, or otherwise affiliated with the Medical Center.

There were challenges to the integration of the two parts of the Planetree program within the Hospital. Both projects were initially announced and developed over a three-year period, and opened within six months of each other. This resulted in some confusion in-house over the independent though interrelated nature of the projects. For example, some employees believed that the Planetree Health Resource Center would house acute care patients instead of library books.

We discovered the importance of having the Health Resource Center librarian available for on-site consultation during renovation to ensure that construction decisions were made in favor of patron access. The librarian's presence among architects and contractors assured that built-in bookshelves were accessible and adjustable for all heights, that high use traffic areas did not overlap, that electrical circuitry and outlet locations met equipment needs, and that plans for the internal reinforcement of the shelving and cabinetry were followed through. Vigilance over these construction details has paid off in many ways, particularly on October 17, 1989, when a 7.1 earthquake centered only 20 miles from San Jose left the Health Resource Center and its collection intact and the patrons and staff safe.

Building a Multicultural Collection

In addition to design, planning, promotion, and fund-raising during the year before the Library opened to the public, the librarian met with health and library professionals at the Hospital and in the community. People were excited at the concept of a health library free and open to the public and many immediately asked what resources would be available for the growing multi-lingual, multi-cultural populations of the county. We were fortunate that in San Jose a Multicultural Health Coalition of health educators, nurses, teachers, and others had been formed under the auspices of a two-year federal grant as the Health Resource Center was under development. Coalition members continue to meet informally and one member serves on Planetree's Community Advisory Committee. This Committee currently includes health educators, an artist, a school librarian, a physician, a banker, and a social worker, among others, and meets several times a year to offer perspective on Planetree's mission to meet the health information needs of the community at large.

Meeting the health information needs of a diverse patronage is an ongoing collection development challenge. Patrons who have difficulty reading English, for example, may also have difficulty reading in their primary language. Videotapes are one response, except for the scarcity of tapes that meet the following criteria: culturally sensitive programming available in languages other than English; current and reliable medical information; and enough production quality to be worth the average cost of $350.

When requesting previews we have found it important to ask such questions as: "Is more than one culture and ethnic group represented in the video?" (particularly important when a videotape or film is translated into another language or an all white cast is dubbed in Spanish) and "What year was this video actually in production?" (release dates are not necessarily indications of the currency of material). Most producers are eager to send previews and are also interested in why tapes may be rejected. We have found it enormously useful to have a bilingual review committee to assist the librarian in making selections of tapes and books that use languages other than English.

There are also difficulties in the availability and accessibility of print material in other languages. Lack of standardization among specialized distributors affects clarity in terms of book description, inventory, and ordering policies. The need for currency of medical information is especially problematic since a distributor may indicate a year in the entry of its catalog that means year last printed, year translated, or, sometimes, year the material was originally produced.

Our familiarity with consumer health literature in English has given us invaluable perspective when reviewing catalogs from other language distributors. Sometimes they do not know what they are offering. One reputable distributor of Spanish-language books listed "Cuando el dia tiene 36 horas" ("The 36-Hour Day"), a classic caregiver's book on Alzheimer's disease, as a time management book under the heading "Self-Improvement."

In addition to carefully perusing catalogs and newsletters from distributors and networking with public librarians and their collections, another source that has worked well in San Jose is to buy books retail at specialized bookstores. With the assistance of a bilingual volunteer, the Planetree librarian purchased general health and medical titles at several Vietnamese bookstores, including Dr. Spock's childcare classic. This has also worked for the Spanish-language collection. Since health and healing in different cultures have unique considerations, we look not only for translations of works we know to be important but also for original materials that would be useful to these populations. Obtaining multi-cultural perspectives, particularly from persons who have a medical background, is a critical step in adding selections to the collection.

The desire for breadth and depth in a Planetree Library extends to materials in languages other than English. However, we have found it complicated to obtain Spanish translations of current medical textbooks that would offer the patron access to more technical information. Some textbooks are offered in Spanish, for instance, but only through foreign sales departments of major publishers, so that orders must be placed directly with distributors in Mexico for titles such as *Cecil Textbook of Medicine* and Lange's *Current Medical Diagnosis and Treatment.*

At the other end of reader sophistication are booklets and handouts in very simple, highly illustrative formats in languages other than English. Straight translations of English materials are rarely effective, particularly if graphics and photographs are not also changed to reflect the particular target culture. We discovered that some of the most effective culturally engaging health information materials for our San Jose patrons were provided by local multi-cultural agencies.

Another critical element in providing health information to underserved minority communities is a bilingual staff. In meeting the demographic needs of the immediate community, the goal for Planetree at San Jose Medical Center is to have at least one Spanish-speaking and one Vietnamese-speaking volunteer available for scheduled hours each week. When approaching a patron who wants assistance in one of those languages, all other staff are trained to say, in that language, "The person who can help you in Spanish works here on Wednesday afternoons. If that is not convenient, you may leave your phone number and someone will contact you soon."

CHAPTER 14
Information Services at the Health Education Center of Pittsburgh

Lois G. Michaels

BEGINNINGS

The Health Education Center in Pittsburgh grew out of the realization that responsible behavior is one of the best hopes for improving health status and containing the continued escalation of medical care costs. Recognition of this potential stimulated efforts in the 1970s to foster more and better education of the public about personal health practices and about involvement in health program development. For example:

- A Presidential Committee for Health Education was appointed in 1971.
- The U.S. Department of Health, Education, and Welfare (now Health and Human Services) established a Bureau of Health Education in its Centers for Disease Control in 1974.
- Congress included health education as one of 10 national priorities in the National Health Planning and Resources Development Act of 1974.
- A private, nonprofit National Center for Health Education was established in 1975.
- Congress called for national leadership and coordination concerning health education in its National Consumer Health Information and Health Promotion Act of 1976.
- The Nation's Forward Plan for Health for 1978–1982 stated: ". . . further expansion of the nation's health system is likely to produce only marginal increases in the overall health status of the American people . . . the greatest benefits are likely to accrue from efforts to improve the health habits of all Americans and the environment in which they live and work."

While organizations, laws, and activities at the national level are important, health education, if it is to make a difference in people's lives, must take place in local communities, with appropriate backup assistance provided by public and private organizations.

In the early 1970s, local and state health education services were unlikely to meet minimum requirements regarding accessibility, acceptability, effectiveness, efficiency, coordination, and comprehensiveness. Business, labor, and industry were hardly talking about wellness at the work place. The media had yet to recognize the revenue potential from health and fitness news, and advertising and marketing health had not yet become buzz words. John Q. and Mary X. Public endured many competing, and sometimes conflicting, exhortations about their health habits, yet they often had difficulty finding easy-to-understand information or advice when they needed it.

Organizations seldom worked together in planning and carrying out health education programs, e.g., health agencies, safety organizations, recreation services, schools, colleges, social service agencies, religious organizations, civic groups, insurance companies, employers, labor unions, consumer groups, and communications media all had their own agendas and no mechanism for collaborations. Health education activities frequently suffered from inadequate analysis of needs, interests, and resources as a basis for program decisions; from selection of inappropriate educational methods; from lack of public involvement in planning and evaluation; and from insufficient funds to support significant activity.

To overcome these deficiencies, the President's Committee on Health Education in 1973 recommended, among other things:

> That a focal point for health education be established in each locality through "Community Health Education Centers" to coordinate and help improve health education programs within the area.

At the same time that the nation's need for improved health education was being noticed, a Task Force of Pittsburgh's local health council, the Health and Welfare Association (now the Health and Welfare Planning Association), recommended establishment of a consumer health education focal point for the region. Its purpose would be to strengthen and coordinate community education about the maintenance of health and the prevention of disease. This recommendation was picked up by a committee of the Comprehensive Health Planning Association of Southwestern Pennsylvania, which developed qualitative and quantitative guidelines for consumer health education. These guidelines were used as the basis of a community organization process involving hundreds of representatives from all segments of the population. The Falk Medical Fund and the United Way of Allegheny County provided money to hold regional hearings about the guidelines and to prepare recommendations for community action.

PURPOSE

As a result of the community planning process, a written model for an organization with a mission to educate the public about what individuals and groups could do to improve health was implemented. The first model for the Pittsburgh Health Education Center evolved from an analysis of needs, interests, and ideas generated at a regional hearing and a community-wide conference attended by over 400 persons. The model was set forth in an eight-page document that concluded:

> . . . the time is ripe for cooperative action between the health education efforts of the schools, public and private agencies, industry and the communications media. Delaying this will prove to be costly, time consuming and of no advantage to the population. It is time for a vigorous and sound community health education effort focused on particular groups and individuals with special needs and varying socio-cultural backgrounds. The Health Education Center. . . provides a mechanism for identifying target populations, establishing priorities and instituting educational strategies in response to community needs. Public and private agencies who have already demonstrated their concerns about individual health, now have the opportunity to pool their resources on behalf of people.

EARLY ORGANIZATION

From the beginning, the Health Education Center's mission was to promote health and prevent disease by encouraging individuals and organizations to voluntarily follow behavior conducive to health. Its purpose was to increase opportunities for people to take responsibility for their own well-being and, by so doing, prove the economic and social advantages of a planned and coordinated community-based approach to health education and promotion.

"Enjoy Life—stay healthy!" was the message in bold letters that greeted visitors to the Health Education Center in its first headquarters in a downtown office building jointly owned by the United Way and the City of Pittsburgh. Colorful murals, live plants, and cheery smiles created an atmosphere of warmth and well-being. The 2,000 square feet of rented space were divided into areas for reception, library, material storage and display, a conference room for meetings of from four to 40 persons, a telephone communication room, work areas for audiovisual screening and educational consultation, and offices for paid and volunteer staff.

A staff of five with skills in administration, fiscal management, health education, and communication was appointed to operate the Center. The core staff was augmented by volunteers and representatives of other agencies organized into an adjunct staff.

From 1976 to 1982, the Health Education Center was a demonstration project of the Health and Welfare Planning Association. In 1983, it became an independent agency with operating funds from the United Way. The commission was reorganized as a board of directors and tax exempt status was obtained. In 1986 HEC became an affiliate in the Blue Cross of Western Pennsylvania Family of Service Companies to bring HEC services to their 2.7 million subscribers. The original functions of program development, communication, and evaluation were expanded to accommodate ongoing and new programs. By the end of the 1980s, the Health Education Center was organized to serve 29 counties in western Pennsylvania with a population of over three million and a radius of 21,912 square miles.

LATER ORGANIZATION

After affiliating with Blue Cross of Western Pennsylvania in 1986, the board and staff went through an 18-month strategic planning process to plan a method for fulfilling our vision for the Health Education Center in the 1990s. This vision included a major emphasis on helping those people most susceptible to preventable disease and disability, particularly low-income groups and minorities, to cope with the complexities of modern life. Staff and programs are organized in four divisions as follows:

1. **Community Wellness:** Health Education Center staff are assigned to reduce risks for preventable disease and disability by providing health education resources to schools and organizations serving youth; increasing the parenting skills of young families regarding discipline, nutrition, and safety; and increasing the ability of older persons to remain independent. Special programs are targeted to building self-esteem for high risk youth, decreasing teenage pregnancy, and reducing infant mortality.

2. **HealthPLACE System:** HealthPLACE, a concept developed by the Health Education Center, has proved to be an effective model for disseminating health information and serving as a technical resource and catalyst for health behavior. Health Education Center is organized to operate HealthPLACE for Blue Cross of Western Pennsylvania in its corporate headquarters in Pittsburgh, and to license the HealthPLACE system to hospitals, schools, and other corporations. The Health Education Center Library is located in HealthPLACE and employees are reached through HealthPLACE at Work programs. Older citizens are also reached.

3. **Community Campaigns:** In keeping with the notion of the community as both a change agent and a target for change in health behavior, the Health Education Center carries out major media events throughout the year. These events call attention to health problems, provide awards for groups addressing the problems, and help to build coalitions to solve health problems. Campaigns are carried out in cooperation with public and private agencies to increase awareness about available wellness and prevention services and to involve all segments of the community in assessing needs and setting priorities. Recent campaigns include reducing smoking in black communities and organizing a community challenge to decrease cardiac disease risks.

4. **New Initiatives:** The Health Education Center has always been organized to attract resources for demonstration projects that will lead toward reaching national priorities in disease prevention. In the 1990s these are being targeted to, among others, smoking cessation among blacks, self-help networks, and injury control.

POPULATIONS SERVED

From the first, Health Education Center programs were organized to serve people where they worked, lived, went to school, and went for medical care. High users of HEC services were the general public and human service professionals. In 1980, the results of a self-care study, supported with funds from the Buhl Foundation of Pittsburgh, identified young people and their families as priority populations. Later HEC studies showed that populations at highest risk for preventable disease and disability included people of low socio-economic status and the elderly.

Health Education Center activities are now organized to reach low-income young and old in a variety of carefully planned, coordinated, and creative ways. Programs are targeted to three population groups—at risk youth, low-income families, and older persons.

PROGRAM SETTINGS

The Health Education Center has traditionally taken its programs to schools, the workplace, where people go for medical care, and the general community. For example:

- **In the Schools**: As lead agency of the Pittsburgh New Futures Wellness Initiative, the Health Education Center is working within high risk neighborhoods and schools to reverse destructive health behaviors of youth. In addition, dynamic presentations on adolescent self-esteem have been given in schools throughout western Pennsylvania, and a special Life Skills Training to encourage children not to start smoking is being implemented in elementary schools.
- **Where People Go for Medical Care**: Under a Healthy Older Persons Project funded by the W.K. Kellogg Foundation, three city communities with large populations of older people have access to HealthPLACE, where they can attend classes, receive personal counseling on prevention, and participate in health screenings. Physicians have a resource through the HealthPLACE nurse and a HealthBOOK to help their patients become partners in care. HealthBOOK is a guide book kept by the patient to record information about physical exams, medications, and tests.
- **In the Community**: A community-wide "Clean Lung Project," supported by the Pennsylvania Department of Health, is encouraging residents in a low-income, mostly black community to quit smoking. With funds from the R.K. Mellon Foundation and the federal programs in the Bureau of Maternal and Child Health Care and Resources Development, the Healthy Families Program trains lay leaders to teach young parents in rural and urban public housing communities health promotion and parenting skills. The curriculum for this project has been adapted for use with the Caring Program. This innovative way to pay for preventive care for

children started by Blue Cross of Western Pennsylvania is being replicated nationwide.

- **At the Workplace:** Taking health education programs into the workplace and getting employers to pay for them began in 1978 with a cooperative program with Pittsburgh Rotary. This led to a series of "Health Promotion in the Workplace, Strategies That Work" conferences that brought national experts to Pittsburgh and encouraged worksite programs in large and small companies. The workplace programs became the basis for Health Promotion Services, Inc., a wholly owned for-profit subsidiary of Blue Cross of Western Pennsylvania.

EXAMPLES OF ONGOING SERVICES

Since first opening, Health Education Center has fostered cooperative programs and services that promote good health. Program areas that have been in continuous service are Tel-Aid, a dial access health information system; a consumer health resource library; professional training, technical assistance, and consultation; risk reduction classes and other interventions; print and electronic media productions; and needs assessments, awareness campaigns, and evaluations. In 1988 many of these services were provided through HealthPLACE. Because of their uniqueness, Tel-Aid, Consumer Health Library, and HealthPLACE will be described.

Tel-Aid

The Tel-Aid telephone tape information system is a consumer education tool available toll-free to three million residents in a three-county area. Beginning with 200 medical tapes, the Tel-Aid Library now includes 653 Tel-Med tapes, 173 Tel-Law tapes, and 40 Tel-a-Teen and 56 Tel-a-Kid tapes. The Pittsburgh Health Education Center's Tel-Aid service grew out of the Tel-Med Program started by the San Bernardino California Medical Society in the early 1970s. This ever-popular system has responded to almost four million calls from Pittsburgh area residents since 1976.

Messages are from 30 seconds to five minutes in length and represent authoritative information recorded by professional actors and actresses using a reassuring and comforting tone of voice. Human service agencies, health-care providers, and special interest groups financially support one or more messages that describe their programs.

In an early telephone survey of a random sampling of 522 Pittsburgh area telephone subscribers, 41 percent had heard of the service, and 15 percent had called for information. On the average, those who called were 33 years old, had lived most of their lives in Pittsburgh, and had an annual income of under $20,000 ($30,000 in 1990 dollars). Three out of four were female, 82 percent were white, and for 48 percent, the highest grade reached had been high school senior. Callers said they had dialed

Tel-Aid an average of 7.5 times each; 92 percent were satisfied with the service, 66 percent reported they had used the information they had obtained from their calls, and 87 percent had told others about the service.

The most frequently requested messages deal with human sexuality, including AIDS. This is not surprising since sex is of universal interest, receiving information on the telephone is private and confidential, and Tel-Aid messages are reviewed for accuracy by a broad range of respected professionals before being put on the line. The system is operated manually for callers using rotary phones. An automated system plays the messages without an intervening operator but the caller must have a push button telephone.

The Tel-a-Teen series was developed with funds from the Pittsburgh-based Hillman Foundation. Tel-A-Teen and Tel-A-Kid are now sponsored by Children's Hospital of the University of Pittsburgh. Teens selected the topics they wanted to hear about and developed a peer teaching model, "Smart Decisions with Tel-a-Teen," that is used in teacher training and for school assemblies. Calling Tel-Aid, when health information is needed, has become normative behavior in our service area.

Consumer Health Library

The Health Education Center began providing library services to health professionals, students, and the lay public when it opened in 1976. Provision of library services was designated by the Center's board of directors as a core service of the organization. In 1981, a resource grant from the National Library of Medicine enabled the Health Education Center to study professionals' awareness of consumer health information (CHI) materials for their patients and clients. A survey of telephone patrons and on-site library patrons provided details on health professionals' use of the Health Education Center's Resource Center, their areas of interest, the material formats they preferred, and the intended use of the materials. Health professionals' demand for information about consumer-oriented materials, their satisfaction with the Health Education Center Library materials, and their satisfaction with the HEC Library suggest that such a resource can be a valuable asset to a community.

Librarians, aware of the growing demand by the public for health information, have made efforts to supply such information directly to consumers. An assortment of consumer health information (CHI) services has been offered by health sciences libraries, public libraries, library networks, and others to encourage consumers to become well-informed about their health. Another way to fill this need is to provide health professionals with consumer health materials that they can share with patients and clients in a variety of settings. While information that a library makes available directly to a consumer can be helpful to that individual, the Health Education Center believes that information given to a professional could help 10 or 20 consumers.

Health Education Center Library services include telephone reference, interlibrary loan, audiovisual rentals, consultations to institutions starting collections, and on-site use of the Library. The collection comprises 650 monographs, 140 journal and newsletter subscriptions, and 3,500 consumer health pamphlets. Through its listing on the Online Computer Library Center (OCLC) database, the HEC collection has been available for interlibrary loan to institutions throughout the country since 1984. In addition, its vertical files house information on 650 other organizations interested in health promotion and a large collection of bibliographies, reports, studies, reprints, curricula, and health education program models. The entire collection is housed at the HealthPLACE in downtown Pittsburgh. It is open to the public and is used by nurses, counselors, school teachers, physicians, health educators, students of the health professions, Blue Cross customers and employees, and the general public.

The National Library of Medicine grant enabled the Health Education Center to accomplish the following:

1. Reorganize the Library to make its collection of free and inexpensive materials more easily accessible. Fifteen hundred pamphlet titles were pulled from the existing vertical files and were placed in a separate file, reorganized alphabetically by subject for easier access.

2. Identify sources of free and inexpensive health education materials, and publish a guide to the local sources so that health professionals can acquire multiple copies of materials. Over 450 organizations that produce or distribute consumer materials were contacted. In September 1982, 4,000 copies of a 50-page directory, *Sources of Health Information Materials in Southwestern Pennsylvania,* were published. Seventy-five organizations were included; the index listed 191 health topics.

3. Enlarge the collection of free and inexpensive health education materials in order to have a current collection of a wide variety of materials. Two thousand new pamphlet titles were added for a total pamphlet collection of 3,500—an increase of 133 percent. Also added were 35 newsletters, 15 journals, and 325 monographs.

4. Evaluate selected items in the collection so that health professionals can choose health education materials more effectively. One hundred pamphlets in 10 risk areas (smoking, drugs, alcohol, stress, pregnancy and infant health, nutrition and weight control, medication use, fitness, safety, and lifestyle) were evaluated using such criteria as appearance, accuracy, readability, and target audience. Evaluators included 35 subject specialists, six librarians, eight health educators, and 10 graphic artists. Results of these evaluations are on file at the Library and are attached to each evaluated pamphlet to aid patrons in selection.

5. Publicize the Library's collection of free and inexpensive health education materials and the guide to their local sources so that health professionals will use the collection. Major promotional efforts included a traveling display of educational and promotional materials; public service announcements; and articles in the HEC newsletter, professional bulletins, and *Pittsburgh Magazine.* Informa-

tive flyers and bookmarks were made available in the Library and at display sites, and were offered to professional organizations.

HealthPLACE

HealthPLACE is a health information and health education resource for consumers. Its main objective is to provide knowledge to consumers enabling them to take active responsibility for disease prevention and health promotion, and to make economical use of the medical care system. HealthPLACE makes it possible for people to adopt a healthy lifestyle, eat wisely, manage stress, exercise regularly, and practice effective self-care. When integrated with a consumer's medical care, optimum health is achieved at minimum cost. HealthPLACE is a unified system with components designed to inform or educate the consumer about one or more aspects of personal health care. By selecting applicable components, HealthPLACE is customized to meet the needs of a particular HealthPLACE sponsor, such as an employer group, rural community, or urban hospital. The components of HealthPLACE are:

- Classes/Workshops/Support Groups
- Displays (Interactive, print, electronic)
- Kiosks (Free-standing, tabletop)
- Resource and Reference Books
- Health Risk Appraisals
- Screenings/Testing
- Health Tip Sheets
- HealthPLACE by Mail
- HealthPLACE at work
- Videotapes
- Newsletters
- Tel-Aid
- HealthBOOK
- Counseling
- Referral
- Software
- HealthPLACE Corner

HealthPLACE assists the consumer in disease prevention and health promotion, thereby supporting the consumer's medical care and improving the health behavior of each HealthPLACE user. In addition, HealthPLACE facilitates the economic use of medical care resources by enabling people to cope with health problems.

Developed by the health and wellness experts on the Health Education Center staff and initially supported by a W.K. Kellogg Foundation grant, HealthPLACE consists of proven health promotion and disease prevention techniques. As new approaches are tested and accepted, they are added to the system. Packages of services are available for specific markets or a customized package of services can be developed based on the specific requirements of a HealthPLACE buyer. HealthPLACE licenses are sold to buyers seeking to establish a HealthPLACE center. The license includes a designated package of services, geographic exclusivity, use of the HealthPLACE logo and trademark, an operations manual, staff training, technical assistance, and inclusion in advertising and promotion. HealthPLACE at Work is sold to employers as an employee benefit at a unit cost per Blue Cross contract. Typically, HealthPLACE at Work includes a health risk appraisal, newsletters, information on local HealthPLACE activities, and HealthPLACE by Mail. HealthPLACE by Mail is marketed as a separate service, as is HealthBOOK, a tool for organizing personal health information and HealthPLACE Corner, a portable information collection.

A health-care provider sponsoring a HealthPLACE center is offering a valuable community service and can expect to generate referrals and good will. Other sponsors, such as employers offering HealthPLACE at Work to employees, can expect a positive impact on the health claims from HealthPLACE users as well as improved employee morale and productivity. Blue Cross/Blue Shield plans sponsoring HealthPLACE have the advantage of an immediately replicable employee benefit, customer service, and community outreach, as well as a revenue-generating product.

In its first year of operation, a center-city HealthPLACE had over 22,000 visitors and three community-based HealthPLACE centers demonstrated the ability to improve the health behavior of older participants.

SUMMARY

A description of the Health Education Center, one of the oldest continuous organizations providing health education and promotion services at the community level, has been provided. Program examples and factors for success have been given. While academic centers for research in prevention have developed since the Health Education Center was founded in 1976, and national goals and priorities have been established, the Health Education Center continues to serve as a community model for the nation.

CHAPTER 15
The King County Consumer Health Information Network

Mary Campbell and Kay Johnson

OBJECTIVES AND ORGANIZATION

The King County Consumer Health Information Network (KCCHIN) is a network of libraries serving the health information needs of consumers located throughout King County, Washington. King County's 1980 population was 1,269,749. Recent estimates indicate that the county's population has grown by 13.87 percent since 1980, to a 1989 population of 1,446,000. Over 40 percent of the population lives in unincorporated areas which cover nearly 90 percent of the county's 2,134 square miles.

From its beginning in 1986, KCCHIN has involved multi-type libraries and library systems. The network includes two public library systems, an academic health sciences library, and 18 hospital libraries. The members are the King County Library System, with 40 community libraries plus its travelling library; Seattle Public Library, with 22 community libraries and mobile service; University of Washington Health Sciences Library and Information Center; and 18 institutional members of the Seattle Area Hospital Library Consortium, Inc.

KCCHIN was developed during 1986 as a one-year model project designed to improve access to consumer health information for the public. Its purpose was to establish a referral and resource sharing network between public, hospital, and academic health sciences libraries. Start-up components included training for library staff, evaluation and enhancement of the two public library system collections, and development of a publicity and promotional campaign.

The mixture of libraries and their respective organizational structures created both opportunities and challenges. The roles and missions for these three types of libraries complement one another. Collection development policies fall within a spectrum from general collection building for lay consumers in the public libraries, to very technical and specific collection development for the research and teaching hospital clientele of the academic health sciences library. The mutual dependence of these various types of libraries stems from the fact that the hospital and academic health sciences libraries receive many requests for information that can be more appropriately handled by the public libraries, while the public libraries need occasional access to technical materials available only in the medical collections.

The motivating factors leading to the formation of this group as a working unit are a tangible result of the demand for consumer health information that has increased beyond the capabilities of any one library to handle. The benefits of working cooperatively to improve the quality of health information services for consumers have far outweighed any of the difficulties encountered.

The combination of mutual needs and the emerging cooperative attitudes provided the backdrop to the receipt of funding from the Washington State Library through the allocation of $88,000 in Title III LSCA funds during 1986. An additional $22,700 was contributed by network members in the form of in-kind contributions. The largest part of the LSCA funds went toward salaries and benefits for a network coordinator and a clerical support staff person hired on a temporary basis specifically for the grant project, and collection development for the two public libraries.

Subsequent to the grant-funded period, King County Library System (KCLS) further developed the concept of providing health and medical information services through the recruitment of a medical librarian to the staff in order to back up the System's public service staff, manage collection development for health materials, and coordinate the KCLS consumer health information program.

RESOURCE SHARING AND ACCESS

The first objective of KCCHIN during the grant period was to improve resource sharing and speed of access to consumer health information for the lay public and health-care providers. This was accomplished through development of a resource directory and implementation of a staff training program. The resource directory is designed to acquaint KCCHIN participants with the resources of other network members in order to improve services to consumers. The resource directory includes information about special collections, database access, hours of operation, electronic mail codes, telephone numbers, and support groups. Information about various services is provided in a handy grid format, showing which services are available, and whether or not there is a charge for the service. Also included in the directory are KCCHIN interlibrary loan and reference referral guidelines, and procedures for handling health information requests.

Guidelines for interlibrary loans among KCCHIN members were developed by a working committee representing each of the network institutional members. Interlibrary loan criteria include directions for handling "rush" requests, priority for filling other interlibrary loan requests, and the agreement to follow American Library Association procedures.

REFERENCE SERVICES

Reference referral guidelines outline the order in which requests should be transferred from one participant to another, the information that should be included in a referred request, and procedures to follow when referring walk-in patrons to public libraries from hospital and academic libraries. These guidelines were also developed by a representative working committee and are included in the directory. Procedures to help prevent misunderstandings and allow for a smooth flow for the request in the shortest time possible are also specified.

Within King County Library System, backup reference services have traditionally been used for questions that cannot be answered with resources available at the local community libraries. The backup sources available include those of the six large resource libraries with their more comprehensive collections, the centralized reference department, and KCCHIN. The Reference Department of King County Library System consists of subject specialists, including the medical librarian, who can access not only the extensive central reference collection, but also a variety of online and CD-ROM database sources. The medical librarian handles health-related questions referred from the community libraries. Requests are submitted in writing or over the telephone, and patrons with medical questions are encouraged to contact the medical librarian directly when necessary. Using the reference referral guidelines developed by KCCHIN, the medical librarian determines when it is appropriate to refer the patron's request to another source of information. The resources of the entire network are extensively used in answering patrons' health-related questions.

TRAINING ACTIVITY

A training program designed to educate librarians working with the lay public about information sources available to meet patron needs and the ethical and legal aspects of offering consumer health information services was also developed during the KCCHIN grant period. Workshops on core medical reference materials, database searching in the health sciences, and medical reference interview techniques were attended by more than 100 librarians from network member libraries.

The training program led to the production of an educational video, *Questions of Health: Trigger Tapes on the Health Care Reference Interview*. Developed by King County Library System staff with extensive input from network representatives, *Questions of Health* presents four paired scenarios of simulated health reference interviews in public library settings. Each pair illustrates a typical problem encountered in the delivery of consumer health information, with the second version of each pair showing improved ways in which a librarian might more appropriately handle the problem. The tape is designed to be used with a discussion group, and comes with a guide for the discussion leader. Discussion topics triggered by the episodes include reference interviewing for highly personal health questions, making the distinction between health information and advice, dealing with the emotional patron, and handling communication problems in delivering information over the telephone. *Questions of Health* continues to be useful for reference training workshops that are offered periodically. It has been successfully used in CHI courses elsewhere in the U.S. and in New Zealand. The video is available for purchase at $30 per copy. An order form is included in Appendix I.

Follow-up needs assessment interviews with reference librarians at some of the libraries have emphasized the ongoing need for staff training in the delivery of consumer health information. Staff members need to be updated in both the use of standard resources for answering health questions and the legal and ethical aspects of delivering consumer health information services.

COLLECTION DEVELOPMENT

A second KCCHIN objective during the grant period was to enhance the quality and depth of lay health collections for consumers and healthcare personnel by evaluating the public library holdings and adding materials as needed. First, an objective and thorough collection assessment program was conducted. Holdings of the Seattle Public Library and the King County Library System were checked using a variety of bibliographies, publisher advertisements, and catalogs. The Western Library Network (WLN), a shared bibliographic utility, was used extensively to compare the collections with published lists of the best or most preferred titles for use with the general public. This study resulted in expenditures of $30,000 for books, $10,000 for videos, and $1,000 for journals divided between the two public library collections.

Criteria for materials selection and future collection development were developed by a joint collection profiles committee, which included representatives from the academic and hospital libraries, as well as from the two public libraries. A core list of titles that should be available in each public library system was produced, and collection profiles and policies were examined. Each public library system determined which materials would be purchased using guidelines developed by the committee. The guidelines addressed such variables as the size of the community library, circulation, geographic location, and subject gaps. A total of 367 new titles were purchased by the two public library systems. Ready access to materials by patrons required purchase of multiple copies of some titles so that they could be placed in various community libraries. The more expensive and technical titles were located at central locations for each system.

Journal purchases were coordinated so as to minimize duplication and increase the range of materials available to patrons. Thirty-six new journal titles were purchased for the two public library systems. Some, such as the *Mayo Clinic Health Letter* and *Medical Self-Care*, are lay publications, while others, including *JAMA* and the *New England Journal of Medicine*, are written for health-care professionals. All of the titles selected are indexed in either the *Consumer Health & Nutrition Index* or Medline online database.

The selection of video materials for public library patrons tends to be somewhat challenging, as the criteria for selection must exclude the dull and didactic. Staff reviewing current videos generally report a 10:1 rejection ratio (one title purchased for every 10 reviewed). Videos selected must have good production quality, be accurate in the information provided, meet an appropriate technical level for consumers, and be up-to-date and free of bias. Budget constraints allowed a cost average of not more than $2 per minute for each video. Sixty-one new video titles were purchased by the two public library systems. Titles were duplicated where necessary in order to provide ready access.

CURRENT PURCHASES

Current collection development for consumer health materials, including pamphlets, books, journals, and audio/video materials, is handled routinely and independently by each of the participating network libraries. Within the King County Library System, budget funds ($5,000–$7,000) are set aside each year to ensure that a minimum number of reference materials is purchased to meet identifiable information needs at the community library level.

The goal of the KCLS consumer health information program is to provide health information in response to health questions at the community library level whenever possible. The 40 community libraries comprising KCLS have a wide array of resources. Some of the libraries are quite large and have fairly extensive health information collections, both circulating and reference. Others are very small, and have only limited resources to serve the health information needs of patrons. Through the network, all patrons can receive the information they need, regardless of which community library they use. Even the smallest of the KCLS libraries keeps an up-to-date vertical file that includes many pamphlets on health topics. These are distributed centrally by a documents coordinator.

Every six weeks the KCLS Collection Development Department distributes an adult purchase list that is forwarded to the centralized Reference Department and to all the community libraries. The list includes annotated titles recommended for purchase at one or more libraries in the system. A section on health and medicine lists titles selected by the medical librarian or reviewed in standard public library sources. KCLS community libraries select titles within their own budget guidelines. A representative committee oversees the purchases, ensuring that collections are balanced geographically and that all recommended materials are made available somewhere within the system. Most of the circulating materials in consumer health subject areas are purchased in this manner.

The KCLS automated circulation system and systemwide catalog provides patrons at all the libraries equal access to circulating materials. Any item in the catalog can be located and either sent to the patron via U.S. Mail, or delivered to and held at a convenient library for pickup. The larger libraries will, naturally, have more of the circulating materials on health topics readily available on their shelves.

Reference materials for consumer health information are also reviewed and included on the adult purchase list. In addition, a core set of reference items is purchased centrally by the medical librarian and made available at the six KCLS resource libraries. The resource libraries are geographically distributed throughout the county, and provide reference services to the smaller community libraries and their patrons. A copy of the core list of reference items is provided in Appendix II. One of the KCLS resource libraries is currently a beta test site for Health Index Plus, an add-on to the CD-ROM-driven public access system, Infotrac, from Information Access Company. Health Index Plus indexes over 100 popular and professional health journals and newsletters, and includes health-related articles from over 2,500 general magazines and newspapers. The full text of the article is included for some titles. An evaluation of patron use and assessment is currently being conducted.

DEVELOPMENT OF A MODEL FOR COOPERATIVE NETWORKING

The third and final objective of the KCCHIN grant period involved development of a model for cooperative networking of health information between public and health sciences libraries that would be disseminated statewide. Presentations about KCCHIN were given at several statewide library meetings during 1986. Brochures describing KCCHIN and its development were distributed, as were copies of the resource directory. Booklists produced through the grant program were made available at all network member libraries and distributed by a variety of local health organizations. A review of KCCHIN was presented at the American Library Association's annual meeting in May 1989.

Since 1986, two additional consumer health information networks have been developed in Washington State. Both the Kitsap County and the Clark County consumer health information networks were initially funded through LSCA grants, using KCCHIN as a model. While KCCHIN has evolved into an informal rather than a formal network, solid networking channels continue to be essential to providing comprehensive service. Resources, both material and human, must be shared in order to effectively meet consumers' health information needs. Members of KCCHIN list their holdings in the Western Library Network for ready access. The Kitsap County Library System (KCLS) medical librarian continues to have contact with members of the Seattle Area Hospital Library Consortium and staff of the University of Washington Health Sciences Library Information Center. KCLS and Seattle Public Library, the two public library systems included in KCCHIN, share reciprocal borrowing privileges and network through exchanged circulation system terminals which allow each library to see immediately what is available in the other library's collection. Interlibrary loans among the system libraries are handled smoothly and efficiently, with no charge to patrons.

PUBLICITY AND PROMOTION

In order to be used effectively, consumer health information services need to be continuously advertised and promoted both to patrons and internally to library staff. Some of the ways this need has been met within KCLS include follow-up assessment interviews with librarians at the community libraries and continuing education opportunities at a variety of settings. Posters advertising KCCHIN and its services have been distributed to all community libraries, as have book, video, and audiocassette lists on health topics. Potential speakers are contacted and made available for programs at community libraries, and KCLS participates in health fairs sponsored by local area hospitals.

Continuing use of network resources has provided the most effective method of keeping network participants together. As new personnel enter into employment in each library, the effort must be extended to ensure that the concept of the network is preserved. A nominal lead institution is needed to monitor trouble spots or emerging needs within the network.

The success of the King County Consumer Health Information Network is best stated by the library patrons who have availed themselves of its services. The many "thank you" notes received by the KCLS medical reference librarian attest to the fact that an important need is being met. The following note was received from a patron whose sister had been diagnosed with Graves' disease: "What a wonderful service! I never expected that the library would research a subject and mail articles to a patron at no cost." A new mother, whose four-month old daughter was suffering from eczema, wrote: "We were so discouraged by the lack of information and support from our daughter's pediatrician. I went to the library hoping to find information on how to care for her, and what type of doctor should treat her. Everyone there did everything possible to help me, but it was really the information you sent that helped us to better understand her situation." And finally, from a young man with reflex sympathetic dystrophy: "In just a week or two I have learned more about R.S.D., and the problems it is causing me, than in the entire last 16 months of asking doctor, after doctor, after doctor." The network continues to operate successfully, providing patrons throughout the county with needed health information. Librarians at the academic health sciences library and at the participating hospital libraries feel confident that when they refer walk-in and telephone inquiry patrons to the public libraries in the community, the patrons will receive the needed service and information.

The public libraries continue to make use of the resources of the academic health sciences and hospital libraries through referral and interlibrary loan channels. This ensures that patrons have access to professional-level materials when such access is required to satisfactorily answer their questions. In turn, the public libraries take responsibility for collection building in the lay health area, ensuring that popular materials will be available to patrons of all the libraries.

The consumer health information network now operates smoothly with little intervention. Mutual benefits to participants ensure ongoing cooperation. Using preexisting channels for activities, such as referrals and interlibrary loans, allows the network to continue to be both active and successful, even after the initial grant support has ended.

███████████

APPENDIX I:
Video Order Form
(please photocopy)

Questions of Health: Trigger Tapes on the Health Care Reference Interview (videorecording).

Produced by:

King County Library System King County Consumer Health Information Network 1986

One (1) video-cassette (18 minutes, VHS), includes guide for discussion leaders.

Intended for reference staff training workshops, this tape presents lay health care reference interviews and explores the sensitivity, legal and ethical issues surrounding this area.

Cost: $30.00

SEND TO: _____

NAME: _____

STREET ADDRESS: _____

_____

CITY, STATE, ZIP: _____

Please enclose purchase order or check with your order. Make check payable to King County Library System.

FORWARD ORDER(S) TO:

King County Library System Medical Reference Department 300 Eighth Avenue North Seattle, WA 98109-5191 FAX: (206) 464-7481

Call (206) 684-6644, Medical Reference, if you have any questions.

APPENDIX II:
King County Consumer Health Information Network Core Health Reference Booklist—June 1989

The following 17 titles are available in each of the six King County Library System Resource Libraries which are geographically distributed throughout King County. According to recent interviews with reference staff, this core list of materials is adequate for answering most of the quick reference questions encountered. The Resource Libraries, along with the centralized Reference Department located at the Service Center, provide referral service to the smaller community libraries.

The core list includes only reference materials purchased on a systemwide basis. In addition to these reference titles, the Resource Library staff select reference and circulating materials necessary to meet the unique needs of their user populations. The variety and depth of materials purchased include both consumer and professional texts and periodicals.

Recent bibliographies for more in-depth reference work are cited on the last page. For additional information, call (206) 684-6644 or write to the medical librarian at King County Library System.

1. *ABMS Compendium of Certified Medical Specialists*, 2nd ed. American Board of Medical Specialties, 1988–1989.
   Updated biannually, this is the only official biographical directory authorized by all 23 medical specialty boards and the American Board of Medical Specialties. Includes such data as board certification, education and training, type of practice, and address and telephone for approximately 350,000 physicians.
2. *American Psychiatric Press Textbook of Psychiatry*. Talbott, John A. et al., eds. American Psychiatric Press, 1988.
   A comprehensive textbook of psychiatry, this source covers most of the general areas of mental health and illness about which public libraries receive questions. While not written for the layperson, the information it presents is clear and will be useful to most patrons.
3. *Cecil Textbook of Medicine*, 18th ed. Wyngaarden, James B. and Smith, Lloyd H., eds. Saunders, 1988.
   This classic text is exhaustive in its coverage of various aspects of internal medicine. Updated approximately every three years, the latest edition includes new sections on AIDS. Well illustrated with photographs, charts, and tables, the book also includes an annotated bibliography for each section within a chapter, making it easy to pursue further information on a topic.
4. *Color Atlas and Synopsis of Clinical Dermatology*. Fitzpatrick, Thomas B. et al. McGraw-Hill, 1983.
   While not comprehensive, this useful text covers most of the common dermatologic problems both clearly and in enough detail for many public library patrons. Color photographs illustrate the variety of skin diseases and disorders.

5. *Consumer Health & Nutrition Index.* Oryx Press, quarterly, annual cumulation. 1985– .
   Indexes 95 consumer-oriented periodicals that have been selected for inclusion based on health-related content, affordability by libraries, and practical nonspecialist approach. Coverage is steadily expanding and currently includes alternative medicine sources as well as general interest magazines.

6. *Current Medical Diagnosis & Treatment,* 1988. Schroeder, Steven A. et al., eds. Lange, annual.
   This standard updated compendium provides the latest accepted standards of diagnosis and treatment for medical disorders. New trends in care are included. Includes useful appendices and an excellent index.

7. *Current Obstetric & Gynecologic Diagnosis & Treatment,* 6th ed. Pernoll, Martin L. and Benson, Ralph C., eds. Lange, 1987.
   Updated every two or three years, this text is an excellent synopsis of both normal and problematic obstetrics and gynecology. Includes many useful photographs, diagrams, charts, and tables.

8. *Current Pediatric Diagnosis & Treatment,* 9th ed. Kempe, Henry C. et al., eds. Lange, 1987.
   This text covers the broad spectrum of disorders and problems of children, from infancy through adolescence, outlining the latest accepted therapies and diagnostic information. Includes information on normal growth and development.

9. *Current Surgical Diagnosis and Treatment,* 8th ed. Way, Lawrence W., ed. Lange, 1988.
   Serving as a ready source of information about diseases managed by surgery, this book is organized primarily by organ system. Clinical findings, diagnosis, complications, treatment, and prognosis are discussed for each condition.

10. *Dictionary of Medical Syndromes,* 2nd ed. Magalini, Sergio I. and Scrascia, Euclide. Lippincott, 1981.
    This specialized dictionary covers approximately 2,700 syndromes, listing both scientific and popular names. Each entry provides information on signs and symptoms, etiology, pathology, diagnostic procedures, therapy, and prognosis. A brief bibliography following each entry identifies the first reports of the syndrome in the medical literature.

11. *Dorland's Illustrated Medical Dictionary,* 27th ed. Saunders, 1988.
    Newly updated to include many recently introduced medical terms, this is considered by many to be the most comprehensive of medical dictionaries available. Includes numerous tables and illustrations and provides pronunciation and etymology for most terms.

12. *Encyclopedia and Dictionary of Medicine, Nursing and Allied Health,* 4th ed. Miller, Benjamin F. and Keane, Claire. Saunders, 1987.
    The beauty of this encyclopedia is that its definitions provide enough background, in clear and straightforward language, to make the concepts understandable to the educated layperson. While it is not as comprehensive as Dorland's, the information it includes is very complete. Includes plates and illustrations.

13. *Harrison's Principles of Internal Medicine,* 11th ed. Braunwald, Eugene et al., eds. McGraw-Hill, 1987.
    This standard text emphasizes detailed coverage of symptoms, diagnosis and diagnostic procedures in internal medicine. It is well-illustrated and includes detailed bibliographies for each section in a chapter.

14. *Marshall Cavendish Illustrated Encyclopedia of Family Health: Doctors' Answers.* Horton, Edward et al., eds. Marshall Cavendish, 1986.
    Published in 24 volumes, this beautifully illustrated and clearly written set is invaluable in the information it provides. Gives brief, easy to understand descriptions of both normal and abnormal functions and disorders of humans.

15. *Melloni's Illustrated Medical Dictionary,* 2nd ed. Dox, Ida et al. Williams & Wilkins, 1985.
    A compilation of approximately 26,000 terms that comprise the common core of information for the health sciences, this dictionary provides brief, accurate, and "to the point" definitions. Illustrations and sections on abbreviations, terminology, and pronunciation enhance its usefulness.

16. *Mosby's Medical & Nursing Dictionary,* 2nd ed. Mosby, 1986.
    This dictionary is revised continuously, with new terms being added even from one printing to another. It presents information clearly and provides many cross-references from definition to definition. Includes extensive appendices and some illustrations.

17. *United States Pharmacopeia Drug Information for the Consumer.* Consumers Union, 1989 (annual).
    Published by authority of the United States Pharmacopeial Convention, this *Consumer Reports* book presents comprehensive, up-to-date information on a wide variety of drug

categories in language understandable to the layperson. Includes an excellent index to both brand and generic names.

Additional reference title selections are described in:

Beattie, Barbara C. "A Guide to Medical Reference in the Public Library." *Public Libraries.* Winter 1988. 172–75.

Gaines, Bob. "Medical Books for Public Libraries." *The Unabashed Librarian 1989.* #71. 13–14.

Perry, Claudia A. "Patron Medical Queries: A Selected List of Information Sources." *Library Journal.* November 1, 1988. 45–50.

CHAPTER 16
Consumer Health and Patient Information Services in the U.S. Department of Veterans Affairs

Iris A. Renner and Janet M. Schneider

VA LIBRARY NETWORK (VALNET)

The VA Library Network (VALNET) is a national network supporting the Veterans Health Services & Research Administration (VHS & RA) health-care system. There are 176 network libraries, staffed by over 315 professional librarians, assisted by more than 300 clerical and technical personnel. VALNET provides educational, vocational, and recreational library services and programs to 193,000 physicians, nurses, dentists, and allied health care professionals; 100,000 students in affiliated teaching programs; and the more than one million inpatients treated each year; as well as supporting 23 million annual outpatient visits. VALNET was established during the 1970s by the VA Central Office Library Division (now Learning Resources Service) to meet the need for a more formalized structure that would promote resource sharing, centralize common performance activities, and encourage innovative cost-effective methods for staff and patient access to materials, information, and services.

Various network activities have been implemented by VALNET. To take advantage of pricing discounts, and ensure availability of information and educational resources to VA staff nationwide, an Audiovisual (AV) Software Delivery System was initiated in 1976, distributing selected VA or commercially produced materials to local, district, or regional delivery sites. VALNET site designations are based on a nationally established VA configuration. In 1982, a similar system for print materials on VA agency priorities, such as AIDS, Agent Orange, and computerization, was established. Coordinated journal collection development and sharing at the district and regional levels has also been encouraged.

Further promotion of networking and resource sharing led to the development of union lists of books, AVs, and journals by VA Central Office Library Division. Each union list is a compilation of the 176 individual libraries' holdings. Union lists are available on microfiche; the union list of periodicals will soon be online through FORUM, the National VA integrated electronic mail and database system. VALNET has also been active in providing expanded access to computerized databases. All libraries have direct access to the National Library of Medicine's (NLM) Medlars system. More than 60 percent also have on-site access to other databases through BRS or DIALOG. Many VALNET libraries also facilitate end-user access to user-friendly databases. Four specially designated libraries also provide DIALOG access to VALNET libraries in their region.

VA Library Services

Individual Library Services within VALNET have many similarities, but also many variations. Each medical center within the VHS & RA health-care system has a Library Service which operates as an independent department. The Library Service is generally organized into separate medical and patients' library sections and may also have a separate Patient Education Resource Center (PERC). The size of staff, scope of collections, and clinical, research, and educational needs of individual medical centers vary greatly, from the smaller library with one professional librarian, 100 journal subscriptions, and less than 2,000 books to the larger library with eight full-time employees, more than 500 journals, 15,000 books, and 1,000 audiovisual titles. Libraries may be affiliated with academic institutions or serve isolated areas.

One common thread, as noted by Diane Wiesenthal in the *VA Practitioner,* May 1987, is that all the libraries are service-oriented. This reflects the desire of all VA libraries to provide the best possible service to the people who comprise each medical center—patients, staff, and students. VALNET librarians work with health-care staff to meet their information and educational needs. Based on each medical center's programs, the Library Service may provide medical care, research, and continuing education information support to medical, nursing, allied health, and management personnel, and to affiliated students. All VALNET libraries provide traditional support, such as reference, bibliographic, interlibrary loan, and circulation services. In addition, many implement special services or programs to serve their clientele, such as the Clinical Medical Librarian (CML) Program and the Literature Attached to Charts (LATCH) Program. Both of these programs utilize the librarian as a patient care team member who responds to specific clinical questions quickly, providing a literature search and relevant articles to team members, or to the patient's chart.

In addition to meeting the information and educational needs of health-care staff, VALNET librarians assist with patient care by supporting patient health education programs and activities. In providing consumer health information, VALNET librarians help veterans and their families learn about their medical care and make informed choices about their treatment. Many VALNET libraries have developed specialized Patient Health Education Centers at their medical centers to meet patient education needs.

These Patient Education Resource Centers (PERCs) may contain classrooms or areas within the library for viewing AV programs at individual study carrels. Health information at a nontechnical level and in a variety of formats is available. Patients may come directly to the library or may be referred by a health practitioner. Also, patients and family members are often introduced to the PERC through other patient education programs and activities. Materials, which include videocassettes, slides, flipcharts, books, pamphlets, models, and simulation games, have been reviewed and approved by involved patient educators, and are linked to the learning objectives of ongoing patient health education programs. Materials may be delivered to patients at bedside directly or via closed-circuit television (CCTV), as well as in the library.

Patient Health Education Program

Library involvement in each medical center's patient education program varies greatly in levels of activities and delivery approaches. The VA System has a long history of promotion of patient health education services, with the first official statement appearing in 1953 when the Department of Medicine and Surgery (now VHS & RA) issued a technical bulletin on the subject. In 1976, the chief medical director designated the Office of Academic Affairs in the VA Central Office as the administrative focus of the Patient Health Education (PHE) Program and charged it with the development of long-range goals and strategies for patient health education in the VA System. In 1980, a national coordinator for patient education was appointed to recommend education policy, provide programmatic expertise and administrative direction, and technical assistance and consultation.

In 1986, the chief medical director approved a patient health education policy which has been published in the VA Policy Manual. The policy states that each medical center should establish an administrative structure to enable it to meet its responsibility to provide patient health education services as an integral part of high-quality, cost-effective care. It is recommended that the responsibility for planning and coordinating patient health education services be in the Office of the Chief of Staff, and delegated to the patient health education coordinator or the associate chief of staff for education or to a facility-based, interdisciplinary patient health education policy committee.

A national patient health education coordinator and seven regional patient health education coordinators, located at VA facilities with enhanced education functions, assist medical centers nationwide in developing effective patient health education programs and strategies. These coordinators act as consultants to individual medical centers, often through PHE committees, and to the approximately 46 facility-based PHE coordinators. Veterans Aministration PHE coordinators and librarians enjoy a collegial relationship, with the librarians identifying, providing, and disseminating information and educational resources, while the PHE coordinators develop or teach others how to develop high-quality PHE programs. Further strengthening this relationship is the learning resources service policy requiring that support for PHE resources, (books, audiovisuals, etc.) must be linked to specific PHE programs with clearly described goals and objectives. This coordinated approach not only reduces duplication of effort but also ensures that patients do not receive conflicting instruction and education materials.

The remainder of this chapter is a case study describing one specific Patient Education Resources Center—the Patient Education Resource Center within the Patients Library of the James A. Haley Veterans Hospital, Tampa, Florida. The development and implementation of the PERC is described in terms of goals and objectives, funding, organization, and services.

CASE STUDY: PATIENTS LIBRARY, JAMES A. HALEY VETERANS HOSPITAL, TAMPA, FLORIDA

Background

The James A. Haley Veterans Hospital is one of the VA's most modern facilities, serving the veterans of central Florida. It operates 681 beds, meeting health needs in the fields of medicine, surgery, psychiatry, spinal cord injury, rehabilitation medicine, neurology, and dialysis. A 120-bed nursing home care unit is located adjacent to the medical center as is the research building, where such projects as the development of an artificial heart are explored. Two full-service satellite outpatient clinics are operated under the jurisdiction of this medical center: in Orlando, 75 miles to the northeast, and in Port Richey, 30 miles to the west. Veterans outreach centers are located in Tampa, Port Richey, and Orlando. The medical center is affiliated with the College of Medicine at the University of South Florida and numerous other institutions, providing residency training programs in most medical and surgical specialties as well as nursing, pharmacy, radiology, social work, dietetics, and others.

The Library Service and the medical center first opened their doors to patients in October 1972. Library Service includes the Patients Library and Medical Library and is adjoined by offices for the chief and for clerical/technical support of the Service. At this medical center, the Patients Library has always been staffed by a professional librarian specifically designated for this area and, with the two libraries being adjacent, can also utilize the assistance of other Library personnel as demand dictates. The resources in 1972 consisted of a general recreational collection of books, magazines, talking books for the blind and physically disabled, and other aids for those patients unable to utilize the traditional resources of the Library. Ward service was provided on a regular basis for those patients unable to visit the Library.

By 1976, the emphasis of the collection was shifting from recreational to health informational literature. As medical staff support grew and patron demands for health information increased, Library staff realized that to fully meet the needs of the medical center would require the development of a health information center within the Library. It was felt that while recreational reading had an important therapeutic value, it had become more important to assist patients in understanding their illness, treatment, and recovery than merely to provide an activity to occupy their time. The change in emphasis here coincided with a national shift recognized and promoted by VA Central Office Library Division. In order to encourage patients' libraries at the local level to adopt the Patient Education Resource Center (PERC) concept, funding for materials, equipment, and furniture to initiate a PERC was made available through Central Office.

A study of the medical center's existing patient education programs and resources was undertaken, with the help of the Hospital's Patient Education Committee and the patient educators. After one and a half years in preparation, a proposal was submitted to VA Central Office in 1985 for a one-time grant to establish a PERC. The proposal was approved and funded.

As a result of this funding, the Library was able to acquire audiovisual hardware and software, books, and anatomical models and charts to enhance the existing collection. LEM carrels were also acquired, providing viewing areas for individuals or small groups in the Library. In conjunction with these acquisitions, the Library underwent a renovation project which reconfigured existing space. Subsequent one-time grant money enabled the Library to acquire additional equipment to broadcast patient education videos on the Hospital's closed-circuit television system (CCTV).

Goals and Objectives

The Patients Library serves as the resource center for patient education programs and activities conducted within the medical center. While maintaining a small recreational collection, including special resources such as large print and talking books, as a therapeutic outlet for long-term and psychiatric patients, the primary and necessary focus is on the health education materials.

The role of the librarian is, of course, still that of a resource provider. The librarian assists individuals in locating information in the health literature, but will not interpret the materials for any individual. Attempts by clients to describe their symptoms, for example, are gently rebuffed, and patrons are directed to their health-care provider. If the individual is a patient in the medical center, and is having obvious difficulties with the materials, the librarian notifies the ward staff of the patient's concerns, comprehension, or communication difficulties. The health-care professionals have appreciated and encouraged this approach, since it eliminates many misunderstandings between themselves and their patients. It also demonstrates to them that the librarian is working with them for the good of the patient by providing accurate information that the patient can understand. Reference questions run the gamut in sensitivity from drug information to penile implants, with each patient's individual needs for confidentiality and discretion observed by the librarian. Inpatients are, for the most part, restricted to their units except for "prescribed" visits, with the result that outpatients and family members are the primary clients within the Library itself. Many of these individuals have been referred for specific materials: for example, surgical patients on their preadmission visit, and the same patients later for other information needs after admission to the medical center.

The Library also supports patients by supplying materials that provide a link to the outside world, and helping them plan ahead for discharge. Resources, such as personal narratives in books or audiovisuals, can aid an individual in finding alternative skills or lifestyles to accommodate illness or disability. Through books and other library resources, the patient can find examples of others who have been in similar circumstances, and which may help the patient gain the courage and confidence to bridge the gulf between the hospital environment and a "normal" life. This is a critical element for an individual who has been suddenly stricken with a major disability, such as spinal cord injury or stroke, or a terminal illness such as cancer. The librarian also refers families and individuals to the medical center's social workers or local support agencies, such as the American Cancer Society, for further information and resources.

The clientele of the Patients Library often has high stress and anxiety levels, and the librarian must exercise additional diplomacy and compassion toward patrons searching for health information which from the patron's viewpoint has the potential to radically change a person's life. Because of the ramifications of disease or disability, the coordination between the librarian and the health care provider is vital to ensure accurate and pertinent information for the patron. Information from the Library can provide a basis for forming questions a patient can ask of his or her provider, for aid in meeting informed consent requirements in patient care, and for supplementation and reinforcement of information received by the patient from health-care providers. The interaction and cooperation of the librarian and the providers ensure quality control of materials held by the Library and provide a mechanism to ensure that the appropriate information is given to the patients and families needing it. The librarian must become an integral part of the multi-disciplinary health-care team, coordinating appropriate resources to be used with the various patient populations and expanding the "traditional" responsibilities of a librarian in a variety of ways.

Patient Education Committee Member

The medical center's patient education programs and activities are organized and overseen by a multi-disciplinary Patient Education Committee, as recommended by the chief of staff. The current Committee membership is comprised of professionals from audiology and speech pathology, clinical bed services, dental, dietetics, library, medical media, nursing, pharmacy, psychology, rehabilitation, satellite outpatient clinics, and social work, with the chief of staff and associate chief of staff for education serving *ex officio*. The Committee serves a facilitating role to providers of patient education, and in an advisory capacity to the director of the medical center in all matters pertaining to patient education. It fosters implementation of patient education; establishes priorities according to existing needs; evaluates ongoing programs and activities; makes recommendations for purchase or development of patient education materials, supplies, and equipment; and approves in-house produced patient education programs, activities, booklets, and instruction sheets.

The current patients librarian assumes an active role as a member of this Committee. Her unique training in the field of information gathering, dissemination, organization and storage makes her an indispensable component in the work of the Committee. She provides current awareness services and other information of interest to Committee members, researches informational requests and stores patient education program course outlines, goals, and objectives in the Library for easy access by medical center staff and Committee members. The patients librarian is able to meet the informational needs of the medical center staff in patient education by providing materials that are helpful to potential educators or referring them to other Committee members for additional information and assistance. For example, in a medical center such as Tampa's, with access to BRS Information Technologies, the librarian provides information on hard-to-find materials via the Combined Health Information Database (CHID). CHID provides online access to citations and some full-text documents of journal articles, fact sheets, brochures, books, and audiovisuals in the health information field. One subfile of CHID is maintained by the VA, and contains more than 80 records describing VA patient health education programs—their goals, objectives, target audiences, evaluation methods, and resources used. This subfile is especially useful for local educators in identifying their counterparts in other VA medical centers as they develop new programs, avoiding "reinventing the wheel" as well as sharing ideas and information. Other online databases, e.g., Medline for professional literature and PDQ (Physicians Data Query) for professionals and laypersons, are also available through the Library. The "Information for Patients" section of PDQ is especially useful in locating state-of-the-art information for cancer patients and their families.

The Committee continually publicizes and promotes the importance of patient education to the medical center staff, holding in-service workshops to train staff in components of the teaching process, e.g., communicating effectively with the patient, writing goals and objectives in a patient education program, teaching methods, and assessing the reading level of patient education materials. The librarian, in addition to providing resources for these classes, also serves as faculty in demonstrating readability tests, discusses the role of the Library and the librarian in the medical center's team approach to patient education, and facilitates small group work.

The librarian is one of the most easily accessible people on the Committee. As such, she serves as liaison for medical center staff who need to contact the Committee about patient education matters, and the Library serves as a focal point for all patient education resources. New health information needs and resources therefore rapidly come to the attention of the librarian as she fulfills her Committee duties and allow her to more quickly meet the information and resource needs of medical center staff. The librarian is able to highlight the Library's services and capabilities and emphasize the cooperative and multi-disciplinary nature of patient education through service on this active, dynamic Committee.

In addition to interacting with local medical center staff, Tampa's Library Service and Patient Education Committee also cooperates with regional and national VA staffs. At the VA Central Office's request, the Patients Library is pilot testing two user-friendly patient health education databases, utilizing a microcomputer with CD-ROM drives. These databases from Information Access Company contain indexes to consumer health literature and health-related articles from newspapers and popular, business, and academic periodicals and are available for trial to all Patients Library patrons. These CD-ROM databases were demonstrated at a recent health fair, and to the regional PHE coordinator who was here assisting the Patient Education Committee in the presentation of a workshop. The coordinator tried the system, and then shared the information with other coordinators nationwide.

Reality Orientation Group Leader

While the majority of patients remain in the medical center for only a few days, some may be hospitalized for considerably longer periods. One unit with many longer term patients is the acute psychiatric ward. The nurse manager of the ward asked the librarian to conduct a weekly group for her patients in order to provide another activity, prevent "hospitalitis," and maintain the patients' focus toward discharge planning. True bibliotherapy for these patients is not possible due to several factors, including the patients' mental status, attention spans, and frequent use of medications affecting vision. For these reasons, the librarian has developed a reality orientation approach, approved by the ward staff, designed to highlight places and events (current or historic) which stimulate patients' thoughts and discussions. Topics range from occupations to travelogues, and political debates to superstitions, with only religious and medical subjects excluded.

The librarian may show a short audiovisual or a book or magazine article of interest to the group. The film or topic is presented by the librarian after a brief introduction and statement about the purpose of the group; discussion by the patients follows. The librarian acts as facilitator, drawing out each individual, guiding the discussion into appropriate channels, and allowing each patient time and opportunity to speak. Patients are assigned to the group by the ward staff and are required to attend as part of their treatment plan. During each session, a staff member from the ward observes the patients' levels of participation, awareness, and interest, as well as relevancy of input to the discussions. This information is later documented in each patient's chart, and used by the physicians and therapists in evaluating the patient's progress toward the goal of mental health.

Discharge Planning Team Member

Due to the patients librarian's active involvement in the medical center's head-and-neck cancer unit, she was asked to participate in its weekly multi-disciplinary discharge planning meetings. The members of the team felt that the addition of the librarian to the meetings would be valuable in helping them to meet the educational needs of the patients and their families. In addition, the librarian would provide the team with medical reference assistance for topics raised during the discussions. Her participation was so successful that she was subsequently asked to join the cardiac/thoracic surgery discharge planning team as well.

At the meetings, the health-care team discusses each patient briefly in terms of his or her physical, social, and emotional status, as well as his or her progress in the course of treatment and future prospects. As the meeting progresses, a patient may be referred to the librarian for materials pertaining to that patient's particular situation. The educator may arrange for a video to be shown via the closed-circuit television system, have materials delivered to the patient's room, or send the patient and/or family to the Library for specific materials. The librarian typically reports to the referring educator to confirm that the patient did see the materials, and to advise the educator as to any interest, confusion, or comprehension the patient may have expressed. This process encourages a good flow of communication among all team members, and ensures quality education reinforced by a variety of methods.

Closed-Circuit Television System Coordinator

In a hospital environment, teaching occurs wherever the patient and educator can meet: in a classroom, dayroom, library, or at the patient's bedside. Since most of these areas do not have easy access to audiovisual equipment, the Patients Library was able to initiate a separate channel and connect its equipment to the existing closed-circuit television system. This was an immediate success with medical center staff; it eliminated the need for them to arrange and transport the equipment and software, thereby producing a tremendous savings in their time and energy. In addition, it afforded more opportunities to provide audiovisual programs to the patients. Initially, the system consisted of one video player triggered manually by the librarian in response to requests from the medical center educators for their classes and for individual patients. As demand for the service grew, the Library requested and received additional one-time funding which added three more players, a character generator, and a control unit. The expanded system now runs 24 hours per day, with videos automatically triggered by the control unit. The character generator allows "pages" of messages to be sequentially displayed on the screen whenever videos are not playing, so that there is a continuous picture on the channel. The librarian uses this capability to "print" a weekly online schedule of programs, lists of upcoming events in the medical center, and other messages of interest to patients.

The programs shown are scheduled by the patients librarian in response to the requests of local educators, e.g., the diabetes clincal nurse specialist, to support classroom and individual/family teaching efforts. Discussions and follow-up measures between the librarian and these educators ensure that the programs meet the needs of the patients and are shown at a proper and convenient time for education to take place. Programs may be requested on an ongoing basis, as for a class held at a particular time each month, or on an individual basis, as a spontaneous presentation. Immediate access to the system via a telephone call to the librarian has won the support of virtually all educators due to the reliability and simplicity of the system. The willingness of the librarian to accommodate as many requests as can be logistically handled has also found much support.

Information Broker/Guest Speaker

Many people come to the Library with health questions that cannot be answered from books, and yet they seem not only unaware of appropriate questions to ask but also how to get the information from their health-care providers. The librarian assists patrons in the Library with methods they can use to communicate more effectively with their doctors and nurses and obtain the information they need to make informed decisions about their health and treatment.

As the medical center educators became aware of the librarian's involvement in this activity, they invited her to address their patient groups on the issue. Topics within the librarian's presentation include appropriate use of the Library in medical matters, e.g., what kinds of information can be found in the Library versus what must be answered by a physician; communication skills and techniques; the importance of taking an active role in one's own health care; and the rights and responsibilities of patients. The information stresses the collaborative roles that patients and medical staff need to maintain and has been favorably received by both health professionals and patients.

Publicity Manager

Utilizing successful marketing techniques, such as flyers in bright colors with eye-catching graphics, to capture attention and encourage further interest, the librarian has developed pamphlets and brochures on a number of subjects. These include "pathfinders," which list the Library's resources on various health topics, describe the closed-circuit television system, and explain the use of the Library and its services. These items are distributed to patients and staff during Library orientations, and to patients' dayrooms and waiting areas. These materials have proved effective in advertising and promoting the Library as well as highlighting the extensive availability of health information to all interested individuals. The medical center's clinical specialists and other educators often distribute these handouts to their patients in order to encourage their questions and active participation in their own health care.

Various groups and committees within the medical center sponsor events during the year in which the librarian is asked to participate and/or provide displays, such as National Nutrition Month activities for employees and patients. For these events, special messages and programs are shown on the Library's closed-circuit television system, bulletin board space and materials are provided, and the librarian assists in distributing materials and highlighting activities and resources, and also participates in closing ceremonies at the end of the month.

The librarian serves as editor of *HealthNet,* a locally produced quarterly health newsletter distributed to patients under the aegis of the Patient Education Committee. This role reinforces her close contact with medical center health educators as she verifies information for inclusion or submission of items/articles for the newsletter. A section on the Library's new resources and services is included in each issue.

CONCLUSION

The librarian in a hospital setting faces a great challenge from the special needs of his/her "captive" clientele. Inpatients are subjected to far greater stresses than individuals who may return to their own homes each night. Dr. Hans Mauksch writes of patients as follows in *Bibliotherapy: Methods and Materials:* "Shucked of his clothes, his identity, and, he feels, his rights, the patient feels lost in the hospital." The library can assist in meeting these needs in several ways. It can provide a constructive means of relieving patient stress through recreational reading or acquisition of knowledge about the patient's health care and treatment, thereby offering the patient the ability to control at least one small segment of his or her life. At Tampa, the Library encourages patients to expand their interests and express their feelings, both of which can aid in relieving anxiety and discomfort. Addressing patients' emotional needs will increase their satisfaction with their health care. The librarian has also discovered that patients will often express despair or frustration with their situation to library staff which has not been voiced to the appropriate health-care providers. In these cases, the librarian notifies the health-care staff involved to apprise them of situations which can often be easily defused through additional counseling or education. This kind of cooperation and coordination among health-care professionals, in which the librarian is included as part of the team effort, demonstrates the medical center's concern for the patient as a total person.

At this medical center, the librarian initially became involved with the health-care team by meeting with the staff members involved and discussing how the Library and librarian could assist not only with the patients' needs, but also with the health providers' needs. Included in these discussions was a firm delineation of what the librarian felt herself qualified to do—provide resources, locate materials for staff and patients, coordinate the delivery of such materials, and provide feedback to the health-care team members about the receipt of requested items when appropriate. With such an understanding well defined, the groundwork was laid to form a noncompetitive, cooperative relationship in which each educator knew not only what the librarian *would* accomplish in a given circumstance, but also what the librarian would *not* do. Initially, this approach demanded a large amount of time and travel around the medical center. But as staff learned of the services available and the willingness of the librarian to assist them, they began to contact her in the Library for further information and orientation. From that point on, the librarian became integrated into activities throughout the medical center, as staff members approached her for various levels of participation. These activities gave her higher visibility, which in turn increased staff requests.

For this kind of approach to work, clear communication and prompt action on the part of the librarian is critical. Once the medical center staff learned that the librarian consistently followed words with actions that were beneficial to them and to their patients, they were delighted to utilize her services. Team members are receptive to including those library services in their programs and activities which can be shown to reinforce their efforts, while not creating extra work for them. In summary, our experience in Tampa has shown us that the tasks of the hospital librarian are to make library services and resources accessible to all patrons, professional staff, patients, and families; to develop and promote a collection of materials that provides therapeutic and educational information to supplement and support the overall mission of the medical center while also helping the individual; and to act as an integral part of the health-care team, providing quality patient care. The successful performance of these tasks has placed this library program in high regard at the medical center, in the community, and at the VA national level.

ACKNOWLEDGMENT

The authors thank Wendy Carter, Karen Renninger, and Diane Wiesenthal, VA Central Office Learning Resources Service, for their assistance and support during the writing of this chapter.

BIBLIOGRAPHY

Bibliotherapy: Methods and Materials. Chicago: American Library Association, 1971.

Lunin, L.F. and Stein, R. "CHID: Combined Health Information Database: A Unique Health Information and Education Database" *Bulletin of the Medical Library Association.* 75 (2) (1987). 95–100.

Schneider, Janet M. "The Role of the Librarian in a Multi-disciplinary Team" *The Journal: Official Publication of the Society of Otorhinolaryngology and Head-Neck Nurses* 2 (Spring 1984). 3–6.

Stout, L. Nan. "Veterans Administration Patient Health Education Policy Statement." *Patient Education and Counseling.* 10 (1987). 301–04.

Van Vuren, Darcy D. "The Veterans Administration Library Network: VALNET" *Bulletin of the Medical Library Association.* 70 (3) (1982). 289–92.

Wiesenthal, Diane. "VA Library Service: The VALNET System and Resource Sharing." *VA Practitioner.* 4 (May 1987). 49–57.

PART III

Program Development and Operation

CHAPTER 17
Development of Consumer Health Library Collections

Alan M. Rees

GENERAL PRINCIPLES OF COLLECTION DEVELOPMENT

According to Wortman,[1] a collection is "a large number of physical materials traditionally found in libraries—books, magazines, maps, video-cassettes, and so forth. A collection also is the information in, or contents of, these things, as well as the information trails into these contents." Collection development, as viewed by Evans,[2] is the "process of making certain the information needs of the people using the collection are met in a timely and economical manner, using information resources produced both inside and outside of the organization." An important component of this process is what Broadus[3] calls "the primacy of the user." Maintaining this primacy requires extensive community analysis, needs assessment, and a responsiveness to present and projected user requirements. As in marketing, the key ingredient of success lies in staying close to the customer.

A collection development policy statement represents a plan of action and information that is used to guide the library staff's thinking and decision making. Katz[4] notes that such a statement is an "effort to bring order, logic and common sense to bear on selection and evaluation view-points." The component steps in collection development and management include analysis and definition of the target population to be served; identification of user needs; selecting the kinds of materials appropriate for a particular collection; assessing an existing collection's strengths and weaknesses; selecting new materials; assuring access to the collection through convenient shelf arrangement, reasonable circulation policy, and photocopy services; reviewing on a regular basis the availability, physical condition, and intellectual quality of the contents of materials; keeping adequate collection usage records to permit future planning and projection of growth; and carrying out an efficient program for weeding, discarding, or storage.[5]

Katz[6] comments that the "librarian who chooses materials is a media czar whose income may be less than that of the television mogul but whose range of choice is more impressive." In this connection, Katz identifies three basic selection philosophies—liberal, traditionalist, and pluralistic. The liberal position reflects social activism and holds that service should reach out to the total community and not just satisfy active users; the traditionalist philosophy stresses continuity rather than change and underscores the need to select quality materials for existing users; the pluralistic position takes a pragmatic middle ground, borrowing from both the liberal and traditionalist positions.[7]

COLLECTION DEVELOPMENT POLICY FOR CONSUMER HEALTH

These general principles apply to consumer health collections. The necessity of community analysis and defining information needs is of crucial importance in arriving at a collection development policy. The component steps are exactly the same as in other library contexts: identification and analysis of target populations to be served; formulation of criteria and guidelines for the selection of appropriate information products and services; facilitating access to the collection; and establishment of a policy for collection weeding and updating.

There is a significant difference between serving a public library community and a patient population within the hospital setting. Analysis of the public library community takes into account demographic variables such as age, sex, and a variety of socioeconomic factors. A similar analysis within the hospital also requires a careful analysis of the patient population in terms of their medical problems. It can be safely assumed that these problems form the basis for the generation of information needs and that attempts to seek information will stem from these medical diagnoses. Data relating to the distribution of diagnoses are readily available in most hospitals from medical records administration. Eliciting the perceptions of need on the part of health-care providers should also form part of the process of establishing need. Of particular interest is the perception of the medical staff with respect to the level of understanding of the patient population, purpose for which the information is needed (diagnosis, treatment, medication, coping), level and type of material that would be most useful, and optimal place and time of information delivery. Information services to patients and their families should obviously be supportive of the mission of the parent institution—namely, provision of quality health care. In general, the needs of consumers in the hospital setting are likely to be more sharply focussed on specific diseases and conditions, treatment options, medications, and problems of coping with chronic diseases. Such a focus must necessarily be reflected in collection development policy. The needs of consumers within public libraries are likely to be more diffused across the entire spectrum of health concerns from wellness to sickness.

QUANTITY CONSIDERATIONS

There is no shortage of health publications suitable for consumer use in the United States. The popular book literature published annually is about 500–600 titles. The publication of pamphlets shows no sign of diminishing, and the federal government, voluntary health associations, and commercial producers continue to distribute a diverse assortment of pamphlets, booklets, and leaflets on most of the common diseases, syndromes, conditions, and ailments. The number of popular health magazines and newsletters now exceeds 100 and *American Health* and *In-Health* (formerly *Hippocrates*) rank among the most successful magazine launches in the past few years. Recent newcomers on the health magazine scene include *Heart Care, Mature Health,* and *Longevity.*[8]

A new phenomenon—the health newsletter—has also taken hold. *The Harvard Medical School Health Letter* has been successfully copied in the form of similar newsletters published by other medical centers, such as Johns Hopkins, Tufts, University of California at Berkeley, Texas, Toronto, and the Mayo Clinic. The *Consumer Reports Health Letter* recently made its debut. In addition, newsletters now exist on specialized topics such as back pain, heart disease, cancer, men's health, women's health, pediatric care, weight loss, executive fitness, diabetes, arthritis, executive health, and nutrition. Consumer advocacy newsletters are published by the People's Medical Society, Public Citizen Health Research Group, the Society for Medical Consumers, and the Center for Science in the Public Interest. Most of these newsletters offer a mix of news notes, short features, summaries of articles in professional journals, book reviews, research reports, questions and answers, tips on self-care, and practical advice. Many newsletters are lookalikes and the market is reaching the point of saturation.[9]

The cost of these publications is not large. The average annual subscription for magazines is about $15–$20, while the average cost of newsletters is about $20–$25. Since much of the content is almost identical in many of these magazines and newsletters, it is quite common for libraries to subscribe to a small but representative number.

QUALITY CONSIDERATIONS

The most critical consideration confronting those engaged in collection development is the issue of quality. This is of the utmost importance in that wrong, misleading, unreliable, and outdated medical information has the potential of causing harm. Quackery is sometimes defined as misinformation, or untrue and/or misleading information about health. The American Council on Science and Health (ACSH) estimates[10] that the total spent by Americans on all types of health fraud is close to $28 billion per year. The ACSH points out that "books and magazines are another source of nutrition and health misinformation. In fact, few of the books in the 'health and diet' section of your local chain bookstore present scientifically accurate information."

There are a number of encyclopedic compilations of medical facts but these have only limited value in that they offer little assistance to individuals attempting to process relevant information for decision making. In contrast, there exist a few books that have proved to be highly successful in sharpening the decision making and problem solving skills of consumers. Two examples of this type of publication are the *The American Medical Association's Family Medical Guide,* with its self-diagnostic decision charts, and *Dr. Spock's Baby and Child Care.* The Spock book excels in helping parents in "trouble shooting" or problem solving by answering basic questions: What is it? What is it called? How serious is it? Do I need to seek professional advice? What can I do? What can I expect? These books serve a triage function by assisting consumers in determining the most prudent course of action—consult a physician immediately or as soon as possible, apply home remedies, or do nothing at the present time.

Unfortunately, the capsule reviews in *Library Journal, Booklist, Choice,* and other library publications are descriptive in nature and provide limited guidance in assessing the value, accuracy, or usefulness of the popular health literature. There are too few instances of critical commentary with regard to accuracy, balance, depth of coverage, author qualifications, or consumer orientation. Although *The Consumer Health Information Source Book*[11] contains critical reviews with commentary on the reliability and usefulness of the book literature it is not published on a regular basis.

Those engaged in selection must make their own decisions on a continuing basis. This is not as difficult as it may appear in that many publications are obviously excellent or manifestly deplorable. Only a minority of books require a judgement call. In this connection, it is important to emphasize that library professionals cannot relinquish the role of judging quality. This is particularly true in view of the intense marketing, promotion, hype, and fanfare that accompany many book introductions. The quality decision is an inescapable professional responsibility that must always be made in relation to the needs and interests of the defined library audience.

SELECTION CRITERIA

But what is "good?" "Good" consumer health information is that which is accurate and useful in explaining diseases and ailments, demystifying esoteric subject matter, imparting a sense of control to patients, and stimulating and enriching communication between patients and physicians. The criteria used in compiling *The Consumer Health Information Source Book* have proved to be highly useful for selection purposes. These criteria are: qualifications of the author; validity and accuracy of the content; quality of the narrative; ease of use; listing of further information resources; physical quality of the book; and consumer orientation. The criteria can be translated into a set of questions that can be matched against each candidate book.

Does the candidate book have:

1. A *qualified author* with relevant credentials?
2. An *informed author* who has researched the topic?
3. *In-depth coverage of the essential aspects?*
4. A *balanced presentation* reconciling diverse viewpoints?
5. A *listing of supporting references and adequate documentation?*
6. *Charts, diagrams and illustrations* that help the reader to better understand the subject content?

7. *Guidance to readers on utilizing problem-solving skills* rather than dictating to them "do this" or "do that?"
8. *An approach that offers insight rather than cures?*
9. *A focus on the sharpening of consumer skills and facilitating of problem solving*

WHAT TO AVOID

In terms of negative criteria, one should avoid the following:

1. Books that tout dubious cures, phony weight loss schemes, unnecessary nutritional supplements, and unauthorized drugs and treatment.
2. Books with exaggerated claims such as "miraculous," "revolutionary," and "breakthrough."
3. Books full of glitz and gimmicks in the form of extravagant terminology and imagery, and inflated prose.
4. Books advocating a "quick fix"—those that offer immediate relief, rapid weight loss, complete freedom from pain.
5. Books by authors with nonrelevant or questionable qualifications from phantom or marginal educational institutions.

A PRESCRIPTIVE OR REACTIVE APPROACH?

A problem in applying these criteria lies in the extent to which one can adopt a judgemental, prescriptive approach in relation to such bestsellers as Harvey and Marilyn Diamond's *Fit for Life*, which sold more than one million copies within a six-week period. Despite its sales popularity, the book was condemned by most health-care professionals as being based upon absurd and unscientific premises. One expert dubbed the Diamonds as "absolute quacks who have been made millionaires by irresponsible talk-show hosts and the gullible public." Likewise, Bernie Siegel's best-selling book, *Love, Medicine and Miracles* has been severely criticized. One reviewer noted that Siegel "draws his inferences from the weakest form of evidence—patient testimonials and clinical anecdotes. Then, he uses scientific studies selectively—and sometimes misleadingly— to support his views."[12] Yet another example of a bestseller based upon dubious scientific evidence is Kowalski's *The 8-Week Cholesterol Cure*, which was on *The New York Times* bestseller list for almost a year. Kowalski's prescription of massive doses of niacin has been denounced by most nutrition experts.

But should one refuse to acquire such books? In view of the media publicity and promotion, countless patrons rush to the library following an author's talk-show appearance and demand to borrow the promoted book. Eric Moon,[13] a former editor of *Library Journal*, urged years ago that librarians should "buy less of the flotsam which is washed up each week or month by promotion-activated demand." But in a democratic and pluralistic society the librarian cannot consistently play censor and refuse to buy *Prevention* magazine. One can, however, offer patrons a choice between such popular, fad works and those that are more scholarly in content. This situation offers an excellent opportunity for the reference librarian to educate the public by pointing to the existence of alternate and more authoritative sources of information.

ALTERNATIVE MEDICINE

Attention also has to be paid to deciding the extent to which publications reflecting alternative viewpoints should be included in collections. Does one acquire materials on chiropractic, holistic medicine, reflexology, chelation therapy, applied kinesiology, iridology, hair analysis, metabolic therapy, colonic irrigation, and acupuncture? In the public library, the answer would be that representative purchases of such materials might be made to achieve a balance and to be responsive to all segments of the community served. Katz considers this to be a pluralistic approach. However, in hospitals controlled by traditional, allopathic medical practitioners, purchases of such materials may not be feasible. The acquisition of publications reflecting an alternative medicine viewpoint could be construed as being counterproductive to the mission of the parent institution. The adoption of a traditionalist philosophy in this connection can be regarded as a reasonable compromise between the liberal and pluralistic selection philosophies.

MIX OF POPULAR AND PROFESSIONAL

The mix of popular and professional is another issue to be addressed. In offering CHI services, the medical library starts with the professional literature and adds a selection of popular works, while the public library begins with the popular literature and supplements it with professional materials. However, professional books are considerably more expensive than popular books and involve a public library in considerable expenditures. The comparative value and utility of professional and popular literature in responding to consumer information requests remains to be explored. The extent that one can rely on either level of medical publications for specific purposes or types of questions remains unknown. Given a small acquisitions budget, in what proportion should the money be spent on professional as opposed to popular works? Can cheaper popular books be substituted for more expensive professional works? Unfortunately, there is no ready answer to this question.

La Rocco describes the operation of a consumer health information service utilizing the resources of the University of Miami's medical school library professional collection. These resources were supplemented by the acquisition of some 100 books, 10 popular periodicals, and a pamphlet collection on microfiche. Kenyon at the College of Physicians of Philadelphia draws upon the 2,100 professional journals currently received at the College and its several hundred thousand professional books and monographs. A small collection of popular materials has been added. Kenyon notes that the popular materials are sufficient to answer approximately 60 percent of the questions received. The remaining 40 percent of the questions are answered by recourse to the professional literature. The questions requiring recourse to the professional literature are in those instances where information is required on advances in medicine, alternative therapies, uncommon diseases and conditions, and details of surgical procedures.

A similar experience is reported by Reidelbach and colleagues at the University of Nebraska but with different percentages. The authors state that "the professional collection has provided a major information resource for the CHIRS program. It often contains the only material available to address the consumer's question." Of the total number of requests filled by the CHIRS program over the past five years, 65 percent of the materials sent were from the professional collection, whereas only 35 percent came from the CHIRS popular collection. This ratio is the reverse of that reported by Kenyon. Moeller points out that at Overlook Hospital the consumer collection is not adequate for 25 to 30 percent of the questions asked. Moeller argues that this is because many users in the hospital setting have illness-specific requests.

These ratios reflecting a 30 to 65 percent reliance in *medical* libraries on the professional literature cannot be applied to public libraries. This is because many of the questions answered by Kenyon and Reidelbach in medical libraries were referred to them only after local popular resources had been exhausted. It is not surprising, therefore, that it was necessary for a large number of these referred questions to be answered from the professional literature. A large number of such referrals can only be answered from the professional literature. It is, however, most likely that as many as 90 percent of the questions in public libraries can be adequately answered utilizing popular materials.

Perry at the New York Academy describes the heavy use of Medline on compact disc, technical publications such as the *Merck Manual* and *Cecil Textbook of Medicine*, and journals such as the *New England Journal of Medicine*. She stresses the value of the professional literature in that "sources geared to the lay public are likely to be concerned with more common disorders and established treatments, so those seeking information on new and alternative therapies may have no choice but to consult the professional literature."

It would appear that the complexity of the professional literature in terms of its suitability to a lay audience has been exaggerated. Much of what is published in professional journals, especially those with a clinical focus, is understandable to the more educated and sophisticated consumer. Within the public library setting, there is a clear demand for the *PDR, New England Journal of Medicine*, and nursing texts. It should also be noted that the line dividing the professional and popular literature is becoming blurred. This is because many of the popular health magazines perform a metabolizing role in breaking down the "undigestible" content of the professional literature into more readily "digestible" articles for popular consumption. Research findings rapidly find their way to consumer magazines in the form of digests prepared for *American Health* and *Prevention*.

CORE LISTS

Great interest has been shown in constructing core lists for CHI materials. There is a continuing fascination in the library profession for such core lists stemming from the notion that one should be able to identify and label the best, undisputed, most authoritative, and most reliable publications. A number of valuable core lists do exist and several are included in this volume as appendices to the chapters by Arcari and Richetelle (Chapter 4) and Perry (Chapter 18). Also of value are the *Consumer Health Information Basic Reference List*[14] compiled by METRO'S Consumer Health Information Task Force; "Medical Reference Tools for the Layperson" published in the Reference Books Bulletin of *Booklist*;[15] and *A Guide to Consumer Health Information* compiled by Moira Bryant at Westmead Hospital in Australia.[16] The ultimate value of these lists is, however, limited by the absence of clearly enunciated criteria, with the result that the basis for the recommendation of any item is not readily apparent. No merit scores are provided and there are few comparisons between similar items.

These limitations are immediately apparent when one examines specific recommendations. For example, the Reference Books Bulletin List recommends the *Merck Index* (a most dubious choice for consumers) and both the *PDR* and *USP DI (United States Phamacopeia Dispensing Information)*, with no guidance as to the comparative value of either. The METRO list chooses the *PDR* over the *USP DI*, and the *Directory of Medical Specialists* over the *ABMS Compendium of Certified Medical Specialists*, without indicating any reason for so doing. Arcari and Richetelle choose the *USP DI* over the *PDR* for their first priority purchases.

The point made here in contrasting the priorities accorded to these comparable publications is that there is no one correct and indisputable selection. What is included in core lists reflects subjective judgment. At present, it would be difficult to achieve a consensus on any specific title. One suspects that some of the popularity of core lists stems from a desire to escape the responsibility of exercising professional library judgment in specific situations.

PRACTICAL CONSIDERATIONS

Some practical guidance can be given with respect to what should be contained within the "ideal" CHI collection. Rather than specifying a list of specific titles, it is more profitable to identify a number of basic categories of materials that should be considered in constructing a CHI collection. Within these major categories, it is possible to list alternate selections of similar and comparable publications. The precise selection will vary according to the available budget, user needs, and individual preferences.

BASIC COLLECTION CATEGORIES

The 13 basic collection categories listed below reflect the usage patterns and question-asking behavior of consumers. Heavy emphasis is necessarily placed upon identifying materials that can respond to user questions relating to signs, symptoms, identification, description, treatment, and prognosis of diseases and syndromes; degrees, licensure and specialty qualifications of physicians; general usage, dosages, side effects, and adverse reactions of drugs; meaning and interpretation of medical tests; health costs and insurance coverage; and alternative medicine. In addition, a number of professional and popular journals are listed together with indexing services that provide subject access. A convenient source of pamphlet materials is also given. The 13 collection categories are:

• Terminology and Definitions
• Provider Qualifications
• Diagnosis and Clinical Medical Practice
• Drug Information
• Alternative Medicine
• Popular Health Guides
• Medical Tests
• Health-Care Costs and Insurance
• Nutrition
• Popular Magazines and Newsletters
• Professional Journals
• Indexing Services
• Pamphlets

1. Terminology and Definitions

American Medical Association. *CMIT: Current Medical Information & Terminology.* 5th ed. Chicago: American Medical Association, 1981. $24.
Dorland's Illustrated Medical Dictionary. 27th rev. ed. Philadelphia: Saunders, 1988. $42.
Glanze, Walter D., ed. *Mosby's Medical & Nursing Dictionary.* 2nd ed. St Louis: Mosby, 1986. $22.95.
Magalini, Sergio and Scrascia, Euclide. *Dictionary of Medical Syndromes.* 2nd ed. Philadelphia: Lippincott, 1981. $59.50.

2. Provider Qualifications

American Board of Medical Specialties. *ABMS Compendium of Certified Medical Specialists.* 2nd ed. 7 vols. Evanston, IL: American Board of Medical Specialties, 1988–1989. $240.

American Medical Directory: Directory of Physicians in the United States. 31st ed. 4 vols. Chicago: American Medical Association, 1989. $400.

Directory of Medical Specialists. 24th ed. 3 vols. Wilmette, IL: Marquis Who's Who, 1989-1990. $295.

3. Diagnosis and Clinical Medical Practice

Berkow, Robert, ed. *The Merck Manual of Diagnosis and Treatment.* 15th ed. Rahway, NJ: Merck, 1987. $21.50.

Braunwald, Eugene and others. *Harrison's Principles of Internal Medicine.* 11th ed. 2 vols. New York: McGraw-Hill, 1987. $110.

Sabiston, David C., ed. *Textbook of Surgery: The Biological Basis of Modern Surgical Practice.* 13th ed. 2 vols. Philadelphia: Saunders, 1986. $129.75.

Schroeder, Steven A., Krupp, Marcus, and Tierney, Lawrence. *Current Medical Diagnosis & Treatment, 1989.* Norwalk, CT: Appleton & Lange, 1989. $32.50.

Wyngaarden, James B. and Smith, Lloyd H., eds. *Cecil Textbook of Medicine.* 18th ed. 2 vols. Philadelphia: Saunders, 1988. $124.25.

4. Drug Information

American Medical Association. *Drug Evaluations.* 7th ed. Chicago: American Medical Association, 1986. $81.

PDR: Physicians' Desk Reference. 44th ed. Oradell, NJ: Medical Economics, 1990. Annual. $39.95.

USP-DI. Volume II. *Advice for the Patient: Drug Information in Lay Language.* Rockville, MD: United States Pharmacopeial Convention, 1989.

United States Pharmacopeia Drug Information for the Consumer. 1990 ed. New York: Consumer Reports, 1988. $27.95.

5. Alternative Medicine

Campbell, A.H., ed. *Natural Health Handbook.* Secaucus, NJ: Chartwell Books, 1984. $13.99.

Grossman, Richard. *The Other Medicines.* Garden City, NY: Doubleday, 1985. $10.95.

Tyler, Varro. *The New Honest Herbal: A Sensible Guide to the Use of Herbs and Related Remedies.* Philadelphia: George F. Stickley, 1987. $18.95.

6. Popular Health Guides

Kunz, Jeffrey, ed. *The American Medical Association Family Medical Guide.* New York: Random House, 1987. $29.95.

Tapley, Donald T. and others, eds. *The Columbia University College of Physicians and Surgeons Complete Medical Guide.* New York: Consumer Reports, 1990. $27.95.

Vickery, Donald M. and Fries, James. *Take Care of Yourself: A Consumer's Guide to Medical Care.* 3rd ed. Reading, MA: Addison-Wesley, 1986. $14.38.

7. Medical Tests

Pinckney, Cathey and Pinckney, Edward R. *The Patient's Guide to Medical Tests.* 3rd ed. New York: Facts on File, 1987. $12.95.

Sobel, David S. and Ferguson, Tom. *The People's Book of Medical Tests.* New York: Summit, 1985. $12.95.

8. Health Care Costs and Insurance

Budish, Armond. *Avoiding the Medicaid Trap: How to Beat the Catastrophic Costs of Nursing Home Care.* New York: Holt, 1989. $18.95.

Hogue, Kathleen, Jensen, Cheryl, and Urban, Kathleen McClury. *The Complete Guide to Health Insurance: How to Beat the High Cost of Being Sick.* New York: Walker, 1988. $24.95.

Inlander, Charles and MacKay, Charles. *Medicare Made Easy.* Reading, MA: Addison-Wesley, 1989. $10.95.

9. Nutrition

Brody, Jane E. *Jane Brody's Nutrition Book: A Lifetime Guide to Better Health and Weight Control.* New York: Bantam, 1987. $12.95.

Carper, Jean. *Jean Carper's Total Nutritional Guide.* New York: Bantam, 1987. $12.95.

Conner, Sonja and Conner, William E. *The New American Diet.* New York: Simon & Schuster, 1986. $18.95.

Yetiv, Jack Zeev. *Popular Nutritional Practices: A Scientific Appraisal.* San Carlos, CA: Popular Medicine Press, 1986. $17.95.

10. Popular Magazines and Newsletters

American Health. American Health Partners. $12. Bi-monthly.

Environmental Nutrition. Environmental Nutrition Inc. $36. Bi-monthly.

FDA Consumer. Superintendent of Documents. $19. 10/year.

Health. Family Media Inc. $15. Monthly.

Health Facts. Center for Medical Consumers Inc. $18. Monthly.

Health Letter. The Public Citizen Health Research Group. $18. Monthly.
Health Tips. California Medical Association. Free. Five topics monthly.
In-Health. Hippocrates Inc. $18. Bi-monthly.
Mayo Clinic Nutrition Letter. Mayo Clinic. $24. Monthly.
Nutrition Action Health Letter. Center for Science in the Public Interest. $20.
    10/year.
PPR: The Child Health Newsletter. Parents' Pediatric Report. $35. 11/year.
Peoples' Medical Society Newsletter. People's Medical Society. $15. Bi-monthly.
Prevention. Rodale Press. $12. Monthly.
University of California Berkeley Wellness Letter. University of California, Berke-
    ley. $20. Monthly.

11. Professional Journals

JAMA: The Journal of the American Medical Association. 48 issues. $66.
New England Journal of Medicine. Weekly. $74.

12. Indexing Services

Abridged Index Medicus. Monthly. $43.
Consumer Health & Nutrition Index. Quarterly. Phoenix: Oryx Press. $89.50.
Health Index Plus. Information Access Company. CD-ROM. $5,000.
Medical Abstracts Newsletter. Monthly. Teaneck, NJ: Communi-Ti Publications.
    $24.95.

13. Pamphlets

CHIS—The Consumer Health Information Service. 1989-1990. Ann Arbor, MI:
    University Microfilms International, 1989. $195.

ELECTRONIC DATABASES

The purchase of compact disc versions of databases often is charged
to the collections budget. A decision has to be made whether, for example, to acquire a CD-ROM version of Medline. This will depend on the
volume of anticipated usage and the extent to which it is necessary to
search the professional literature. In most consumer health library situations, the number of times that such searches are performed is limited.
In special situations, such as at the New York Academy of Medicine,
Medline on CD-ROM is offered on a self-service basis and is well used.

The availability of Information Access Company's *Health Index Plus*,
a user-friendly database on CD-ROM, offers a great potential for consumer health libraries. This index provides access to the full text of more
than 100 popular magazines and newsletters and a number of professional

journals. An expanded version of *Health Index Plus* is IAC's *Health Reference Center*, which in addition contains CD-ROM consumer summaries of select articles in a number of professional journals, the full text of several medical reference books, and disease summaries. Yet the cost of $6,000 for *Health Index Plus* and $12,000 for *Health Reference Center* place them beyond the reach of most consumer health library budgets, which will probably continue to rely upon printed subject indexes such as the *Consumer Health & Nutrition Index* ($89.50) and subscriptions to a select number of magazines and newsletters. The cost of subscribing to all of the 100 popular journals covered by *Health Index Plus* and the *Consumer Health & Nutrition Index* is no more than $2,000. In the hospital environment, *Health Reference Center* has great promise as a support of patient and health education programs.

CONCLUSION

The selection of materials in the field of medicine poses some formidable challenges. Much of the material published is of questionable value and verges on the fraudulent. While it is easy to detect outright quackery, many publications are ostensibly plausible. A large number of authors have dubious qualifications which at best are not relevant to the topic discussed. Such opportunistic authors, lured by the size of the consumer market, pander to the public's insatiable desire for rapid results, painless cures, magic potions, and quick fixes. One must also guard against the militant crusaders motivated by missionary zeal to promote their cause. Another challenge lies in the rapid obsolescence of the library collection. Much of the material published becomes rapidly outdated in the light of medical research and discovery with the result that the necessity to weed becomes urgent.

In selecting the optimal mix of materials to comprise a consumer health collection, there is little that is mechanical, routine, or unexciting. The challenge is ever present to keep up with the swiftly moving frontiers of medicine on the one hand and the increasing sophistication of library users on the other.

REFERENCES

1. Wortman, William A. *Collection Management: Background and Principles.* Chicago: American Library Association, 1989. 15.

2. Evans, G. Edward. *Developing Library and Information Center Collections.* Littleton, CO: Libraries Unlimited, 1987. 13–14.

3. Broadus, Robert N. *Selecting Materials for Libraries.* New York: H.W. Wilson, 1981. 30.

4. Katz, William. *Collection Development: The Selection of Materials for Libraries.* New York: Holt, 1980.

5. Wortman, William A. *Collection Management: Background and Principles.* 10–11.

6. Katz, William. *Collection Development: The Selection of Materials for Libraries.* 3.

7. Katz, William. *Collection Development: The Selection of Materials for Libraries.* 16–19.

8. Rees, Alan M. "Characteristics, Content, and Significance of the Popular Health Periodicals Literature." *Bulletin of the Medical Library Association.* 75 (4), October 1987. 317–22.

9. "Health Magazines and Newsletters" in Rees, Alan M. and Hoffman, Catherine. *The Consumer Health Information Source Book.* 3rd ed. Phoenix: Oryx Press, 1990. Chapter 5. 43–52.

10. *Special Report: Quackery and the Elderly.* New York: American Council on Science and Health, 1990. 1.

11. Rees, Alan M. and Hoffman, Catherine. *The Consumer Health Information Source Book.* Phoenix: Oryx Press, 1990.

12. Jarvis, William. "Book Review: Love, Medicine and Miracles." *NCAHF Newsletter.* 12 (40), July/August 1989. 2.

13. Moon, Eric. "View from the Front." *Library Journal.* 89, February 1, 1964. 57.

14. Courtney, Diane and others. *Consumer Health Information: Basic Reference List.* Brooklyn, NY: N.Y. Metropolitan Reference and Research Library Agency (Metro.) METRO Miscellaneous Publication No. 39. 1988. 12p.

15. "Medical Reference Tools for the Layperson." Reference Books Bulletin. *Booklist.* December 1, 1988. 620–24.

16. Bryant, Moira. *A Guide to Consumer Health Information.* Westmead, Australia: Westmead Hospital HealthLink, 1988. 52p.

CHAPTER 18
Reference Sources and Services

Claudia A. Perry

With the heightened interest in health issues nationwide, reference queries on health topics are on the increase. While most reference librarians in public libraries lack a background in the health sciences, many medical reference queries from the lay public tend to fall into fairly predictable categories that do not require extensive subject expertise. Knowing what to expect should help generalist librarians meet many of their users' health information needs.

This chapter is intended for the reference librarian in the public library or general academic library setting. It will discuss the role of the librarian, the reference interview, types of users and questions, reference sources and referrals, and the reference policy. Chapter 7 on "Community Access to Health Information: The Role of the New York Academy of Medicine" addresses the provision of reference service to the public in the context of a medical library setting.

Medical information is available both in sources geared to the health professional and in those written specifically for the health consumer. The quantity and quality of health-related materials written for the lay public have increased substantially in recent years. These titles are much easier for the average user to understand, but even the most authoritative work for a general audience must necessarily lag behind the publication of professional medical titles. Ideas filter down from the professional to the popular literature. Sources geared to the lay public are likely to be concerned with more common disorders and established treatments, so those seeking information on new and alternative therapies or rare diseases may have no choice but to consult the professional literature. There is undoubtedly a place for consumer health materials, particularly in a circulating collection, but it is this author's belief that standard medical works should also be found in every library. A basic list of recommended titles is included in the section below on reference sources, and the discussion which follows will assume the availability of many of these sources in the reference collection.

MEDICAL QUESTIONS AND THE ROLE OF THE REFERENCE LIBRARIAN

There are probably more similarities than differences in the handling of medical and general reference queries. While larger and more specialized medical libraries will always have the advantage of a better selection of sources from which to choose, this same size advantage holds true for almost any type of question. Staff at smaller libraries must refer a great many reference queries on a wide range of topics to other sites or organizations. At the same time, careful interviewing and the creative use of standard reference works can be a major help in pointing users in the right direction. One should not underestimate the proportion of questions which can be at least partially answered with the help of a medical dictionary and the *Encyclopedia of Associations.*

Katz defined the reference interview as "a dialogue between someone in need of information and someone—the librarian—able to give assistance in finding it."[1] This characterization of the reference role is as important to bear in mind when answering medical reference questions as it is in any other library context. Experienced reference librarians have usually developed a set of skills in eliciting user requirements, clarifying the reference question, and then interpreting the query so that it can be answered using the available sources. Librarians are not, and should not be expected to be, experts in law, medicine, gardening, or plumbing. Library staff often need to insist that they are not able to interpret medical information, diagnose an illness, or choose between two therapies. These activities are the responsibility of a health-care professional. Adherence to such professional limitations is no different than refusing to recommend a particular car model for purchase or refusing to advise clients on their legal rights. Rather, the librarian's objective is to be viewed as helping users to find the information they need. This is a major challenge in itself.

The standard approaches used by a reference librarian are quite similar whether or not a question relates to health issues. Nonetheless, it is important to note that the volume of medical literature is vast and growing faster than that of many other subjects. Keeping up with medical advances is a daunting task for most health professionals, and it is not surprising that members of the lay public often need assistance navigating through the mass of information currently available. Fortunately, bibliographic access to the professional medical literature is among the best developed in any field of knowledge, and new access and delivery mechanisms are being introduced at an unprecedented rate. These continuing innovations promise to make it increasingly easy to find medical information. In addition, new publications specifically geared to the layperson are making it simpler for nonspecialists to identify and understand relevant materials. But, regardless of the availability and quality of source material, the role of the librarian in assisting users will remain important.

THE REFERENCE INTERVIEW

Just as in any reference interaction, librarians faced with a medical question must try to understand what the client actually wants or needs to know. This task requires the librarian to determine who is asking the question, the intended use of the information, and his or her present state of understanding and knowledge. Although stereotyping should be avoided, the categorization of different types of users and their queries provides a useful way to begin to develop a reference strategy. Different groups will have particular concerns, time constraints, and requirements which can substantially affect their information seeking behavior, the amount and depth of information desired, and the ways in which they can best be assisted. These individual differences must be carefully ascertained during the reference interview.

In the *Handbook of Medical Library Practice,* Lucretia McClure lists some of the goals of the reference interview. Among the information to be gathered during the interview process are the following:

1. Clear definition of the question.
2. Motivation and objectives of the user.
3. What the user already knows about the subject; his or her ability to suggest synonyms or other terms for the disease, process, drug, or the like.
4. What the user needs to know about the subject; how to narrow the question if a great deal of information is available; how to broaden the scope if little information is available.
5. Sources already consulted by the user, if any.
6. Status of the user.
7. Amount and level of material needed.
8. When the information is needed.
9. Time period to be covered.
10. Languages acceptable to the user.
11. Form in which the answer is expected.[2]

While the above list was generated specifically for a medical library setting, it is a valuable checklist for all reference professionals. In using this framework, several differences between health professional library users and lay library users should be borne in mind.

To a much larger extent than those with a medical background, lay clients may not have a clear idea of what information is needed, how much information is available on the topic, or even if the words they are using are spelled correctly. The client's lack of knowledge may require the librarian to engage in active detective work. In what part of the body is this disorder observed? Does it affect a particular age group? What condition was the drug prescribed to treat? With careful questioning, it may be possible to match clues and identify the nature of the problem involved, but if the spelling of a drug name or disease is ambiguous, library staff should insist that the client verify the information with his or her physician or pharmacist. Medical terminology can be confusing, so it is better to verify facts than to risk presenting a client with the wrong information.

Just as in the general reference situation, inquiries for health information are often couched in excessively general terms. Katz comments, "this is such a normal condition of the reference interview that too many librarians fail to consider its implications. The interview, at least from the point of view of the user, should be of assistance not only in finding an answer, but in formulating the question itself."[3] The user who states, "I'd like to read all the information you have on heart disease" may really be concerned with the impact of diet on cholesterol levels. By elaborating upon a request and responding to careful questioning, the client may be able to provide the librarian with a clearer sense of the information sought. The negotiation of the reference question can be viewed as a collaboration in which both the librarian and the client play an active and equally important role. Taylor differentiates between four progressive levels of question formation in the library context. These range from the initial visceral need, to the conscious, the formalized, and finally the compromised need. "At the fourth level the question is recast in anticipation of what the files can deliver. The searcher must think in terms of the organization of particular files and of the discrete packages available—books, reports, papers, drawings, tables, etc."[4] Although the client will have the best sense of what it is that he or she needs to know, the reference librarian usually knows far more about what information is likely to exist and how to locate it. Many clients underestimate the volume of health information available. In such a case the initial question may need to be reworked to avoid an overwhelming deluge of information. The volume of medical information is so large that it is literally impossible, for example, to fill a request for everything there is to know about cancer.

Alternatively, a query may be couched in terms so specific that answers are not likely to be found. It may not be possible to find out the average cost of a gall bladder operation in New York City, but statistics for the eastern part of the United States may be available. Statistical queries are a prime example of the sort of question which may have to be substantially amended so that they can be accommodated with respect to available library resources, no matter how extensive the collection may be. Statistics for very specific geographic areas or very recent periods of time are unlikely to be available in print. Clients can be referred to appropriate agencies or organizations which may maintain files of such data, but the information required may not yet be published for general distribution.

Further, the cognitive and educational levels of the individual, as well as the depth of subject knowledge, may well affect the nature of the questions which are asked and the way in which the reference librarian can answer requests. Individuals with little knowledge of a topic frequently require background information before they can ascertain what it is they really want to know. Librarians who have taken the time to clearly understand the needs and expectations of their clients will be more effective in helping users clarify their needs and thereby identify the most appropriate information.

GENERAL REFERENCE TECHNIQUES

The same interview techniques useful in the general reference interview are appropriate when handling medical queries. Katz reviewed the use of "open" questions, expanding the "closed" query, using a "why" question, making the person feel at ease, and listening, among other approaches.[5] Sensitivity to the client and attentive listening are particularly important when dealing with very personal requests. The client may be reluctant to provide potentially embarrassing details, particularly if others are waiting to consult with the librarian. Clients may feel more comfortable talking about their questions away from the reference desk. Locating a ready reference health collection within sight of the reference desk, yet sufficiently removed so that it provides some privacy, may be a way of encouraging this sort of usage.

One must be careful not to appear intrusive, but knowing the intended use of the information can be an important factor to consider in negotiating the reference query and formulating a search strategy. A patient contemplating surgery would certainly want the most recent materials available, while a malpractice attorney would be interested in the state of the literature at a particular point in time. A student writing an extensive research paper on a drug would probably need to consult the journal literature, while a parent concerned about the adverse effects of aspirin on children would be well-served with a drug handbook. Intended use can affect the recency and amount of material needed, as well as the degree of detail and the level of sophistication which are most appropriate.

It is usually helpful to determine how much the requester already knows about the topic, as well as the date and source of that information. This provides an important starting point for the research, particularly if it is a topic unfamiliar to the librarian. One might ask if the client has already visited any other libraries, or consulted any other sources. Were these useful? What other types of materials might now be appropriate? Is it necessary to find more current information, or is information needed in greater depth? Although it is difficult to generalize, one might expect that a user who has already visited another library or libraries has established an information base on which to build, while those who have just begun their information search may need to start with more fundamental sources. At the same time, just because clients have made the effort to visit a larger library following a trip to the local branch library does not necessarily mean they have actually used the more basic sources available and are ready for more specialized titles. In referring a client to another library, subsequent interactions would be facilitated if the referring librarian recorded what sources have already been consulted.

If neither the client nor the librarian know much about the topic, some background reading is in order. *The Merck Manual of Diagnosis and Therapy,* a medical dictionary, or a basic medical textbook like *Cecil Textbook of Medicine* can provide an information base on which to build. Finding (or not finding) an entry in one of these works can provide a sense of how common or rare a condition might be, how much information there might be about it, and where else information is likely to be found.

Readers' satisfaction with the information provided in the *Merck Manual* can reflect their understanding of medical language and the degree of detail which may be appropriate for their needs, particularly if they are having trouble explaining what they want. The *Merck Manual* uses accurate medical terminology but it is clearly and concisely written, and understandable to a fair proportion of general library users. One might ask, for example, "Is this the sort of information you were looking for, or do you need something a little easier to understand? Do you need more specific information than we find here?" From user reactions, the librarian may be better able to gauge a reader's expectations and capabilities. One who understands the entries in the *Merck Manual* may be prepared to read a more specialized medical textbook or articles in the professional journal literature, perhaps with the aid of a medical dictionary. One who finds it confusing will probably be better satisfied with a title from the consumer health literature. Alternatively, the librarian may wish to begin with a comprehensive lay source, such as the *American Medical Association Family Medical Guide*, or the *Columbia University College of Physicians and Surgeons Complete Home Medical Guide*, and from there progress to more specialized sources. In any case, the interaction should be considered an ongoing one.

Conducting research on health-related topics can be time-consuming and sometimes difficult, so it is especially important for librarians to check back with users to see if additional help is needed, and to encourage them to return for more assistance as appropriate. The librarian might suggest several titles initially, while perhaps considering alternative strategies should the initial suggestions prove inadequate.

If specific titles on a topic do not immediately come to mind, beginning the interaction with one or more medical textbooks or comprehensive health titles geared to the consumer at least signals to the reader that the librarian is trying to be helpful. As already mentioned, these sources can provide useful background information which can help the requester to further refine the question and the librarian to plan an appropriate strategy. Such an approach can be especially important for librarians in the early stages of developing their expertise on health-related topics.

After consulting a comprehensive source, the search may be extended in a number of ways. A more detailed overview may be available in a specialty textbook, a specialized consumer title, or in a monograph on the topic. Depending on the needs of the requester, these sources may be quite sufficient. One should be aware that in view of delays in publication and the rapid rate of progress in the field of medicine, books by their very nature are outdated as soon as they are published. If currency is an issue, an additional step will be required. This involves recourse to journals.

As in most of the sciences, the journal literature plays an extremely important role in medicine. If the most current information available is needed, the client will have to consult indexes to the periodical literature, such as *Index Medicus* or *Cumulative Index to Nursing and Allied Health Literature*. Due to the availability of abstracts and the capacity for browsing, access to a CD-ROM version of Medline (the online form of *Index Medicus*) can be of particular assistance. This is discussed below in the section "Online and CD-ROM Sources.")

While some of the journal literature of medicine is indeed intimidating, many of the periodical titles geared to nurses and family practitioners can be readily understood by the lay public. Review articles even in more specialized journals often offer an accessible and up-to-date overview of a particular topic which can be extremely useful to the layperson. Review articles are listed in a special section in the printed *Index Medicus*, and can be specifically identified in Medline.

Even if the journal collection of the library is limited in size, identifying relevant articles on the topic of interest can be an important step in meeting the client's information needs. Of course, if this is to be helpful, librarians must be prepared to assist users in obtaining copies of the articles from other libraries or through interlibrary loan. Librarians may also need to educate their users so that they do not expect instantaneous answers to their medical questions. It may help to mention that even in the largest medical libraries, referrals and interlibrary loans are often necessary because of the vast size of the literature.

TYPES OF USERS

Lay clients with inquiries concerning medical topics typically fall into three broad groups: students, those engaged in work-related research, and those seeking information for personal reasons. Members of the first two groups will often state their requirements directly: "I'm writing a report on alcoholism," or "I need to find everything that's been written by Dr. John Smith," for example. The third group—patients or family members of patients—may have more difficulty explaining their needs to a librarian. Such individuals may be reluctant to reveal potentially embarrassing personal information to a stranger, and may be less sure what it is that they need to know.

Student Users

The explosion of interest in health-related topics throughout the culture seems to have been reflected in students' choices for research projects. Katz remarked that "in almost any type of library the student population constitutes from 50 to 80 percent of the users"[6] so it is scarcely surprising that students, ranging from grade school through graduate school, form one of the largest single groups seeking medical information. Students may be looking for quick answers to factual questions, researching a paper, or possibly both. If writing a paper, they may be required to include specific types of references in their bibliographies (e.g., five recent articles, no more than three books), which may severely limit the permissible sources that can be used. They are typically under time pressures, and may need assistance in narrowing a topic so that it can be reasonably handled within the designated time. While many clients may underestimate the volume of health information, students in particular may need to rework their initial question so that it can be accommodated within the resources of the library and the constraints of their project. It may be necessary to demonstrate the magnitude of the literature in order to convince some individuals that it is just not possible to summarize the state of knowledge on a topic like AIDS in 10 pages or less.

As with any assistance to students, the librarian must bear in mind the educational function of a research assignment in that an important reason for such a project is the development of library skills. More than with other groups, it is important that students be instructed in the use of a source so that they can conduct their own research. Even if the reference tool is difficult to use, the librarian should not be expected to find the answer, but rather to assist the student in finding it. While this approach may appear to be time-consuming, the skills learned should be transferable so that in the long-run both students and librarians will be better served by such a philosophy. It is recommended that the type and levels of service provided to different categories of users should be specified in the library's reference policy, and in particular that service levels to students be addressed.

Work-Related Research Users

Representatives of corporations conducting research for an employer form another substantial category of seekers of health information. Health is big business, not only for those directly concerned with the delivery of health care, but in many cognate areas as well. Publishers, writers, attorneys, marketing consultants, medical equipment manufacturers, personnel directors, social workers, representatives of advertising firms and insurance companies, and nonprofit agencies may all have occasion to seek health information in the library. While these various individuals may have vastly different needs, they often share certain characteristics.

Corporate representatives may be several steps removed from the original requester of the information and under severe time pressures. Without a full understanding of the reference question, they may have a tendency to focus on specific words or phrases rather than on terms of equivalent meaning. Accustomed to certain levels of service in their corporate libraries, business clients may expect librarians to conduct extensive research on their behalf. In response, librarians may need to be more assertive than usual in dealing with requests from the business sector, and to develop specific policies guiding their handling of such requests.

More than other groups, business clients are likely to be willing to pay fees for such specialized assistance, which is usually needed on a rush basis. Corporate users may be especially interested in requesting a mediated online bibliographic search or in obtaining photocopies of specific articles. Time is apt to be a more important consideration than cost in meeting their requirements. The increasing availability of fax machines in libraries and businesses may intensify the pressure for an immediate response. If the library has not developed a fee-for-service component, it may be useful for reference staff to compile a referral list of individuals or organizations that supply such specialized services.

The nature of the information needs of business users is also often distinctive. In contrast to students, for example, an attorney's request for *everything* that is known about the adverse effects of a drug or procedure may be precisely what is required for use in a malpractice case. Obtaining such a large volume of information is a separate problem, but it is important to be able to differentiate between those instances where comprehensiveness is an actual requirement, and those where a general request stems from a lack of precision. Malpractice attorneys often need older information dating from the time of the incident that forms the focus of the lawsuit. This requirement is in contrast to those of most other users, who usually need more current information. Consequently, the characteristics and needs of the library's user population can affect not only collection development decisions but also retention policies. Libraries serving a large population of malpractice lawyers might wish to ensure that superseded editions of important medical texts are retained rather than discarded.

Other groups have their own special needs. Writers and representatives of publishing firms may need to verify difficult bibliographic citations or track down the address and phone number of the publisher of a particular book or journal for permission to reproduce a chart or illustration. Advertising firms may need to verify a particular claim for the efficacy of a drug to use in a product advertisement. Marketing consultants may seek statistics on the prevalence of a specific disease, or lists of names and addresses of medical specialists. Some of these types of requests are not strictly health-related, but they may be perceived as such.

Some clients may not realize that the publisher of a medical book or journal, for example, will be listed in standard directories, and will claim they have a medical request. In such a case, the library may have only the most basic collection of medical sources, and yet will be able to answer the question by looking in a title such as *Books in Print* or the *Serials Directory.* Answers to other frequent "medical" questions may also be found in standard nonmedical reference sources. The *Encyclopedia of Associations* can provide the addresses and phone numbers of organizations that may supply health-related statistics or that publish and sell membership directories of medical groups. Other questions frequently received from the corporate sector may be at least partially answered with the help of the Yellow Pages, the *United States Government Manual,* the *Statistical Abstract of the United States,* or a variety of business sources. An important point is that librarians should not assume that the requests of business clients cannot be handled by the library simply because the collection of medical titles is limited, nor that business clients will know best which source will meet their needs, despite what they may claim.

Clarifying the initial query is extremely important, particularly in those instances where the individual delegated to visit the library has only the vaguest sense of what information is needed. An extreme example of such a scenario would be when a messenger arrives at the library equipped only with a request, scribbled on a scrap of paper, which the librarian is expected to fill. As is the case with students, a clearly articulated reference policy can help to guide decisions on how much assistance library staff should be expected to provide the corporate library user.

Personal Users

A third major category of requesters are those who seek health information for personal reasons. These may include patients concerned with a particular medical problem, friends and family members of a patient, and individuals who have an interest in a topic. A diagnosis may lead individuals to seek information concerning the likely course of a disease, alternative treatments, or specialists to consult for a second opinion. Friends and relatives may wish to gain a better understanding of a patient's disease, or explore ways in which they can help someone adjust to a health problem. Announcements on television or radio, or articles in newspapers and magazines, frequently prompt clients to read more about a particular health topic.

This latter group of requests can be alternately one of the easiest to satisfy or one of the most frustrating. A large proportion of the news stories reported in the media are taken from either *JAMA* (*Journal of the American Medical Association*) or the *New England Journal of Medicine*. For this reason it is strongly recommended that libraries make an effort to subscribe to these titles. Unfortunately, newspeople are usually reporting from a press release or prepublication copy of the most recent issue of these journals, which is unlikely to be received by the library for several days. If the client wants to read the full article on the same day that it was reported in the media, the *New England Journal of Medicine* is available in an online full-text format through BRS Information Technologies. Otherwise, he or she will have to wait until the library's copy is received and processed.

In other cases it will not be so clear as to when a particular news story was announced. It is much easier to track down an important recent research study if the client brings in a copy of the source in which it was quoted, than if it is known only that there was a radio report about a new treatment for a disease several weeks ago. In anticipation of such requests, it may be useful to maintain a clipping file of current health news stories, and to keep a copy of the most recent issues of these two major medical journals on reserve at the reference desk.

Most articles in newspapers and in popular magazines do not provide the full citation of research studies when reporting on medical topics. An article at most may refer to "a recent study by Dr. Sally Smith in the *Annals of Internal Medicine.*" Without knowing the lag time in publication of the popular magazines in which the medical paper was mentioned, it can be quite difficult to track down the original source. Authors' conceptions of "recent" may vary considerably, or the research study may not yet have been indexed in the medical literature. Even if the journal has been indexed in an online source, there is generally a delay of several months between online availability and the publication of a citation in printed indexes such as *Index Medicus*. Then too, the client's memory of the news story may be faulty. A ready reference search of Medline is probably the easiest way to determine if a citation can be readily identified. This type of question is tailor-made for the use of a CD-ROM version of Medline. If the citation cannot be found quickly, the client may be best advised to wait several months and then to try scanning the indexes again. If the library does not have an extensive journal collection, the reference librarian should be prepared to refer clients to other libraries once a citation has been identified, or to make information available concerning interlibrary loan policies and procedures.

Although clients often want to track down a specific research report, book, or article, particularly if it contains information on a very recent development in medicine, in other cases a general overview or similar document on the same topic will suffice. Such requests may be handled in much the same manner as inquiries from patients.

The reference interview is important for most reference inquiries, but particularly so with patients and family members. Patients may remember only a portion of what their physician has told them,[7] or may carry only a misspelled diagnosis or drug name recorded on a slip of paper. They may be distressed about a particular diagnosis or reticent to reveal personal details. More likely, however, they are anxious to know more about their problem and will be extremely grateful for whatever assistance the librarian can provide. Studies have indicated that many patients are dissatisfied with the amount of information they receive from their doctors,[8] which leads them to seek information elsewhere. Some may be frustrated because of their difficulties in obtaining appropriate information, but others are highly motivated to find out whatever they can, even if the information is difficult for them to understand.

As mentioned earlier, it is first necessary to clarify the question. If the information cannot be readily found in a standard medical text, the correct terminology may become apparent by cross-checking such details as the part of the body affected with the name of the drug or disease or by scanning key words in a CD-ROM version of Medline. If the terminology is in doubt, the client should verify the information with his or her health-care professional.

Reference interviews with patients and family members are often best conducted away from the reference desk to afford some privacy in the interaction. Librarians should strive to convey a courteous, concerned, and professional manner, especially when dealing with sensitive topics. Requesting information on the treatment and implications of a sexually transmitted disease like genital warts, or a urological problem like penile induration, may be rendered less difficult for the user if the librarian responds with a nonjudgmental, matter-of-fact approach, while still conveying the desire to be helpful. Finding an initial source, and using that as a springboard for further discussion, can be one way of defusing a potentially difficult interaction. By focusing on the text, librarian and client may be able to deal more easily with personal details. If the client is still hesitant to discuss the problem, the librarian might wish to suggest a number of potentially relevant sources, perhaps at varying levels of difficulty and specificity, which can be perused by the user in private. Grouping together a collection of health-related reference titles, which clients can browse without asking for specific assistance, may also help the client who is uncomfortable in verbalizing his or her information need.

In some reference interactions, clients may claim that information is needed for a friend. While at times this seems to be a cover to prevent embarrassment concerning sensitive topics, in other instances it is undoubtedly true. Working people or the homebound may have problems in visiting the library, particularly if hours are limited, and may ask a friend or family member to visit the library on their behalf. Libraries located in cities with large immigrant populations may be used by those seeking information for relatives in other countries. Moreover, many individuals wish to learn more about a friend or relative's illness simply for their own peace of mind. Even if one suspects that the "friend" approach is merely a ruse, this need not substantially change the handling of the interaction. The client's statements should be taken at face value, although one might also wish to provide every opportunity for privacy.

Delegated searches for information are inherently more difficult than interactions directly with the actual requester of the information. Just as with corporate representatives, individuals conducting research for a friend may know little about the reference question. In such cases it is often difficult to determine what information is needed, how much, and whether the information identified has answered the user's actual question. It may prove useful for the visitor to photocopy selected sections from a number of titles, and to be certain to note the identifying bibliographic information on each photocopy as well as what sources were searched. Relevant circulating materials, if available, can supplement reference sources. The librarian might also wish to provide the names, addresses, and telephone numbers of organizations that may be able to furnish additional information in the event that insufficient information has been identified. Even with a delegated query, attempts should be made to determine the client's characteristics and purpose in seeking information.

REFERENCE SOURCES

Space limits the discussion of specific sources in this chapter. A selection of standard reference sources that should prove useful in answering many of the more common health-related questions encountered in libraries is listed in Appendix I. Annotations describing each of these titles, their use, and relative merits have appeared elsewhere,[9] and may be supplemented by information in a number of professional sources.[10] The reader is also referred to the *Consumer Health Information Source Book,* 3rd edition, for additional valuable suggestions from the consumer health literature.[11]

The titles are grouped by type of source, and certain titles are starred for first purchase. In many cases, particularly for smaller libraries, purchase of one source within a category should be sufficient to handle a fair proportion of questions within its scope, although many sources listed in a particular category are complementary in their coverage. The list emphasizes professional medical sources over consumer health sources, and should not be viewed as comprehensive.

ONLINE AND CD-ROM SOURCES

The increasing availability of a wide variety of health-related materials in online and CD-ROM formats is an invaluable aid to the reference librarian in every size library. Although cost may be a limiting factor, online availability permits library staff to access sources which may be requested too infrequently to justify purchase, vastly extending the scope of the collection. Furthermore, the health-related databases produced by the National Library of Medicine (e.g., Medline, Dirline, Toxline, Health Planning and Administration, Bioethicsline) tend to be relatively inexpensive when compared with databases in other fields.

A useful overview of relevant databases is provided by Jo Anne Boorkman,[12] although new sources are announced regularly. The coverage of medical databases provided by BRS Information Technologies is particularly extensive. These include databases of the professional medical literature, such as Medline and the full text of *New England Journal of Medicine,* as well as those sources more geared to the layperson, such as CHID (Consumer Health Information Database). A recent entry into the field is Health Periodicals Database (HPD), produced by Information Access Company (IAC) and available online through DIALOG and CompuServe. A CD-ROM version of the database is called Health Index Plus. HPD indexes an extremely wide range of health-related articles, from the professional literature as well as from popular health and general interest magazines. Many of the articles are available in full text. One expects that this and similar databases, particularly those available on-site in CD-ROM, will continue to grow in importance in the provision of health-related information in both public and academic library settings.

The costs of online access make it necessary to explicitly discuss the conditions of providing online reference service to clients, preferably in a reference services policy statement. Librarians will want to consider the issue of ready reference use of online sources as well as the handling of more extensive searches, possibly on a cost-recovery or fee-for-service basis. Regardless of one's perspective on the fee-for-service controversy, libraries that do not provide some mode of access to online sources in the 1990s—if only by referral to another library—are neglecting their responsibilities to their clientele.

The availability of health-related databases on CD-ROM can be a particular boon to both librarian and client. Medline was one of the first databases to be widely marketed in this format, and like its online counterpart, tends to be reasonably priced in comparison with other sources. Although one must commit to a fairly substantial investment of equipment and a database subscription, CD-ROM access removes the inhibiting "ticking clock" cost factor from each search interaction, and permits one to readily check the client's terminology in the initial stages of the reference interview. In this manner, one can easily identify synonyms and preferred Medical Subject Headings (MeSH), limit a broad concept to its constituent parts, or scan abstracts for a relevant article. Alternatively, if no mention can be found of a particular word, there is an excellent chance that it may be misspelled, and will need to be verified from the original source.

Medline on CD-ROM allows the client to browse through the medical literature far more quickly and easily than through printed indexes. The availability of abstracts provides immediate feedback on the potential relevance of an article, substantially reducing frustration. Online or CD-ROM access to Medline is also particularly useful in finding information on very new concepts, because of the capability of searching key words in addition to subject headings. CD-ROM Medline may be one of the single most valuable sources currently available for assisting the library client with health-related requests.

REFERRALS

As has been mentioned, no single library, particularly if its resources are limited, will be able to meet all the health-related information needs of its users alone. Consequently, an awareness of the resources of other libraries, organizations, and institutions is an essential aspect in reference assistance. *The Encyclopedia of Associations, United States Government Manual,* and Jean Carper's *Health Care U.S.A.* are valuable resources for referral information. Health-related organizations and government agencies often distribute free or inexpensive materials in their areas of interest. They may staff information hotlines and maintain files of hard-to-find statistics. The United States government collects a major portion of the health-related statistics publicly available, and also publishes a large number of health-related publications. This information will be available in U.S. Depository libraries, which are open to the general public by law.

Requests for physician referrals and credentials are among the most common health-related inquiries in libraries. Although often developed as a marketing strategy, hospital referral hotlines nonetheless can meet very real needs of prospective patients. Librarians distributing these numbers should note that physicians referred by these services are usually affiliated with the participating hospital, and that clients may wish to verify credentials independently. Hospitals may also staff information hotlines and maintain patient information centers which distribute free informational brochures. These can be useful as alternatives or supplements to the information found in the library.

As previously mentioned, well-developed interlibrary loan policies and procedures are often necessary if clients are to obtain copies of materials not held by their local library. Knowledge of collection strengths and access policies of nearby libraries, as well as the local availability of databases in CD-ROM format, can substantially extend the librarian's ability to assist clients. Reference staff may also wish to stay abreast of alternative sources for online searches, document delivery, and other fee-for-service assistance, particularly if these services are not offered by their own library.

REFERENCE SERVICE POLICIES

Reference policies are of importance in any library, for a variety of reasons which can only be briefly touched upon here. Different user groups may need various kinds of assistance. Students, for example, will benefit from a greater emphasis on instruction in library use, while clients with a one-time need may be better served by being provided with a specific answer to a question. Space does not permit an extensive discussion of the advantages and content of reference service policies, particularly since other sources[13] treat the subject in depth, but the availability of such a document may be especially valuable in the context of reference assistance on medical topics.

The difficulties that many clients experience in conducting research on medical topics may lead to expectations for more individualized assistance than library staff usually are able to provide. Business clients may be especially demanding and more willing than other groups to pay for service. Will the library provide extended reference for a fee? How much information should be provided to the homebound client who is unable to visit the library precisely because of his or her medical condition? Librarians should not discriminate, but various client groups do have very different needs which should be considered separately. Once written guidelines for reference assistance have been agreed upon, it is especially important that they be implemented consistently, so that clients who have been told by one staff member that they must conduct their own research, or that drug information is not provided over the telephone, are not able to cajole other librarians into providing such service. Failure to implement policy consistently can lead to a host of problems on subsequent interactions.

The costs associated with online searches and interlibrary loan, two services which are particularly important in meeting medical information needs, must be considered in decisions concerning the ways in which these services are to be made available. If services are provided for a fee, will rush requests be given priority over others, or will all requests be handled on a first-come, first-served basis? What sort of information will be provided over the telephone or by fax? For fear of misinterpretation, many libraries limit the types and amount of medical information provided over the telephone but place no restrictions on use of materials on-site. The availability of fax technology may reduce the problem of misinterpretation of information, but creates new pressures to provide specialized reference assistance that incurs costs. Most libraries charge for photocopies. Will they continue to do so if the photocopy is sent by fax? If so, how will money be collected?

Apart from costs and levels of service is the issue of content. Libraries are intended to encourage the free dissemination of information, but concerns over explicit medical illustrations or potentially alarming prognostic information may prompt some individuals to wish to censor these materials. Issues such as censorship, imposition of fees, and differential service levels are certainly not unique to medical reference, but they may be particularly noticeable or frequent in this context. Prior consideration of the types of issues which may arise in the reference interaction, and written guidelines concerning how they are to be handled, can be of vital importance in ensuring that appropriate and consistent levels of reference assistance are provided to all clients.

CONCLUSION

The provision of reference assistance to those seeking health-related information can be one of the most rewarding categories of service librarians can provide, and it is unlikely to decrease in importance in the years to come. While a basic knowledge of sources is of course helpful, most medical questions from the lay public do *not* require extensive subject expertise. In fact there are more similarities in the handling of medical and general reference queries than there are differences. But the vastness of the medical literature and the difficulties that many experience in conducting medical research do make the role of the reference librarian particularly important in this context.

Careful interviewing, an awareness of the different needs of various types of users, and the creative use of a basic collection of medical reference sources will help reference staff to respond to a large proportion of health-related inquiries. Some of these questions are likely to raise concerns about such issues as the levels of service to be provided to various client groups and the problems of cost involved with access to medical information, which can be anticipated by the development of a clearly defined service policy. But regardless of the size or the quality of the collection and the expertise of staff, referrals to other institutions, agencies, and libraries will be essential for some proportion of health-related inquiries in even the largest libraries. In order to respond to such requests, an awareness of the availability of other health-related information sources and services and the ability to make appropriate referrals are likely to be among the most important skills the reference librarian hoping to assist the lay client can develop.

REFERENCES

1. Katz, William A. *Introduction to Reference Work.* 4th ed. 2 vols. New York: McGraw-Hill, 1982. 2:41.

2. McClure, Lucretia. "Reference Services: Policies and Practices" in *Handbook of Medical Practice.* vol. 1. 4th ed. Chicago: Medical Library Association, 1982. 140.

3. Katz, William A. *Introduction to Reference Work.* 2:43.

4. Taylor, Robert S. "Question-Negotiation and Information Seeking in Libraries." *College and Research Libraries.* May 1968. 182.

5. Katz, William A. *Introduction to Reference Work.* 2:46–50.

6. Katz, William A. *Introduction to Reference Work.* 2:10.

7. Ley, Philip. "Patients' Understanding and Recall in Clinical Communication Failure" in Pendleton, David and Hasler, John, eds. *Doctor-Patient Communication.* New York: Academic Press, 1983. 94.

8. Freimuth, Vicki S., Stein, Judith A., and Kean, Thomas J. *Searching for Health Information: The Cancer Information Service Model.* Philadelphia: University of Pennsylvania Press, 1989. 131; Scholmerich, J., Sedlak, P., Hoppe-Seyler, P., and Gerok, W. "The Information Needs and Fears of Patients with Inflammatory Bowel Disease." *Hepato-gastroenterology* 34, August 1987. 182–85.

9. Perry, Claudia A. "Patron Medical Queries: A Selected List of Information Sources." *Library Journal.* 113, November 1, 1988. 45–50.

10. Bain, C.A., ed. *Health Information from the Public Library: A Report of Two Pilot Projects.* Albany, NY: University of the State of New York, State Education Department, New York State Library, Cultural Education Center, 1984; Brandon, Alfred N. and Hill, Dorothy R. "Selected List of Books and Journals for the Small Medical Library." *Bulletin of the Medical Library Association* 77, April 1989. 139–69; Roper, Fred W. and Boorkman, Jo Anne. *Introduction to Reference Sources in the Health Sciences.* 2nd ed. Chicago: Medical Library Association, 1984.

11. Rees, Alan M. and Hoffman, Catherine. *The Consumer Health Information Source Book.* 3rd ed. Phoenix, AZ: Oryx, 1990.

12. Boorkman, Jo Anne. "Online Bibliographic Databases" in Roper, Fred W. and Boorkman, Jo Anne, eds. *Introduction to Reference Sources in the Health Sciences.* 2nd ed. Chicago: Medical Library Association, 1984. 63–86.

13. Katz, Bill, ed. *Reference and Online Services Handbook.* 2 vols. New York: Neal–Schuman, 1982-1986.

APPENDIX:
Selected List of Reference Sources

AUDIOVISUAL MATERIALS

National Library of Medicine Audiovisuals Catalog. Bethesda, MD: National Library of Medicine. Quarterly; annual cumulation.

DICTIONARIES

*It is recommended that the current edition of at least one unabridged medical dictionary should be available in public libraries of any size.

Dorland's Illustrated Medical Dictionary. 27th ed. Philadelphia: Saunders, 1988.

or

*Stedman, Thomas Lathrop. *Stedman's Medical Dictionary.* 24th ed. Baltimore: Williams & Wilkins, 1982.

Taber, Clarence Wilbur. *Cyclopedic Medical Dictionary.* 16th ed. Philadelphia: Davis, 1989.

Magalini Sergio, and Scrascia, Euclide. *Dictionary of Medical Syndromes.* 2nd ed. Philadelphia: Lippincott, 1981.

DIRECTORIES

*American Board of Medical Specialties. *ABMS Compendium of Certified Medical Specialists.* 2nd ed. 7 vols. Evanston, IL: American Board of Medical Specialties, 1988. 1989 supplement. Biennial.

or

Directory of Medical Specialists. Chicago: Marquis. Biennial.

American Hospital Association Guide to the Health Care Field. Chicago: American Hospital Association. Annual.

American Medical Directory. 31st ed. 4 vols. Chicago: American Medical Association, 1988.

American Men and Women of Science. 17th ed. 8 vols. New York: Cattell/Bowker, 1988.

Encyclopedia of Associations. Detroit: Gale. Annual.

*Carper, Jean. *Health Care U.S.A.* New York: Prentice-Hall, 1987.

Kruzas, Anthony T., Gill, Kay, and Backus, Karen, eds. *Medical and Health Information Directory: A Guide to Associations, Agencies, Companies, Institutions, Research Centers, Hospitals, Clinics, Treatment Centers, Educational Programs, Publications, Audiovisuals, Data Banks, Libraries, and Information Services in Clinical Medicine. Volume 1: Organizations, Agencies, and Institutions. Volume 2: Libraries, Publications, Audiovisuals, and Data Base Services. Volume 3: Health Services.* 4th ed. Detroit: Gale, 1988.

Medical Device Register. Stamford, CT: Directory Systems. Annual. Volume 1: *U.S. and Canada;* Volume 2: *International.*

DRUG INFORMATION SOURCES

Drug Facts and Comparisons. St. Louis: Facts and Comparisons, Lippincott. Annual hardcopy or monthly loose-leaf or microfiche updates.

Handbook of Nonprescription Drugs. 8th ed. Washington, DC: American Pharmaceutical Association, 1986.

PDR: Physicians' Desk Reference. Oradell, NJ: Medical Economics. Annual.

*Reynolds, James E.F., ed. *Martindale: The Extra Pharmacopoeia.* 29th ed. London: Pharmaceutical Press, 1989. Available online through DATA-STAR.

USP DI: United States Pharmacopeia Dispensing Information. Volume I: *Drug Information for the Health Care Professional.* Volume II: *Advice for the Patient: Drug Information in Lay Language.* Rockville, MD: United States Pharmacopeial Convention. Annual. Bimonthly *USP DI Update* also available.

Zimmerman, David R. *The Essential Guide to Nonprescription Drugs.* New York: Harper and Row, 1983.

HANDBOOKS, MANUALS, TEXTBOOKS

*Berkow, Robert, ed. *The Merck Manual of Diagnosis and Therapy.* 15th ed. Rahway, NJ, 1987.

*Braunwald, Eugene et al., eds. *Harrison's Principles of Internal Medicine.* 11th ed. 1 or 2 vols. New York: McGraw-Hill, 1987.

or

*Wyngaarden, James B. and Smith, Lloyd H., Jr., eds. *Cecil Textbook of Medicine.* 18th ed. 2 vols. Philadelphia: Saunders, 1988.

The following two sources are recommended by purchase only by larger libraries, or in those sites where demand is substantial:

Diagnostic and Statistical Manual of Mental Disorders. (DSM-III-R). 3rd ed. rev. Washington, DC: American Psychiatric Association, 1987.

The International Classification of Diseases, 9th Revision, Clinical Modification: ICD-9-CM Annotated. 3 vols. Ann Arbor, MI: Commission on Professional and Hospital Activities, 1986.

INDEXES TO PERIODICAL LITERATURE

*Abridged Index Medicus (AIM) or *Index Medicus (IM).* Bethesda, MD: National Library of Medicine. Monthly; annual cumulation. Available online (Medline) on BRS, DIALOG, NLM and other systems, and in CD-ROM format through a variety of vendors.

*Consumer Health & Nutrition Index. Phoenix, AZ: Oryx Press. Quarterly; annual cumulation.

*Cumulated Index to Nursing and Allied Health (CINAHL). Glendale, CA: Glendale Adventist Medical Center. Bimonthly; annual cumulation. Available as an online database on BRS, DIALOG, and DATA-STAR.

MEDICAL GUIDES—POPULAR

*Kunz, Jeffrey R. M. and Finkel, Asher J., eds. *American Medical Association Family Medical Guide.* Rev. and updated. New York: Random House, 1987.

*Pinckney, Cathey and Pinckney, Edward R. *The Patient's Guide to Medical Tests.* 3rd ed. New York: Facts on File, 1986.

*Tapley, Donald F. et al., eds. *Columbia University College of Physicians and Surgeons Complete Home Medical Guide.* New York: Crown, 1985.

REFERRALS

Consider also hospital referral services, medical societies, and particularly the directories listed above. Clients are also well-advised to independently verify the credentials of hospitals or individuals by using these directory sources.

*Dietrich, Herbert J. and Biddle, Virginia H. *The Best in Medicine: Where to Get the Finest Health Care for You and Your Family.* New York: Harmony Books, 1986.

*Pekkanen, John. *The Best Doctors in the U.S.: A Guide to the Finest Specialists, Hospitals and Health Centers.* New York: Seaview, 1981.

*Sunshine, Linda and Wright, John W. *The Best Hospitals in America.* New York: Henry Holt & Company, 1987.

STATISTICS

Consider also contacting the sources or agencies listed below the tables in the *Statistical Abstract of the United States,* or organizations listed in the *Encyclopedia of Associations.*

American Statistics Index. Washington, DC: Congressional Information Service. Monthly; annual cumulation.

*Bureau of the Census. *Statistical Abstract of the United States.* Washington, DC: U.S. Government Printing Office. Annual.

National Center for Health Statistics. *Health: United States.* Public Health Service. Washington, DC: U.S. Government Printing Office. Annual.

World Health Statistics Annual. Geneva, Switzerland: World Health Organization. Annual.

PART IV

International Scene

CHAPTER 19
Consumer Health Information Services in Canada

Joanne Gard Marshall

INTRODUCTION

In the 1970s, Canadian health sciences librarians were inspired by the same idealistic spirit as their colleagues to the south to support the consumer health movement through the provision of consumer health information (CHI). The purpose of this chapter is to review developments in the provision of CHI in Canada in the context of the Canadian health-care system, a system which has developed quite differently from that of the United States during the last few decades. This context is essential to understanding the development of consumer health information services in Canada.

THE CANADIAN HEALTH-CARE SYSTEM

Since World War II, Western democracies have enacted legislation and developed policies that provide for at least some of the people's basic needs according to the economic tenets of the Keynesian welfare state. In the case of Canada, a country of 26 million people, a mix of universal and employment-related social programs have emerged. These programs include national health insurance; unemployment insurance; monthly family allowances; old age security; guaranteed income supplement for older Canadians who qualify for it; and Canada pension based on employment contributions. These programs, especially national health insurance, have been extremely popular in Canada. As a result, even though there is constant talk in the media about threats to our social programs, Canadian politicians have remained wary about tampering with them. Some of the differences that presently exist in the Canadian and American health-care systems can be traced back to more fundamental historical and political disparities. Unlike the United States with its revolutionary roots, Canada enjoyed a peaceful departure from its colonial past. Canada's formal relationship with Great Britain evolved through a series of constitutional acts, the most recent being the patriation of the Canadian constitution in 1982. A theory of Canadian-American differences has been proposed by Lipset;[1] it contrasts the social democratic and collectivist core values held in Canada with the more liberal and individualist values held in the

United States. In comparison with the centrality of the Bill of Rights in the American Constitution, Canada has been much slower to enact legislation touching the rights of individuals. Prime Minister Diefenbaker introduced a Canadian Bill of Rights in 1960 which applied to federal law, but it was not until 1982 that the Canadian Charter of Rights and Freedoms was passed as part of the Constitution.

Although Canada and the United States have diverged in recent years in their approach to reimbursement mechanisms for health care, they share a common history in the development of the health professions. Canada went through a period of consolidation of the medical profession in the nineteenth and early twentieth centuries under the influence of the Flexner report[2] that resulted in the development of university-based medical education and medical science in both countries. In 1912, the Canada Medical Act standardized the licensing of physicians across Canada, thereby confirming the solo practice, fee-for-service model of medical care based on individual cure that is found in the United States. The shared experience of Canada and the United States in the rise of medicine as a profession has had lasting effects, as evidenced by the fact that medical schools in both countries continue to be accredited by the same group. Because of the similarity in their educational experience, Canadian-trained physicians are not considered to be foreign medical graduates in the United States. In recent times, the influential report on medical education entitled, "Physicians for the Twenty-First Century," known as the GPEP report,[3] included participation by both U.S. and Canadian medical schools. Like the United States, Canada has also seen the rise of a variety of allied health professions in recent years.

The Canadian government's move towards the provision of national health insurance began in earnest after World War II. Although universal health insurance had been suggested much earlier, it was the government's recognition of the need for improved hospital facilities across the country that finally led to the acceptance of federal-provincial cost sharing for health services.[4] Hospital insurance was first introduced in 1947 in the province of Saskatchewan where a strong tradition of agrarian cooperatives existed. Gradually other provinces enacted universal hospital insurance plans until all provinces were included by 1961. Saskatchewan was also the first to enact universal medical care insurance in 1962, despite a bitter doctor's strike. The federal Medical Care Act of 1968 subsequently enacted additional federal-provincial cost sharing for physicians' services in all of the provinces.

At the present time, health care is a provincial responsibility with cost sharing contributions from the federal government. As Vayda and Deber point out, since health care is provincially administered in Canada, a national health-care system per se has never existed. Instead, each province is required to provide universal health insurance to its citizens under the terms of the federal-provincial cost sharing arrangement. Vayda and Deber emphasize that the Canadian health-care system contains various features that are also found in the systems of the United States and the United Kingdom. Like the U.K., Canada has a government-run insurance plan but, like the U.S., patients have a free choice of physician and the physician is paid on a fee-for-service basis. As in the United States, recent trends in health care have included increasing competition of physicians with other health professionals, growing skepticism about medical treatments, and a rise in medical consumerism.

In recent years, the United States has shown a particular interest in the Canadian health-care system.[5] This interest has been due, in large part, to the fact that the Canadian system appears to have been able to control health-care expenditures while at the same time eliminating problems of uncompensated care, the burdens of catastrophic illness on families, and the problems created by large groups of uninsured. In a recent study, Evans, Lomas, Barer et al.[6] point out that before 1971 Canadian and American health-care costs both consumed about 7.5 percent of the respective national incomes. By 1987 the Canadian share had stabilized at 8.6 percent, but the U.S. share continued to rise with estimates for 1987 in excess of 11 percent. The cost savings in the Canadian system appear to come from lower administration costs in a universal, tax-based system and the control of hospital costs through provincial budgets.

Relman[7] has raised the issue of whether better cost control and universal coverage have affected the quality of care and general availability of elective services in Canada. But a subsequent study published in the *New England Journal of Medicine* by Anderson, Newhouse, and Roos[8] found that, "elderly Canadians were as likely, if not more likely, than their U.S. counterparts to have access to acute care hospitals and the high-technology services available in them." When the authors explored a seeming difference in access by U.S. seniors to cardiovascular surgery, they found that the difference in access was accounted for by one single procedure, coronary bypass surgery. In other respects, older Canadians had even greater access than those in the U.S. to high technology procedures.

Despite the relative financial stability of the Canadian health-care system, there continues to be great concern about the substantial cost of health-care services. Programs in quality assurance and workload measurement similar to those underway in the U.S. are being implemented in an effort to maintain quality while controlling costs. Periodic skirmishes continue to break out between physicians and goverment ministries, particularly about the resources allocated to health care in the provinces and the issue of extra-billing beyond the government rates. Evans, Lomas, and Barer et al. note, however, that in Canada there is actually less intrusion into individual physician practices than in the United States where managed care systems and prospective payment have been used in an attempt to control the cost of physicians' services.

Given the tenor of the times, there will likely continue to be challenges to the universal health insurance system in Canada. Most recently, the proposed federal-provincial Meech Lake accord dealing with constitutional reform includes a clause which, because of its loose wording, has the potential to undermine the present system. Clause 106a states that the federal government will compensate provincial governments that choose not to participate in national cost-shared programs that fall into areas of exclusive provincial jurisdiction (such as health care), if the province carries on a program or initiative that is compatible with the national objectives. If the Meech Lake accord is approved with this clause, it would presumably be possible for provinces to modify their health-care insurance plans substantially while still maintaining "programs that are compatible with national objectives."

HEALTH INFORMATION SERVICES IN CANADA

Many of the initiatives in CHI in Canada are being taken by librarians who have traditionally provided information services for health professionals; therefore, it is important to understand the resource base from which Canadian health sciences librarians operate. In many ways, the health-care system previously described has served the Canadian populace well. But the lack of centralized responsibility and funding for health care has made it difficult to develop a coordinated national system for the delivery of health information similar to the Regional Medical Library (RML) Program supported by the U.S. National Library of Medicine (NLM). Efforts to evaluate and coordinate library services can be traced back to a report on medical school libraries prepared by Beatrice Simon.[9] Simon recommended that a national resource centre for medical literature be established. After considerable debate, the Association of Canadian Medical Colleges (ACMC) commissioned a second report, prepared by John B. Firstbrook,[10] that resulted in the establishment of the Health Sciences Resource Centre (HSRC) at the National Science Library in 1968.

The National Science Library, which has since become the Canada Institute for Scientific and Technical Information (CISTI), continues to house HSRC. CISTI has a broad mandate to provide integrated information services to Canadian researchers in all areas of science, engineering, and biomedicine. CISTI does not have a mandate to organize library networks similar to the RML's funded in the United States. Anyone in Canada with a need for specialized scientific information can use CISTI directly.

HSRC operates under the same broad mandate as CISTI, offering reference service, computer searches, and a variety of other services to health professionals and librarians across the country. Again, HSRC has no mandate to coordinate health library networks, although the staff make referrals to the closest Medlars centre and produce several directory-type publications. HSRC does a great deal with a very limited staff. In addition to offering reference and referral services, HSRC is the Canadian coordinator for Medlars, the online service of NLM. In this capacity, HSRC staff issue NLM codes and provide support and training for Canadian Medlars users. HSRC has had an advisory committee since 1978 that consists of representatives of various types of libraries and professional organizations.

The 16 medical school libraries continue to be the backbone of the information delivery system for health professionals in Canada with the CISTI collection as a backup resource. The directors of the Canadian medical school libraries meet annually as the Special Resource Committee on Medical School Libraries (SRCMSL) of the Association of Canadian Medical Schools (ACMC); however, no funding has been made available to this group to officially coordinate a national health information service. In 1987, SRCMSL and the Canadian Health Libraries Association published a survey of health science library collections and services in Canada,[11] but again, the recommendations relating to initiatives at the national level proved difficult to implement. There have been two other reports in Ontario that have examined the feasibility of government-supported health library network development,[12] but the recommendations of these reports were not implemented. SRCMSL members have expressed an interest in consumer health issues in the past. In 1982, a list of consumer health titles in the medical school libraries was produced by the group.

While funded efforts at the provincial and national government levels have not been forthcoming, there has been considerable support of library network services for health practitioners through professional organizations, such as the College of Family Physicians of Canada and the College of Physicians and Surgeons of British Columbia. Health sciences librarians, particularly those located in medical schools and hospitals, have become very adept at networking through local or regional groups in order to meet the information needs of their users. Sometimes this activity is taking place, at least in part, through the local chapters of the Canadian Health Libraries Association/Association des Bibliotheques de la Sante du Canada (CHLA/ABSC), which was founded in 1976. In other cases, medical school libraries have taken the lead in establishing formal networks based on a cost-sharing consortium approach. In 1984, a special issue of *Bibliotheca Medica Canadiana,* the CHLA/ABSC journal, published descriptions of 12 different library network initiatives across the country.[13]

CONSUMER HEALTH ACTIVITIES IN CANADA

The nature of the health-care system has had an impact on the information needs of consumers and the priorities of consumer groups. Some of these priorities are evident in the activities of the Consumers' Association of Canada (CAC), an organization that has actively promoted consumer access to health information. CAC has provincial Health Committees and a national Health Council. In 1974, the Association issued the Consumer Rights in Health Care document which emphasized the individual's right to be informed about all aspects of health care. In 1989, a CAC Policy Statement on Consumers and Health Care[14] was issued. The Policy Statement's basic principles are:

1) The consumer interest in enhancing, maintaining or regaining health status should be given the highest priority in health care.

2) The consumer interest in health care consists of the recognition of a number of basic rights of health care consumers, in the removal of impediments to the realization of these rights, and in positive reforms to create a consumer-oriented health-care system. The consumer interest includes health promotion and disease/accident

prevention as well as rehabilitative, curative, supportive and educational health-care services. All levels of government should work together to establish, and to allocate resources for, a long-term plan of health care for Canadians.

The Policy Statement goes on to specify the rights of health-care consumers. Among the primary rights is equal access to quality health care regardless of economic status. While the original Consumer Rights in Health Care[15] included a section on the right to be informed, the 1989 policy document goes further to state that consumers have a responsibility to seek information in a number of areas:

* About preventative health care
* About their own diagnoses and specific treatment programs
* About the policies and procedures of the health-care facility or program
* About the specific costs of procedures, services, and professional fees undertaken on their behalf

The emphasis in the CAC Policy Statement on preserving the universal access and on consumers' responsibilities to participate in the planning and evaluation of the health-care system through informed consumer representation is a reflection of the context in which Canadian consumers operate. Another emphasis found in the CAC document is that of health promotion and illness prevention. Under the leadership of the Health Services and Promotion Branch of Health and Welfare Canada, Canadians are initiating many health promoting activities in an effort to reach the World Health Organization goal of health for all by the year 2000. The framework for health promotion set out in *Achieving Health for All*,[16] commonly known as the "Epp report" after Jake Epp, then Minister of Health and Welfare, is being used to guide these activities.

All of the components of the framework shown in Figure 19-A require the effective dissemination of information to health-care providers, consumers, and policy-makers. Within the framework, there is a recognition of the need for individuals to promote their personal health through self-care. But there is also a clear indication of the importance of family and other support groups at the community level and of the need for public policies at various governmental levels that promote healthy environments. As a result of this framework, efforts to improve population health in Canada are being aimed as much at community groups and legislative bodies as they are at individual consumers of health services.

One of the initiatives of the Health Services and Promotion Branch has been the funding of research papers on various components of the framework. This initiative illustrates the importance given to information and knowledge as a basis for health-care activities. Summaries of the research papers have been released under the title, "Knowledge Development for Health Promotion: A Call for Action."[17] The results of Perrault and Malo's[18] review of the self-care literature have particular relevance for librarians interested in CHI, even though libraries as dissemination points are not specifically mentioned in the report. The authors recommend the establishment of storefront self-care resource centres as clearinghouses for

FIGURE 19-A: A Framework for Health Promotion

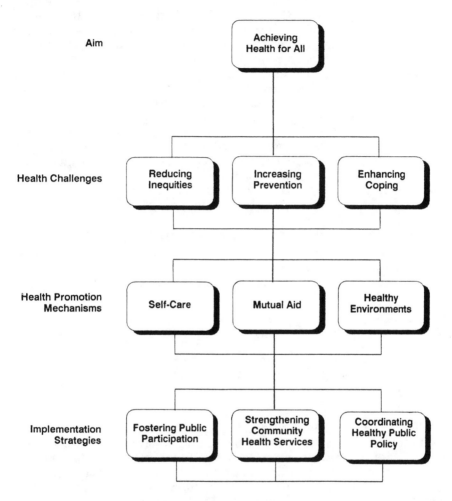

self-care literature and material; a computer network for self-care; and a self-care task force. The Health Committee of CAC (Ontario) is currently undertaking an assessment of consumer health information needs as a basis for preparing a proposal for a consumer health information service.

CONSUMER HEALTH INFORMATION SERVICES IN CANADIAN LIBRARIES

Priorities in the health-care system and the nature of health sciences library services have both had an impact on CHI services in Canadian libraries. As a result of priorities in the health-care system, wellness information tends to be emphasized along with illness information in CHI collections. A recent study of health information services in Ontario public libraries defined CHI as ". . . the provision of information related to personal health care, the health-care system, self-help groups, disease prevention and health promotion, and health policy and environmental health issues."[19] This study found that health questions accounted for about 8 percent of public library reference questions. The public librarians who responded to the survey commented that health enquiries came in daily and steadily and that health materials were heavily used. Librarians' estimates of the types of questions received are shown in Table 19-1. While the largest proportion of the requests dealt with disease or treatment information, there were also substantial proportions of questions dealing with health promotion, health policy and the environment, and the health-care system. The low proportion of questions on self-help groups may be an indication that consumers are using the provincially-funded consumer information services for such referrals.

TABLE 19-1: Types of Health Enquiries Received

Type of question	Mean %	Median %	S.D.
Disease or treatment	41.7	35.0	17.8
Health promotion/prevention	23.9	20.0	13.8
Health policy/environment	13.5	10.0	8.7
Health care system	10.2	10.0	10.9
Self-help groups	6.4	5.0	4.4
Other	3.8	0.0	10.6

N=75

The types of problems reported by public librarians in providing health information reflect some of the priorities that need to be addressed in the future if librarians are to play a significant role in this domain. The problems reported are shown in Table 19-2. The most frequently reported problem was the incomplete or unclear query from the requester. This may be a reflection of the difficulty that consumers have in expressing health information needs clearly because of the medical terminology required. It may also be that consumers feel more comfortable making an indirect request when the information required is of a personal or confidential nature. In any case, this finding suggests that public librarians, and probably librarians in general, need to develop special reference interview skills for consumer health questions.

The second most frequently reported problem, missing or unavailable sources, points to a continuing difficulty with theft and mutilation of health materials in public libraries. While this is a problem that librarians face in all parts of the collection, the librarians' responses indicated that this problem is especially acute for health-related materials. Educating users about the responsible use of shared resources such as library collec-

TABLE 19-2: Frequency of Problems Reported by Librarians

Rank	Type of Problem	n	%	Mean	SD	N
1	User presents incomplete or unclear query	33	44.0	2.56	.76	75
2	Source is missing, unavailable	28	37.9	2.76	.95	74
3	Library does not own the source	22	29.7	2.81	.71	74
4	Librarian/user does not know enough	11	14.9	3.19	.77	74
5	Source does not exist (not yet published)	14	20.0	3.26	.88	70
6	Librarian fears wrong answer, advice	12	16.7	3.36	.92	72
7	Librarian unsure about conflicting sources	8	11.5	3.40	.86	70
8	Librarian unsure about referral procedures	6	8.2	3.69	.88	74
9	Librarian has difficulty using sources	1	1.4	4.0	.62	74

Note: the first two columns represent the number and percentage of librarians who described the problem as occuring "often" or "very often". Item means and standard deviations are provided on the basis of a 5-point scale where 1=very often, 2=often, 3=occasionally, 4=rarely and 5=never. N=the total number of librarians answering the question.

tions is an ongoing social task, but it seems wise for librarians to recognize this problem. Depending on the circumstances, the library administration may be able to make some decisions about the physical placement of health materials in the building and to make allowances for this situation in the collections budget.

The study also revealed that few public libraries had strong collections of health materials. Not owning the sources was the third most frequently mentioned problem by the respondents. Almost half of the respondents (49.3 percent) described their collections as "basic" and another 36 percent as "moderate." Only 8 percent of the librarians described their library's collections as "comprehensive." A checklist of 68 health sources was included in the survey and the average number of sources checked as being in the collection was 19 (S.D.=8). Many of the public librarians reported that they could not purchase medical textbooks because of restrictions in their collections policies, even though such textbooks were considered to be excellent sources for many questions.

An interesting result was that the librarians generally reported that they felt confident about their ability to access health materials (providing they were available in the collection) and that they were not especially worried about being asked for medical advice or interpretation. The latter difficulty has often been expressed in the past. But it seems, from this survey at least, that librarians are very clear about the difference between providing information from authoritative sources and providing advice or interpretation and that they feel able to handle such requests appropriately.

In the questionnaire the librarians were asked about the relative importance of various CHI continuing education topics. Assistance in using health reference materials was rated "most valuable" by the greatest number of librarians, followed by collection development, the health reference question interview, and the ethical and legal aspects of providing CHI.

TABLE 19-3: Number of Librarians Rating Educational Program Topics as "Most Valuable"

Program topic	n	%
How to use health reference materials	40	53.3
Collection development	24	32.0
Health reference interview	20	26.7
Ethical and legal aspects	7	9.3
Community health resources	4	5.3
Introduction to health care system	3	4.1
Other	1	1.3
TOTAL	99*	132.0*

----

*Note: The respondents (N=75) were asked to number each topic in order of how valuable it would be where 1="most valuable". Some respondents marked more than one program topic as "most valuable" which explains the total in the Table. Several librarians commented that all of the program topics were important.

While there was some CHI referral activity between the public libraries and other types of libraries (73 percent of the respondents reported giving referrals and 53 percent received them occasionally), the study concluded that a more formal arrangement would be useful. Ninety percent of the public librarians supported the development of a network arrangement between public libraries and other hospital and academic health sciences libraries in the province.

Unfortunately, the lack of coordination of health sciences library services at the provincial and national levels in Canada has made it difficult to obtain funding for cooperative projects between hospital and medical school libraries and public libraries. Most CHI projects developed by health sciences librarians have been pilot projects without continuing funding or projects initiated with limited funds in individual libraries. As a result, CHI services have frequently been dependent upon the energy and enthusiasm of one or more dedicated librarians in particular settings. Despite some of the obstacles facing Canadian librarians, there has been a continuing interest in providing CHI services over the years.

During the reasonably affluent times of the 1970s and early 1980s, a number of projects were initiated in response to the general movement towards medical consumerism in North America. One especially innovative project investigated the use of Telidon, the Canadian version of videotex, for disseminating health information.[20] Another project included the provision of health information for patients and families and collaboration with the public library as part of a hospital-based clinical librarian service.[21] A review of some of the early Canadian CHI activities was published in a special issue of *Bibliotheca Medica Canadiana* in 1980.[22]

In 1981, CHLA/ABSC established a Consumer Health Committee that in 1984 published "Guidelines for the Role of Health Sciences

Libraries in the Provision of Consumer Health Information."[23] The purpose of these guidelines was to provide support for librarians who wanted to offer information services to the consumers as well as the providers of health care and to give some guidance to librarians in planning their CHI activities. The CHLA/ABSC Committee worked closely with the Medical Library Association Ad Hoc Committee that had been set up in 1980 to examine the role of the librarian in providing CHI, and similar approaches were developed by the two committees. Following the development of the guidelines, the CHLA/ABSC Committee intended to continue collaborating on national-level activities, but this proved to be difficult to coordinate and the Committee was eventually disbanded.

The preparation of this chapter has provided the author with an opportunity to review the history of CHI services in Canada and to investigate the current state-of-the-art. Background for the following discussion of current activities was obtained by reviewing the Canadian library and information science literature and writing a letter of enquiry about CHI activities to the local chapter presidents of the CHLA/ABSC in July 1989. The chapter presidents were asked to send copies of the letter to librarians in their area who were involved in CHI activities. The following is a representative rather than a comprehensive review of activities in Canada.

The Health Libraries Association of British Columbia (HLABC), a chapter of CHLA/ABSC, has been active in CHI activities since the early 1980s when members of their Health Education Committee produced a selected list of consumer health materials.[24] Recently the Consumer Health Committee chaired by Margaret Price developed a machine-readable database of consumer health materials with provincial Ministry of Health funding. Future updates to the database are planned and a public library union list is being considered. The group also participated in a major health conference in late 1989 in Vancouver entitled 2001: A Health Odyssey, presenting a workshop on locating CHI materials.

Albertans are clearly enthusiastic about CHI because they have given the theme, Health Information for All, to the CHLA/ABSC annual meeting being held in Edmonton, Alberta in June 1990. The theme builds upon the World Health Organization goal of health for all by the year 2000, which is currently guiding health care policy in Canada and many other countries. Alan Rees will present a continuing education course on consumer health information services at the meeting and a panel of experts will discuss consumer health and health promotion. CHLA/ABSC members from Alberta who responded to the call for information about consumer health services emphasized the cooperation that exists between health libraries and both community information services and public libraries in the province. Members of the Northern Alberta Health Libraries Association (NAHLA), a chapter of CHLA/ABSC, recently presented a brief to the premier's Commission on Future Health Care for Albertans that cited the need for better informed health-care consumers.[25]

An especially innovative project is The Health Connection, a health information centre located at the Rockyview General Hospital in Calgary,

Alberta. The Health Connection is funded by the Hospital auxiliary with support from the community. The centre provides access to books, videos, recent articles on health topics, listings and referrals to community organizations and agencies, public lecture programs, computerized health and risk analysis, and medication counselling. Access to the medical library for more advanced information is also available.

The theme of cooperation between libraries and community information services is common in many Canadian communities. In Ontario, the Ministry of Culture and Communications funds such information centres. Sometimes these centres are formally associated with the public library and other times the information centre and the library cooperate as independent organizations. At the North York Public Library, the LINK Community Information Centre used a SEED grant from Employment and Immigration Canada to develop a computerized database of community services. This LINK service includes information on health and health-related issues such as personal and family adjustment, children's services, and the environment. In Hamilton, Ontario, the Regional Municipality, the public library, and the Community Information Service have developed a master plan for the provision of information services. Peter Loades, science, technology, and business librarian at the Northern District Branch of the Toronto Public Library (TPL), has produced a useful guide to over 200 popular health books at TPL. The latest edition of this booklet, dated November 1988, was produced after an earlier, shorter version prepared in 1987 generated considerable interest.

In Orillia, Ontario, a librarian at the Huronia Regional Centre, a provincial Ministry of Community and Social Services facility for the developmentally disabled, has been very active. Maureen Maguire writes columns in two in-house publications of her Centre, one aimed at family and friends of Huronia Regional Centre clients and the other for staff. Since the Centre is in the process of downsizing and settling residents in the community, Maureen stated that family support for their programs is very important. In her columns, she tells family, friends, and staff about books and other resources that are available to them in her library as well as other helpful materials that are being published or available in the local public library.

Several hospital librarians, including Louise Lin at St. Joseph's Health Centre in London, Ontario and Tsai-O Wong at Mississauga Hospital in Mississauga, Ontario, reported that they had obtained small grants from sororities or other service groups to start a consumer health collection. Since most hospital libraries do not have allocations in their budgets for consumer health materials, the librarians often find it necessary to look to special funding sources for these collections. Freedman[26] has described a pilot project for a Seniors Health Information Program at the Elizabeth Bruyere Health Centre in Ottawa, Ontario. At McMaster University Health Sciences Library, a reference staff member maintains a collection of consumer health pamphlets from various health-related community agencies which are useful for health professionals, students, and health-care consumers in the hospital and outpatient clinics.

One of the most collaborative consumer health projects in Ontario is InfoHealth of the Kingston Public Library, which began in 1985. The goal of the project is to increase the accessibility, accuracy, and amount of current health information available to the general public in the Kingston area. The public library maintains a union list of consumer health books in the Kingston area libraries which is updated annually. The simple, but effective pamphlet that describes the service states that InfoHealth is a community service using the combined resources of the Kingston Public Library, Queen's University Health Sciences Library, and the libraries of the Kingston General Hospital, Hotel Dieu Hospital, Kingston Psychiatric Hospital, and St. Mary's of the Lake Hospital. InfoHealth offers in-person or telephone reference service, referral to appropriate agencies or institutions, access to the union list of materials, borrowing of materials directly or through interlibrary loan, online searches, and photocopying. The Library is accessible to the physically disabled and can be contacted through its "Visual Ear" by deaf and speech-impaired persons possessing TDD equipment.

We are fortunate that Frances Groen, life sciences area librarian at McGill University, has had a continuing interest in CHI. Groen[27] presented a thoughtful discussion of the legal and ethical aspects of providing health information in the *Canadian Library Journal*. She contended that there is a need to answer basic questions about the role of the library and the librarian as they pertain to the provision of medical, consumer health, and patient information. D. Elizabeth Christie,[28] also from Montreal, conducted a survey of 17 Montreal medical libraries about the role of the library in CHI. She found general support for the idea, although few of the libraries were actually providing services to patients in 1986. In particular, the respondents were anxious to work with health professionals and public libraries to provide effective service.

In the mid-1970s, a Montreal suburb was the site of the federally funded Health Workshop that involved the provision of health promotion and illness prevention services by community nurses. As part of this project, M.A. Flower developed a consumer health collection which was later transferred to the Nursing and Social Work Library at McGill University. The late Wendy Patrick, who was in charge of the collection at McGill, had a strong interest in CHI and wrote about the collection in *Bibliotheca Medica Canadiana*.[29] The Health Workshop represented many of the ideals in the Framework for Health Promotion. The goal of the combined nursing and information service was to assist individuals and families to deal with situations of daily living in a healthy way with an emphasis on health promotion and prevention.

Another indication of nurses' interests in CHI is the Women's Health Centre being established in the Nurses' Library at the Montreal General Hospital. The librarian, Barbara Covington, reports that the service was developed in response to the Department of Nursing's annual strategic planning event, during which a task force was set up to develop women's health care at the Hospital. The goals of the task force were: 1) to assess the services currently provided to address women's health needs for health promotion and health education; 2) to explore current trends in women's health care as a basis for determining priorities for action; 3) to monitor the disposition of funds by the Hospital for women's health programs; and 4) to heighten awareness of women's health issues among Hospital staff and the community. The Women's Health Centre in the Nurses' Library is part of this plan and provides pamphlets, booklets, and books addressing women's issues. Particular concerns of the task force include sexuality, violence, poverty, aging, and attitudes of health-care providers towards women.

Some libraries, such as the Jewish General Hospital in Laval, Quebec have developed specialized collections. Irene Shanefield, librarian at the Jewish General Hospital, reported that her library had one of Canada's most comprehensive international collections of accessibility guides for the disabled traveller. Information on accommodation, access to historical sites, restaurants, public institutions, and transportation is provided for consumers with mobility limitations. A booklet published by Transport Canada, which lists all of the Canadian guides in the collection and addresses of where the guides can be obtained, is available from the librarian.

Another group that reflects the priorities in Canadian health care is the Disability Resource Library Network (DRLN) created in 1984. DRLN is a Toronto-based association of librarians that "represents the first formalized attempt in Canada at resource sharing in the field of disability and rehabilitation."[30] The membership of DLRN includes specialized health sciences libraries in hospitals, nonprofit organizations like the Ontario March of Dimes and the Canadian Rehabilitation Council for the Disabled (CRCD) and coordinators of specialized collections for disabled persons at the public libraries. The CRCD has developed a Rehabilitation Classification Scheme for cataloging its books and pamphlets and and a companion Rehabilitation Thesaurus that is used by many of the DLRN members. Jaeggin states that DLRN maintains its national contacts through CHLA/ABSC, the National Library of Canada's Services to Handicapped Persons Department, and the Canadian Library Association's Interest Group on Library Services to Disabled Persons. Jaeggin ends his description of DLRN on a positive and possibly a prophetic note when he comments that even though DLRN must limit its face-to-face contacts to those resource centres operating in the Toronto area, the network of contacts is much wider. The possibility of electronic networking and resource sharing developed by DRLN provides a useful model for the development of CHI services.

THE FUTURE CHALLENGE

This chapter has summarized past and present CHI activities in Canada. Considerable attention has been given to explaining the context of the Canadian health-care system and the structure of health information services which have determined the opportunities and constraints facing librarians with an interest in developing CHI services. The future challenge for Canadian librarians will be to recognize and respond to the differences in health-care consumerism in Canada and to develop complementary resources and services. With the current initiatives being undertaken by the federal and provincial governments in health promotion, a tremendous opportunity now exists for librarians to become more actively involved in the dissemination of health information to consumers. The theme of the 1990 CHLA/ABSC meeting, Health Information for All, truly represents the goals and aspirations, if not the reality, for Canadian health sciences librarians at this point in their history.

REFERENCES

1. Lipset, Seymour Martin. "The Value Patterns of Democracy: A Case Study in Comparative Analysis." *American Sociological Review.* 28, 1963. 515-31.

2. Flexner, Abraham. *Medical Education in the United States and Canada: A Report to the Carnegie Foundation for the Advancement of Teaching.* Bulletin No. 4. Boston, MA: Updyke, 1910.

3. *Physicians for the Twenty-First Century. The GPEP Report. Report of the Panel on the General Professional Education of the Physician and College Preparation for Medicine.* Washington, DC: Association of American Medical Colleges, 1984.

4. Vayda, Eugene and Deber, Raisa B. "The Canadian Health Care System: An Overview." *Social Science and Medicine.* 18(3), 1984. 191-97.

5. Andreopoulos, S. *National Health Insurance: Can We Learn from Canada?* New York: John Wiley, 1975; Fein, R. *Medical Care, Medical Costs: The Search for Health Insurance Policy.* Cambridge, MA: Harvard University Press, 1986; Inglehart, J.K. "Canada's Health Care System. *New England Journal of Medicine.* 315, 1986. 202-08.

6. Evans, Robert G., Lomas, Jonathan, Barer, Morris L. et al. "Controlling Health Expenditures—the Canadian Reality." *New England Journal of Medicine.* 320(9), 1989. 571-77.

7. Relman, Arnold S. "American Medicine at the Crossroads: Signs from Canada." *New England Journal of Medicine.* 320(9), 1989. 590-91.

8. Anderson, Geoffrey M., Newhouse, Joseph P., and Roos, Leslie L. "Hospital Care for Elderly Patients with Diseases of the Circulatory System: A Comparison of Hospital Use in the United States and Canada." *New England Journal of Medicine.* 321(21), 1989. 1443-48.

9. Simon, Beatrice V. *Library Support of Medical Education and Research in Canada.* Ottawa: Association of Canadian Medical Colleges, 1964.

10. Firstbrook, John B. *A National Library Resource Centre for the Health Sciences in Canada: The Report of a Committee to the Association of Canadian Medical Colleges and to the Committee on Medical Science Libraries of the Canadian Library Association.* Ottawa: Association of Canadian Medical Colleges, 1986.

11. Flower, M.A. *Libraries without Walls: Blueprint for the Future. Report of a Survey of Health Sciences Library Collections and Services in Canada.* Toronto: Association of Canadian Medical Colleges and the Canadian Health Libraries Association, 1987.

12. *Medical Information Network for Ontario: Determination of Need.* London: School of Library and Information Science, University of Western Ontario, 1973. Demonstration model grant No. 27, Ontario Department of Health; *Report of the Ontario Council of Health on Library and Information Services.* Supplement No. 4. Toronto: Ontario Department of Health, 1970.

13. "Special Issue on Networks." *Bibliotheca Medica Canadiana.* 7(2), 1985. 57–82.

14. *Policy Statement on Consumers and Health Care.* Ottawa: Consumers' Association of Canada, 1989.

15. "Consumer Rights in Health Care." *Canadian Consumer.* 4, April 1974. 1–3.

16. *Achieving Health for All: A Framework for Health Promotion.* Ottawa: Health and Welfare Canada, 1986. Also printed as a supplement to the *Canadian Medical Association Journal,* March 1, 1987.

17. *Knowledge Development for Health Promotion: A Call for Action.* Ottawa: Health Services and Promotion Branch, Health and Welfare Canada, 1989. Ministry of Supply and Services Canada Cat. No. H39-147/1989E.

18. Perrault, Robert and Malo, Clare. "Self-Care: A Review of the Literature" in *Knowledge Development for Health Promotion: A Call for Action.* Ottawa: Health Services and Promotion Branch, Health and Welfare Canada, 1989. 127–34. Ministry of Supply and Services Canada Cat. No. H39-147/1989E.

19. Marshall, Joanne G., Sewards, Caroline, and Dilworth, Elizabeth. *Health Information Services in Ontario Public Libraries: Final Report of a Project Funded by the Faculty/Student Research Program of the Ontario Ministry of Culture and Communications.* Toronto: Faculty of Library and Information Science, University of Toronto, 1989.

20. Taylor, Margaret P.J. "The Role of Videotex in the Dissemination of Health Information." *Bibliotheca Medica Canadiana.* 6(1) and (6)2, 1984. 59–61.

21. Marshall, Joanne Gard. "The McMaster Health Sciences Library and the Hamilton Public Library" in Rees, Alan. *Developing Consumer Health Information Services.* New York: Bowker, 1982. 154–71.

22. "Special Issue on Consumer Health." *Bibliotheca Medica Canadiana.* 5(2), 1980. 112–30.

23. "Guidelines for the Role of Health Sciences Libraries in the Provision of Consumer Health Information." *Bibliotheca Medica Canadiana.* 6(2), 1984. 69–72.

24. Health Education Committee, Health Libraries Association of B.C. "Consumer Health: A Selected List." *Bibliotheca Medica Canadiana.* 5(2), 1983. 58–68.

25. Schoenberg, Peter, Slater, Linda, Sutherland, Leslie et al. "Information: A Priceless and Cost Effective Resource: Brief to the Premier's Commission on the Future Health Care for Albertans." *Bibliotheca Medica Canadiana.* 11(1), 1989. 49–52.

26. Freedman, Zelda. "Setting Up a Seniors Health Information Program (SHIP): A Pilot Project." *Bibliotheca Medica Canadiana.* 11(2), 1989. 97–100.

27. Groen, Frances. "Provision of Health Information Has Legal and Ethical Aspects." *Canadian Library Journal.* 40(6), 1983. 359–62.

28. Christie, D. Elizabeth. "A Role for the Medical Library in Consumer Health Information." *Canadian Library Journal.* 42(3), 1986. 105–09.

29. Patrick, Wendy. "The Health Workshop: The Concept and the Collection." *Bibliotheca Medica Canadiana.* 9(2), 1987. 114–18.

30. Jaeggin, Robert B. "Disability Resource Library Network." *Bibliotheca Medica Canadiana.* 9(3), 1988. 155–57.

CHAPTER 20
Consumer Health Information Services in the United Kingdom

Robert Gann

THE BRITISH NATIONAL HEALTH SERVICE

The National Health Service (NHS) is Great Britain's most cherished institution. The principle of free treatment at the point of need is dear to the hearts of the British public, and is not to be violated even by Conservative politicians. It is also an extremely efficient way of managing a national health system, leading to far lower administrative costs than health-care delivery systems in the United States or most other European countries. Health-care staff (doctors excepted) have always been low paid, and there is still a sense of vocation in working for the health service. As a result nurses in particular have an almost saintly image (they are usually dubbed "angels" by the popular press).

The negative side of this warm relationship between the British people and the NHS is that for the most part patients are absurdly grateful for the treatment they receive, treatment for which they may have paid through a lifetime of taxes. It is only very recently that British patients have started to behave like empowered health consumers and come to expect services which are more sensitive to their needs. Above all they are seeking information. It is no longer good enough in our society for consumers to receive more information about the operation of their new washing machine than the operation of their own body. In part this change has been due to an increasing consumerism in British society, in part due to an erosion of professional mystiques (fueled by the powerlessness of the medical profession in the face of the AIDS crisis) and partly because of official policies which are encouraging a culture of openness and consumer sensitivity in the NHS (a health service glasnost).

The informed participation of patients in their own care has no basis in law in the U.K. A Patients Charter was issued in 1987 by the Association of Community Health Councils (consumer watchdog bodies operating within the NHS) which urges the provision of information as a basic right. The Charter states that all people have a right "to written information about the health services, including hospitals, community and general practitioner services. . . to be informed about all aspects of their condition and proposed care, unless they express a wish to the contrary. . . to have access to their own health care records." This document was not taken particularly seriously at the time but it is interesting to see how "informed consumer choice" is rapidly becoming the new orthodoxy in policy statements from the Department of Health, particularly in the recently announced reforms of the NHS, as announced in the White Paper review *Working for Patients.*[1]

THE NHS REFORMS

Traditionally patients have had very little basis for choice within the NHS. They register with a general practitioner (GP) who acts as the gatekeeper to all health care received under the NHS. The patient consults the GP who may give self-care advice, prescribe medication, or refer the patient to a physician or surgeon for hospital treatment. Currently the patient needing hospital treatment almost always attends his or her local District General Hospital, unless the condition demands treatment at a specialist centre of excellence. Both at the primary care and hospital levels the patient has few genuine options. GPs are forbidden by law to advertise, and most GPs are chosen on the basis of geographical convenience or personal recommendation. Changing GPs is certainly possible but in reality it is a bureaucratic and sometimes acrimonious procedure. Technically GPs can refer a patient to any NHS hospital in the U.K. but this is not widely known and GPs tend to refer patients to local hospital doctors (consultants) known personally to them. In any case, patients (and their GPs) would not have the information to enable them to make a choice between one hospital or consultant and another.

Working for Patients sets out to change all this. GPs are to be given cash-limited practice budgets with which to "buy" treatment for their patients, either in the form of drugs or treatment at the hospital of their choice. Practice budgets will be based on the number of patients in the practice and GPs are to be encouraged to "compete" for patients, providing brochures giving information on the services available. Hospitals now have the option of opting out from direct control by local health authorities and setting themselves up as self-governing trusts. They would still be obliged to provide free health care to the local community but would have much greater independence. As money comes with patients there would also be an incentive to attract patients to hospitals through the provision of high quality care. No NHS reform would be complete without an attempt to tackle the deeply entrenched problem of lengthy waiting lists for surgery. It is not uncommon for a patient to wait several years for surgery for a nonurgent, yet painful and debilitating, condition such as an arthritic hip. Now GPs are being urged not simply to refer patients to their local hospital but to "shop around" for treatment where the waiting list is shortest.

There are areas in the White Paper which give cause for concern, and there has been considerable opposition from such strange bedfellows as the Labour Party and the British Medical Association. There seems to be little incentive for health promotion and preventive medicine programmes such as cervical screening. Limited practice budgets may make it difficult for high cost patients (such as AIDS patients receiving zidovudine) to secure the treatment they need. Self-governing hospitals will no longer be accountable to the community they serve. But there are undoubtedly enormous possibilities for information services.

The ideology behind the White Paper is one of individual consumer choice; without information to enable a comparison of the options available there is no possibility of this choice being a reality. In one area the White Paper is quite specific. Hospital patients should have:

> Clear information about the facilities available. . . and clear and thoughtful explanations of what is happening—on practical matters such as where to go and who to see, and on clinical matters such as the nature of the illness and its proposed treatment.

HEALTH INFORMATION IN THE U.K.

In the U.K. the responsibility for providing information on health issues to the general public rests with a variety of organisations.[2] Community Health Councils were set up in 1974 as "patients' watchdogs." Based in every District Health Authority (DHA) in the U.K. (200 in all), they provide information on local health services and patients' rights, and handle complaints. Their power is undoubtedly limited by the fact that they are funded by the very health service which they seek to monitor, giving rise to the accusation that they are more often lapdogs than watchdogs. Within each DHA there is also a health education or health promotion department, with a responsibility for promotion of good health and prevention of illness in the local community. Increasingly health promotion departments are adopting a wide variety of approaches, including sophisticated marketing techniques and "community development" work with local self-help groups. Outside the NHS and within the specific field of disability there has developed a network of over 100 DIAL groups (Disablement Information and Advice Lines). The importance of DIAL is that these independent advice services are run by disabled people for disabled people. DIALs are based on the Citizens' Advice Bureau model. CABs are generalist advice services usually with a paid coordinator and a number of volunteers, and are to be found in almost every town in the U.K. First set up during World War II, there are now 900 CABs, utilising 23,000 volunteers and answering two million enquiries a year. The most common enquiries relate to social welfare, consumer issues, debt and housing.[3]

Some of the most exciting activity in the area of information provision has come from self-help groups for specific health problems. The U.K. has a rich heritage of voluntary activity in the sphere of health and welfare, and since the 1960s this philanthropic tradition has been complemented by a boom in the number of true mutual aid groups formed by people with a common problem. Growth has been particularly strong in the areas of disability, women's health, and, more recently, HIV/AIDS. The self-help group database maintained by Help for Health in Southampton (the most comprehensive in the U.K.) includes details of over 1,000 national self-help groups for health problems, with over 2,000 groups in the local Wessex area.[4] Probably the most sophisticated consumer health information service in the U.K. is run by a voluntary agency, BACUP: British Association of Cancer United Patients. BACUP was set up by a doctor who discovered, when she was diagnosed as having cancer, the lack of information experienced by many patients.[5] BACUP's Cancer Information Service now provides nationwide free-phone access to a panel of trained cancer nurses, who answer enquiries with the support of an extensive databank of information on cancer incidence, treatment, and resources. Established in 1985, BACUP now has a staff of 20 and answers 22,000 enquiries a year. The careful monitoring of enquiries is producing some fascinating insights into the characteristics of callers to the service.

Another nongovernmental organisation which has made a significant contribution to the health information scene in recent times has been the national HIV/AIDS support organisation, the Terrence Higgins Trust. As in the United States, a voluntary agency has been able to move quickly, and without an official body to satisfy has been able to fill an urgent need for nontechnical and explicit information on HIV and AIDS. AIDS stands as the supreme example of the importance of information to health. In the absence of a vaccine or a cure, improved public knowledge is the only effective weapon against the virus. In the U.K. the crucial role of information was underlined in 1987 by the delivery to every home in the country of a government leaflet entitled "Don't Die of Ignorance." The AIDS experience is also a paradigm of the changing relationship between health professionals and patients. Doctors are powerless in the face of a major public health crisis. For their part, people with AIDS are often extremely well informed and obviously highly motivated to learn as much as possible about advances in management of the condition. The British daily newspaper, *The Independent*,[6] carried an interesting feature a while ago in which a GP described how he learned much of what he knows about AIDS from a patient who had access to the fast developing information networks in the United States.

In the U.K. each of the major professional groups in medicine has its own College (the Royal College of Surgeons, the Royal College of Physicians, the Royal College of Nursing, the College of Speech Therapists, etc.). These bodies exist to protect the interests of members, provide information services, training programs, etc. But until the 1980s there was no equivalent body for the other partner in health care, the patient. In 1983 a new nonprofit body, the College of Health, was established. Like its parent body, the Consumers Association, the College of Health is funded by membership subscriptions and has some similarities to the People's Medical Society in the United States. A quarterly journal for health consumers (*Which Way to Health*) is published and the College is also an effective pressure group. In July 1984 a new telephone information service for the public was launched. Called Healthline, the service was modelled on Tel-Med in the United States and offers a bank of several hundred audiotapes accessible over the telephone.[7] It is fair to say that Healthline has not been as succesful as has been hoped. Only available at certain times of day and not adequately publicised it soon faced competition from the growing number of commercially based phone-in tape services such as Healthcall and Self Helpline. These could afford extensive marketing and technology which allows 24-hour access without the need to speak to an operator (a significant consideration when dealing with embarrassing topics).

LIBRARY AND INFORMATION SERVICES

In the library and information world, the public library sector, with the advances in community information services in the 1970s, has made a great contribution to the provision of information about local organisations and resources. A good example is West Sussex County Library Service, where a comprehensive directory of resources called Contact West Sussex has been developed, linked to collections of health-related material in public library service points throughout the county. The directory is published annually and contains details of about 500 voluntary groups concerned with health matters in West Sussex, and also 250 voluntary and statutory agencies offering help with social problems. There are major health information collections in 12 branch libraries on 84 medical and related subjects, and the index to these collections is included in the directory. Over 250 directories have been distributed to libraries, health professionals, social workers, and voluntary agencies throughout the county. Worthing Library has provided the location for the largest collection, drawing together health books from different areas of the classification scheme in a single place (many of the relocated books doubled their issue rates) and taking out subscriptions to newsletters and bulletins from a number of voluntary groups.

Another model service based in a public library is Healthpoint Dorset, an information center housed in the central public reference library in Poole, Dorset. In keeping with current emphasis on cooperative planning and funding of consumer health information services.[8] Healthpoint is receiving financial support from the national Office of Arts and Libraries (OAL), Dorset County Library, local health authorities, and commercial sponsorship largely from a pharmaceutical company, Lederle. Healthpoint opened in February 1989 and has resources comprising two full-time staff, a collection of books, magazines, articles, and newsletters, and also holds the Help for Health database, Helpbox. Leaflets form another important element of the collection. These are not always easy to store and display, but as many as possible are on show to allow readers to help themselves. Healthpoint is located in a separate room at the main entrance to the lending library; all visitors to the Library pass Healthpoint, but they can use the health information collection without having to enter the main Library. On average 200 people a month make enquiries to the staff and a similar number browse in the centre without making a specific enquiry. Healthpoint is also an important county resource for branch libraries throughout Dorset. Branch libraries either contact Healthpoint directly with enquiries or give Healthpoint details direct to the enquirer.

The third major initiative with a public library input is Health Matters in Milton Keynes. Milton Keynes is a new city in the Midlands and, as a new development, lacks established social and support networks.

Information on health matters was seen to be a specific need and in 1989 the most comprehensive health information "shop" in the U.K. was opened (although Health Matters had been operating for 14 months in temporary premises). Health Matters is a cooperative venture, receiving funding from Buckinghamshire County Library, local health authorities, the Community Health Council, and Milton Keynes Development Corporation. The shop itself is in a covered shopping mall, close to a major food supermarket. The front is completely glazed and the visitor looks in to see the main collection of books (around 500 volumes), leaflets, and current journals. There is an attractive display area, and a children's corner with books and toys. Once again, the Help for Health database is taken on subscription, although Health Matters is unique in developing its own user-friendly DBASE/Clipper environment for the database. Staffing consists of one full-time librarian, some CHC staffing, and a team of volunteers. In addition to the information service, Health Matters offers space to self-help groups for events and talks. As an integral part of the local voluntary sector, Health Matters also participates in a wide range of community events, health fairs, etc.

While public librarians have always been mindful of their responsibility to the public, they have not always been confident in handling medical information. For their part medical librarians may have had the subject knowledge but until recently few have been ready to open up their resources to the public. Although this is beginning to change, with information services starting in hospitals (Frenchay Hospital in Bristol) and in community health centres (in Nottingham), for many years the only libraries within the NHS actively involved in the provision of consumer health information were the Health Information Service at the Lister Hospital in Stevenage (managed by Sally Knight) and the Help for Health Information Service at Southampton General Hospital (managed by Robert Gann). The Health Information Service (HIS) was the first into the field by a short head in the late 1970s. The information service arose from Sally Knight's own interest in consumer health information, and in particular her editing of *Popular Medical Index,* an index (unique in the U.K.) to health-related articles in the general press and to popular medical books. In 1982 Hertfordshire County Library provided additional funding to employ a member of staff specifically to support Sally in the development of the HIS, and last year an HIS development officer was appointed to develop outreach services, in particular in GP practices.

The project to provide patient libraries in GP practices in Hertfordshire also has funding from the Office of Arts and Libraries. Currently there are seven participating practices and a waiting list of a further 12 wanting to join the scheme. Budgets ranging from £600 to £1000 (depending on the size of the practice) have been provided to participating practices by Hertfordshire County Library, using funding from the OAL. A GP from each practice accompanied the development officer on a book buying trip and collections of 100–150 books have been assembled, reflecting the social, age, and sex profile of the practice. A union catalogue of holdings in all practices is being developed by HIS. The books will be available on an open access basis in the waiting and reception areas, and a simple loan system is administered by the practice receptionist. An important part of the project will be the evaluation of the service. All loans over a six-month period will be monitored, and an assessment made of the most popular titles and subjects. In addition, a questionnaire is to be administered covering patients' satisfaction with books read, and their overall information seeking behaviour.

The core of the HIS information centre at Lister Hospital is a collection of some 3,000 subject files made up largely of cuttings from medical and popular journals. There is also a library of popular medical books and the Helpbox database is taken on subscription from Help for Health. HIS has always received its largest proportion of enquiries directly from the public and total enquiries per month now average 280. HIS was the subject of a detailed British Library/College of Health evaluation in 1987.[9] This study reviewed the U.K. and U.S. literature on consumer health information services, and went on to evaluate the service provided by HIS. Perhaps the most interesting aspect of the report is the extensive quotation from a series of group discussions held with patients, members of voluntary groups, and health professionals. The discussions revealed a widespread dissatisfaction with information giving and evidence of poor communication when information is given verbally, without written back-up ("I can never remember one otomy from another otomy" said the wife of one surgical patient). Following the group discussions, use made of HIS was monitored for a month, and a comparison made with use of Help for Health over a similar period. The findings showed HIS to be be providing a more detailed service to a clientele largely made up of members of the public contacting the service by personal visit or through the public library service. Help for Health on the other hand was providing a quick, high turnover service to professionals and consumers who largely contacted the service on a phone-in basis. The average amount of time spent on an HIS enquiry was 30 minutes; for Help for Health it was five minutes. However, the report concluded that the services were becoming more similar all the time, and between them they offer the model for development of CHI services in the U.K.

Help for Health was established following a research project funded by the British Library which drew attention to the wealth of support available to patients and the lack of an effective mechanism for communicating this information. The report recommended the establishment of an information centre and enquiry service. The recommendation was accepted and funding is now the responsibility of the Wessex Regional Health Authority as part of its Public Affairs Service. Although based in a district general hospital, the service receives the majority of enquiries from members of the public and health professions in the community, from throughout Wessex and beyond. Over 900 enquiries are answered each month. The largest number of enquiries now comes directly from the public, either from people seeking information about their own health and illness, or acting as carers on the part of others. The leading professional users are health visitors but there is also extensive use by ward nursing staff, district nurses, general practitioners, social workers, and health promotion officers. Use by hospital doctors remains low, though the hostility expressed towards the service when it started has been replaced for the most part by indifference.

A significant factor in the increase in credibility and status in the eyes of doctors has been the appearance of Help for Health's regular column "What Your Patients May Be Reading" in the *British Medical Journal*. This has also been a major source of free review copies of books for the information service. Particularly gratifying has been the good use of the information service made by self-help groups. We expect a lot from groups, using their publications and putting people in touch with them for free support and counseling. It is good to be able to offer something in return by opening up information resources which would otherwise be closed. Self-help groups are experts in their own right and deserve access to the latest "professional" literature on their particular sphere of interest.

Help for Health has undoubtedly the largest collection of consumer health literature in the U.K., including a lending library of several thousand books, subject files of leaflets and articles, and subscriptions to 150 self-help periodicals. The most important resource is a database of self-help groups and publications which will run on any PC/MS-DOS microcomputer. The database includes details of self-help groups, pressure groups, community projects, etc., on a national level (1,000 groups), as well as details of several thousand self-help publications. The database is available free of charge to health promotion departments and libraries within Wessex, and on a subscription basis to authorities elsewhere. Twenty other health authorities are now subscribing to the subscription version of the database (called Helpbox), enabling them to establish similar services to Help for Health without reinventing the wheel. The availability of the database is undoubtedly a major factor in the blossoming of new consumer health information services in the U.K. over the past two to three years. Helpbox is in use in a number of interesting settings, one of these being the Self Help Team in Nottingham. Here an information officer forms a key member of a team offering information and practical services to local self-help groups. There is a twin center information service, with collections in the Self Help Team offices and in a busy inner-city health centre used by local health professionals, consumers, and groups.

Help for Health continues to look to the future by developing information services which respond to contemporary consumer needs. In 1988 additional funding was made available by the Department of Health to establish Wessex Waiting Line, a phone-in service on waiting times for treatment throughout the Wessex Region. At present the service is only marketed to GPs (although enquiries from patients which do come in are answered) and it allows GPs to "shop around" for treatment where the waiting list is shortest.[10] We are currently exploring options for making the waiting list database more fully available to the general public, including the possibilty of a Healthcall-type taped information service. Obviously this is exactly the kind of service envisaged to support the internal market concept which is central to the NHS White Paper.

The Wessex Waiting Line service raises interesting issues in the politics of information in the new consumer conscious NHS. How far does the information give patients any real choice, given that attendance at another hospital may involve costly travel, no visitors, and treatment away from the support of their community? But on the other hand, information on waiting times is in the public domain and opinion polls suggest that a vast majority of patients would be happy to travel to a more distant hospital if they could be treated more quickly. The increasing medical consumerism in British society poses new dilemmas and offers new opportunities for information services, but ultimately it should be the patient who decides how to use the information that is becoming increasingly available.

REFERENCES

1. *Working for Patients.* Cm555. London: HMSO, 1989.

2. For a more detailed review see Gann, R. *The Health Information Handbook: Resources for Self Care.* Aldershot: Gower, 1986. 2nd ed., Faber, 1991.

3. Citron, J. *Citizens Advice Bureaux: For the Community, by the Community.* London: Pluto Press, 1989.

4. Gann, R. "Self Help Is at Hand." *Nursing Times.* 84 (10), 1988. 61–62.

5. Clement-Jones, V. "Cancer and Beyond: The Formation of BACUP." *British Medical Journal.* 291, 1985. 1021–23.

6. Williams, J. "AIDS in a Time of Ignorance." *Independent.* March 21, 1989.

7. Rigge, M. "Healthline: A New Service from the College of Health." *Health Libraries Review.* 3, 1986. 1–10.

8. "Health Information Services." *Health Libraries Review.* 6, 1989. 83–88.

9. Kempson, E. *Informing Health Consumers.* London: British Library/College of Health, 1987.

10. Laurance, J. "Hospital Waiting Lists Rise Again." *Sunday Times.* November 13, 1988. 1–2.

CHAPTER 21
Health Link: An Australian Consumer Health Information Service

Moira L. Bryant

The consumer health movement is a relatively new development in Australia and Health Link was the first comprehensive, hospital-based consumer health information service to be established. The service is based on ideas gathered from similar services elsewhere in the world but has been adapted and developed to meet the requirements and expectations of its Australian users. In order to understand the services which Health Link provides, it is necessary to describe the current Australian health-care system and the health status of the population, because these factors can play a part in the development of medical consumerism in a society.

THE AUSTRALIAN HEALTH-CARE SYSTEM

Australia has a federal system of government formed from six states and two territories. Both federal and state governments have traditionally borne a substantial responsibility for health services; currently, health care is a mixture of public and private provision. The Federal Department of Community Services and Health is responsible for the planning and development of a range of national health and welfare policies and provides hospital, medical, and pharmaceutical benefits to the individual. State and territory governments receive general revenue grants for health from the Commonwealth government and supplement these with state revenues to provide public health, hospital, and community health services.

During 1984, Medicare was introduced. This is a universal health insurance system which entitles all 17 million citizens access to the public health-care system through their payment of a 1.25 percent health insurance levy on taxable incomes. The balance of the cost of the scheme is financed by general income tax. Approximately half of the population have still retained private health insurance coverage[1] which can provide reimbursement towards the cost of private hospital accommodation, the services of the doctor of choice in public hospitals, and also dental and ancillary services.

Expenditure on health-care has grown substantially in the last 20 years in both the public and private sectors. Total health expenditure in 1985–86 was A$18.5 billion.[2] Health (13 percent) is the third largest item of federal expenditure after Social Security and Welfare (29 percent) and Assistance to State and Territory Governments (16 percent). Defense and Education consume 9 percent and 7.5 per cent, respectively.[3] However the share of the Gross Domestic Product [GDP] spent on health care in the last five years has remained fairly constant at 7.6 percent. Both federal and state governments have reduced health-care programmes and cut hospital expenditures. Australia is spending less on health-care than a number of similar countries. The per capita health expenditure in 1984–85 for Australia was stated to be US$737, compared with US$1776 in the United States, US$728 in New Zealand, and US$456 in the United Kingdom.[4] During 1984–85, 94 percent of the total health expenditure was spent on institutional and noninstitutional services, 3 percent on administration, 1.5 percent on research, and less than 1 per cent on health promotion activities.[5]

POPULATION: MORBIDITY AND MORTALITY

Most Australians reside in cities. Since more than 80 percent of the population live on the coastal fringe, geographic access to health-care facilities is a problem for only a relatively small proportion of the populace. During the 1980s, Australians had the same mortality and morbidity patterns as other parts of the Western industrialized world; the major causes of death were mainly linked to ischemic heart disease, cancer, and accidents.[6] A 1977 survey[7] indicated that a relatively large proportion of the Australian population (45 percent) was affected by one or more chronic conditions at any one time. Nearly 2 million people are classified as disabled and 1.2 million (8.6 percent of the population) are classified as handicapped.[8]

Despite the gradual disintegration of traditional tribal society, the majority of the Aboriginal population, either by choice or necessity, live a separate existence from the rest of the population in economic and physical environments which are so poor that their present health status is much worse than the national average. Beck[9] notes that the disease patterns of Aboriginal children, with high infant mortality and gastrointestinal problems, resemble those of Third World countries. Amongst the adults, diseases of Western industrialized societies, especially alcoholism and diabetes, predominate.

The population of Australia is aging. A post-World War II migration boom resulted in an influx of migrants from the United Kingdom and Europe. These citizens will increasingly require considerable resources from the health and welfare systems, particularly institutional care. An aging population and increased unemployment in the general population result in a diminishing tax base from which the Medicare levy can be collected. Since the mid-1970s a larger proportion of migrants has come from Asia and the Middle East. Many Middle Eastern women are illiterate in their own language and do not communicate easily in English.

This causes problems with the delivery of health services as women are traditionally the carers in the family unit.

TRENDS IN HEALTH CARE

Australia has experienced a crisis in its balance of payments as a result of a worldwide, long-term decline in the prices for primary goods. Health care has been a prime target for government measures to implement expenditure control in view of mounting budget deficits and an economic recession. In line with other countries there is increasing concern about the quality, quantity, and effectiveness and efficiency of health-care in view of rising costs. The escalation of costs has been influenced by increased salaries and high technology medicine together with the higher health expectations of the general public.

"The current issues in Australian health policy about the role of government and the cost and form of services are common to all Western industrialised countries."[10] Some of these current issues in Australian health policy are cost control, which is to be obtained through increased rationalization and efficiency; rationing of services in the public system, which results in waiting lists for elective surgery; rationing of services in the private sector, which means higher costs to individuals; and the ratio of public and private responsibility with regard to the provision of health services.

The "managerialist" approach to health services, which has become increasingly apparent in recent years, aims at obtaining more value for money. Administrative costs have been reduced and the federal government has explored the idea of implementing Health Maintenance Organizations, in the hope that they will encourage the use of less expensive preventive health-care rather than high cost technological medicine, and has also set aside $5 million to sponsor research into the feasibility of Diagnostic Related Groups reimbursement systems.

Public hospitals are the most expensive health-care service in Australia. They consume 70 percent of government money spent on health, whereas community health and domiciliary care receive 5 percent of the budget.[11] A recent move in the state of New South Wales resulted in the creation of Area Health Boards which integrated community and institutional services. It was hoped that one result would be a reduction in health costs as a result of increasing competition between hospitals and community health services as they compete against each other for a portion of the area budget.

It has become increasingly apparent that some health services have been provided in inappropriate and uneconomic environments. There are trends towards a greater provision of palliative care and hospices, and greater use of hostels and small group houses for various groups which were previously institutionalized, because it is argued that community care is cheaper and more humane.

The increasing awareness of the relationship between disease and lifestyle and an increase in treatment costs encouraged federal and state governments to expand and improve health promotion and education activities in the 1980s.[12] The National Health Promotion Program provides federal funding for projects of national significance which promote better health and prevent illness. The Victorian (State) Health Promotion Foundation currently distributes $23 million per annum, which has been raised by a wholesale levy on the sale of tobacco products. This is used to replace tobacco company sponsorship of sporting and cultural events and to substitute health promotion messages in place of tobacco advertising at these events. However, less than 1 percent of total health expenditure is allocated to health promotion and current preventive measures probably appeal most to the middle and higher socio-economic groups.

Australia seems to be following the United States example in the provision of health care. The government is increasingly withdrawing from the health-care industry and allowing private interests to move in.[13] There is a growing interest by foreign companies, such as the Hospital Corporation of America, in running private hospitals and day surgery centres in Australia. Much of the profits from these enterprises returns to shareholders in the United States. Both government and private corporations are seeking increased cost effectiveness and the losers could well be the financially unattractive groups of patients, such as the poor, the old, and the chronically disabled. However "these trends towards commercial rationalisation are much further advanced in the U.S.A. than here in Australia."[14]

THE CONSUMER HEALTH MOVEMENT IN AUSTRALIA

The consumer health movement is based on the concept that members of the general public are capable of coping with many health matters themselves. However, in order to make decisions and participate in our own health care, information is needed. This information can assist in making informed choices about lifestyle to improve one's health. It can also foster an understanding of medical procedures and conditions, help us choose between treatment options, and forge linkages with others in similar situations. Sometimes this knowledge can empower people to question health-care policy and priorities of service and to bring about changes so as to make the health system more responsive to consumers.

The health-care delivery system of a country influences the development of medical consumerism in that society. In Australia health care is largely provided by government, with the result that consumers have a more limited choice of services than in the United States. Medical consumerism is still in its infancy.

Australia is experiencing, however, some of the trends that are taking place in the United States, such as cost containment. However, in Australia much of the high-technology equipment and procedures are available only in public hospitals and the government often carries out preliminary evaluation of them in a very limited number of sites. After the evaluation is completed, there can still be rationing of the availability of these high tech procedures among public hospitals, which restricts the access of those in need. As there are relatively few large private hospitals in Australia, this places further limitations on the number of alternative sites at which high technology procedures can be carried out.

In Australia, there is still a low level of complaints against doctors. As doctors are less fearful of possible litigation they are less likely to carry out procedures simply to protect themselves against possible malpractice claims. However, fewer specialists are entering the field of obstetrics because this is perceived as the speciality which is most prone to future litigation. There is less aggressive marketing by private hospitals which are mainly used as alternative locations for care by those wanting to circumvent public hospital waiting lists and to receive treatment from the doctor of their choice. Few private hospitals provide total health-care services and so do not offer the range of options such as courses, programs, and information services.

In some sections of Australian society there is an increasing interest in health promotion and self-care. The "prudent" diet, health food stores, concern about food additives, awareness of personal cholesterol levels, attendance at exercise classes, and greater interest in holistic practitioners and alternative therapies are evidence that some are accepting a greater personal responsibility for their own health. Conversely, it is still difficult to convey preventive messages about the benefits of pap smears, breast self-examination, sunscreens and good nutrition, and the dangers of drinking and driving to other groups of the population.

INFORMATION NEEDS AND THE AVAILABILITY OF CONSUMER HEALTH INFORMATION IN AUSTRALIA

The majority of Australians seek only limited types of consumer health information. They do not consider the quality and cost of the care which they receive, do not "shop" for health care, and are not forced to make decisions about how to access, utilize, and pay for health care. If they do seek information, it is usually information which will help them maintain and improve their health, understand an illness and its treatment, and cope with chronic conditions.

The Australian scene has many similarities to the British scene, as summarized by Rees,[15] who states:

> It is interesting to note that the British consumer health information activity avoids confrontation of the type common in the United States and focuses instead on promoting self-care, facilitating referral to self-help groups, supporting health education, improving doctor-patient communication, and providing coping information with regard to illness and treatment. There is an almost complete absence of information relating to evaluating the qualifications of competing medical practitioners, monitoring mortality statistics of hospitals and other indicators of quality, comparing costs, pursuing instances of malpractice, and exercising freedom of choice in seeking health-care. . . . Medical consumerism in Britain, unless a person is one of a small number with private health insurance with a measure of choice, concentrates on making the most effective use of the National Health Service.

Selected consumer health information is available from a variety of sources in Australia. A number of organizations have responded to public demand for information about health and illness and have developed consumer health information services as part of their overall work. Some services such as the Disability Information and Resource Centre in Adelaide, South Australia, and the national office of the Association for the Welfare of Children in Hospital in Sydney have developed library and information services to meet the needs of special groups. State health departments provide pamphlets on general health topics. The various branches of organizations such as the National Heart Foundation and the Cancer Councils distribute literature by mail and answer queries by phone. However, many people are unaware that this information is available. Women's magazines have articles on health and the soap "A Country Practice" is one of the longest-running and most popular programmes on Australian television. "Choice" the magazine of the Australian Consumers' Association, includes reports on health-related subjects from time to time and two health newsletters are now available by subscription. These are *The International Health Reader* which is edited by a Sydney G.P. and an Australian edition of the *University of California, Berkeley, Wellness Letter*. During 1988, a telephone service with recorded health messages was launched as a commercial enterprise but the high cost of such calls has made it an unattractive proposition for most people. Few public libraries have attempted to address the growing need for consumer health information in any systematic manner. Community information centers are sometimes an access point for general consumer health information, and women's health services place great importance on providing information to their clients. Some hospitals and health centers provide displays of health materials for patients, relatives, and staff, and at Flinders Medical Center in Bedford Park, South Australia, an information service is incorporated in the Health Promotion Unit.

BACKGROUND TO HEALTH LINK: WESTMEAD HOSPITAL'S HEALTH INFORMATION CENTER

Health Link is the Health Information Service of Westmead Hospital. Westmead Hospital was opened in 1978 and is a 998-bed teaching hospital attached to the University of Sydney. The Hospital provides referral services for the 1.5 million residents of the Western Metropolitan Region of Sydney. Westmead Hospital and its community health centers are units of the Western Sydney Area Health Service [WSAHS] which was created during 1988. WSAHS covers the five Local Government Areas [LGAs] of Auburn, Parramatta, Holroyd, Baulkham Hills, and Blacktown. The geographic area is a mixture of urban and suburban, with large tracts of housing, both old-established and new residential areas, two commercial centers, pockets of industry, and a northern section with a more rural character. Large sections of the area were developed during the last 15 years because the western region of Sydney had large amounts of land available for residential subdivision. The area has a poor public transport system and many residents travel long distances each day to their place of employment.

According to the 1986 census figures, 550,000 people (10 percent of the population of New South Wales) live in the WSAHS region and one-quarter of the population was born overseas. In many households, Arabic, Maltese, Serbian, Croatian, or Spanish is the language of communication. 18.5 percent of the residents are in the 10–19 age group and only 7.5 percent (which is less than the state average) are aged over 50. Overall, by New South Wales standards, the residents have a good level of income, which has partly been aided by a growth in female employment. However, there are areas where many single parent families live and recently there has been a marked influx of Aborigines into the region, which is placing a strain on all social services. Rapidly rising interest and mortgage rates over recent years make it more difficult for families to balance the household budget. Statistics reveal that residents of the area, especially in Blacktown, have an excessive mortality caused by heart attack, and various projects have been funded by the New South Wales government and the National Heart Foundation to address this major health problem.

WHY A HEALTH INFORMATION CENTER?

The Westmead Hospital/Australian Medical Association Library, like most hospital libraries, was developed as a medical library for use by health professionals. Access is not available to the general public. The growing number of requests for information by patients and relatives confirmed the belief that a specialized collection in a more informal setting should be assembled with the needs of the general public in mind. The Library staff believed that a separate health information center was a better arrangement than to provide public access to the medical library in that a medical library can be a very daunting place and that better service can be offered in an alternate location.

In February 1983, under the direction of the social work student supervisor, an information booth was set up for 12 days in the main foyer of Westmead Hospital. This project was aimed at assessing the informational and service needs of the Hospital population. The information requested by the booth users fell into three main categories: health promotion, medical enquiries, and hospital resources.

In July 1983 the head of the Health Promotion Unit surveyed all heads of departments, both medical and paramedical, together with the assistant directors of nursing, as to their anticipated use of a proposed Health Information Center. The staff recorded a 90 percent approval for such a concept and envisaged referring patients and relatives to the Center for specific health information.

In many areas of the Hospital there was a growing recognition of the need to reinforce information that had been given verbally to patients, so as to increase their understanding and their compliance with treatment. It was known that individual staff in various clinical and nursing areas were gathering information to give patients and relatives when the need arose.

However, there were many problems with such an informal approach: the provision of material was dependent on the enthusiasm and dedication of clinical staff; there was no evaluation of the quality of material; there was some duplication of resources and effort; and there was no definite access point for information.

During 1984 an initial Hospital Health Promotion Grant was obtained from the New South Wales Department of Health to assist in financing the establishment of a Health Information Center. Westmead Hospital assumed full financial responsibility for the service from July 1985. Since its inception, the Center has been staffed by a full-time medical librarian and, in its early days, was administered by a multidisciplinary steering committee.

HEALTH LINK

When Health Link opened in March 1985 it was a new concept for Australia—an organized health information service within a hospital setting, the role of which was to provide credible health information covering self-care, health education, and self-help in response to inquiries by patients, relatives, staff, and the general public; and to support the patient education activities of the Hospital. Such a service would be a concrete example of the Hospital's commitment to meeting the information needs of its community.

Health Link is situated on the corridor which runs between the two ward blocks and is open 9 a.m. to 4 p.m., Monday to Friday. The Center is equipped with a computer workstation, reception desk, photocopier, easy chairs, and revolving pamphlet stands containing paediatric, nutrition, and general health material. The collection of books is housed for easy access, not in bookshelves, but in a series of custom-built transparent plastic containers. These stand on top of low filing cabinets holding the pamphlet collection, which has been organized into specific subject packets. An effort has been made to provide a quiet, comfortable, nonthreatening atmosphere in which users can read the available information. This information is available to enquirers at a time when they are ready to assimilate it.

ACHIEVING SERVICE OBJECTIVES

The main objective of Health Link is to provide a collection of accurate, easily understood medical and health-related information for the general community and to people who have been referred by health professionals. When a person comes to Health Link requesting information on a specific topic, this is provided either from a collection of pamphlets stored in a subject packet, or from a relevant book. We do not discuss symptoms or treatment, nor do we give advice or interpret material.

One of the objectives is to provide written information which can reinforce the information which has been given verbally by health professionals, especially at a time when an individual's motivation to learn is strongest, either as a result of their own illness or that of a relative. By providing accurate information it is possible to strengthen patient-doctor relationships and communication in that a better informed patient is more likely to take responsible action. The importance of patients discussing with their doctor matters they do not understand is stressed.

Health Link has a referral role. It assists in disseminating information from national organizations such as the National Heart Foundation, Cancer Councils, and the Australian Arthritis Foundation. By building up good links with medical, nursing, and allied health professionals within the Hospital, it is possible to refer enquirers to more appropriate support where necessary. If it has not been possible to satisfy a request for information, or if an enquirer seems especially worried, an effort is made (with the consent of the enquirer) to advise the particular doctor. In addition, we refer people to community agencies and support groups and provide information about health education or health promotion programs held in the Hospital or at local community sites.

Pamphlets on a wide range of topics are freely available. People are welcome to browse or to sit and read the reference resources. The librarian is always available to find suitable material for enquirers. Copies of popular health books in the collection may be purchased from Health Link. It became evident, soon after the Center first opened, that people were eager to buy books, particularly those on sensitive topics, from the Center, rather than from the Hospital bookstore. During 1988–89, $10,000 worth of printed health resources was sold at Health Link. Although it is not possible to borrow books from the collection, a small collection of videos has been assembled at the suggestion of the parenting educator. These videos can be rented from Health Link by people attending her classes in the Hospital.

In order to encourage greater awareness amongst health professionals and other information providers of the range of resources and sources of assistance which are available, Health Link has published two editions of "A Guide to Consumer Health Information." Over 3,000 copies of these bibliographies of locally available consumer health information materials and support organizations have been distributed to general practitioners, public libraries, and other services in Australia and New Zealand.

COLLECTION DEVELOPMENT

All the books and pamphlets in the collection have been circulated for review by appropriate Hospital staff. This screening process is time-consuming but is considered to be very important to a hospital-based service because it ensures the medical accuracy and currency of the information which is supplied to the general public. Some material is not included in the collection because treatment protocols, especially in the United States, can be different with the result that such information would only cause confusion. The review process has also made health professionals more aware of resources which could be relevant to their patients, and our records sometimes show a marked increase in the volume of enquiries by patients for an item after a specialist has reviewed it. The collection is constantly being reviewed and enlarged. It currently consists of 4,000 individual reference pamphlets, which are collected into 700 subject packets, and a reference collection of 400 books.

Over the past five years there has been a marked increase in the number of book titles relating to consumer health information available in Australia. However, the range is much smaller than that available in the United Kingdom or United States; many titles never reach Australia. This is partly due to the fact that Australia forms a closed market for most books published overseas. This stems from an arrangement whereby an overseas publisher assigns to an Australian agent exclusive rights to sell and distribute books in Australia. The agent is often an Australian subsidiary of the overseas publisher. This means that Australian retailers can only buy copies of those books from that agent, who can prevent the sale in Australia of any other edition, or even any edition at all. As a result, overseas books usually cost a great deal more in Australia and are frequently not available for a long time after their original publication. Libraries are not affected by the closed market, since the importation provisions of the Copyright Act of 1968 only relate to books imported for commercial purposes. Currently there are discussions taking place about possible deregulation of the Australian book trade.

In the earlier stages of building the collection of reference books it was necessary to include many American titles, but it has since been possible to replace many of these with locally published material. This is usually preferable because local titles are generally less expensive to obtain, are more readily available to the enquirer, and are likely to be more relevant in content.

However, because of the relative smallness of the Australian population, the number of people diagnosed with certain conditions is much smaller and, as a result, support networks are often much less organized. To meet this need, a concerted effort was made to request suitable printed resources from support groups and organizations listed in the *Encyclopedia of Associations*[16] when it proved impossible to trace a similar group in Australia. Sometimes, when providing printed material they also gave details of an Australian group. As a result it has been possible to build up a very wide-ranging consumer health information collection.

The New South Wales Department of Health has translated many of its free health pamphlets into 17 other languages ranging from Arabic to Vietnamese. A copy of each of these translations is included in the collection. These are more likely to be requested by a health professional for a client rather than by the client themselves. However, during the various Health Awareness Weeks which are held throughout the year, Health Link distributes material in the Hospital relating to the selected themes in a variety of languages.

Ideally, when applicable, we aim to have information available for the English-speaking enquirer at three levels. A free, concise pamphlet or fact sheet which would cover the main points of a topic, a more detailed booklet which can be read at Health Link or purchased for a small charge, and a comprehensive book which enquirers can either purchase from Health Link or can request from their local public library. As we are servicing a constantly changing clientele, and because Health Link has only one staff member, it is not logistically possible to lend resources from the collection. The information resources fall into two major categories: basic everyday information relating to health education and self-care, and illness-related information which assists patient education and self-help.

We know that many personal factors can influence the incidence of chronic diseases and that preventive health practices can lessen the likelihood of these conditions developing. Health education information encourages people to adapt their lifestyle to lessen the likelihood of being affected by certain illness and to maintain or improve their health status. The literature confirms that people treat many minor complaints at home and that the measures they take are often safe and appropriate.[17-20] However, they need self-care information in order to know what is the appropriate action to take.

When someone receives a diagnosis of an illness, both the patient and his or her relatives often need information to help them understand the condition in order to adjust to the changes which the illness can bring about and to be actively involved in the treatment and rehabilitation process. Patient education resources can give an explanation of an illness, of medical procedures, or of a treatment regimen, and can reinforce information and advice which has already been given verbally by health professionals. Self-help information puts people in touch with the range of services available to them in the community and with organizations which can provide practical and moral support. Health Link has compiled a state-by-state database listing of many organizations and support groups within Australia. Some of this information was included in the second edition of "A Guide to Consumer Health Information."

BIBLIOGRAPHIC CONTROL

The resources of Health Link have been arranged in 24 sections based on a customized classification scheme and thesaurus. Some sections relate to various systems of the body, for example, cardiovascular system, endocrine system, and digestive system. Other sections cover particular topics, for example, women's health, men's health, mental health, and mental illness. Each resource is indexed under the most specific term available rather than by broad subject areas. This ensures that the enquirer receives the most relevant information.

The classification scheme and thesaurus were derived after discussions with the Hospital specialists. It soon became apparent that they favored easily understood terms, for example, "Heart attack" rather than "Myocardial infarction," and English rather than American spelling or terms, such as "Motor neurone disease" rather than "Amyotrophic lateral sclerosis." However, whenever possible each term in the thesaurus has been cross-referenced in the computer database to the equivalent MeSH subject heading so that resources could easily be identified by those accustomed to searching by MeSH terms.

USERS AND USAGE

Between March 1985 and July 1989, more than 26,000 people visited Health Link seeking information, an average of 6,000 to 7,000 per year. Westmead Hospital also incorporates a 190-chair clinical dental school in one wing of the building. The Health Link librarian replaces between 1,000 to 1,500 pamphlets on general health matters each week in two more revolving pamphlet stands in the foyer of the dental school. This would imply that the service is also providing access to general health information for many more people than actually visit Health Link.

Everyone who comes to Health Link is offered assistance in finding material to meet their needs and all enquiries are categorized in order to provide an on-going record of usage and demand. Users are assigned to one of three categories: Inpatients, Staff, and Other (which includes outpatients, patients' relatives, and members of the general public). The largest group of users (66 percent) are those classed as "Other." Staff use has accounted for 30 percent of enquiries. Staff seek information for their self-care, self-education, and patient education activities. The resources which health professionals seek for patient education or health promotion might either be used in their present format or can become the basis for developing their own programs or resources. Social workers find the material very useful to gain an understanding of a client's condition and difficulties, and dieticians and physiotherapists regularly refer to Health Link resources during patient education programs.

There has been relatively little use of the service by inpatients (4 percent). This is consistent with the results of a project in Ontario, Canada,[21] and perhaps is not surprising both because patients are generally discharged from the hospital as soon as possible and since, while in the hospital, they are often too unwell to seek information, or are busy with tests. It is more likely to be the patient's relatives who are looking for information in that they want to be better informed in order to reduce their own anxiety and to be able to care for the patient. It has been observed that the majority of users of Health Link are female and often appear to be enquiring on behalf of someone else. This could well be because women are usually responsible for the health and care of children and of sick and elderly relatives.

Since the service opened in March 1985 each user has been assigned by the librarian to one of three categories: those who come prompted by a particular query (54.6 percent), those who were browsing (37.6 percent), and those seeking information about the Hospital and its services (7.8 percent). The findings indicate that the majority of people are seeking specific health information, but a large number wish to browse and help themselves to the free material. It seems likely that some of the "browsers" visit with a particular query in mind but "self-select" the information they require without assistance from the librarian.

Health Link users frequently volunteer the reason why they are seeking information and this can assist in the selection of the most appropriate material. Sometimes the enquirer does not want to bother a medical professional in that they believe in initiating self-care prior to deciding whether they need to consult a doctor. Sometimes, the enquirer is planning to see a doctor but is looking for background information in order to understand the terms which might be used and to ask relevant questions. Some enquirers have been given information verbally by a health professional but now wish to clarify what they have been told. Some enquirers would like to understand the difficulties facing a relative or friend but are reluctant to consult the doctor. Sometimes the enquirer wishes to contact other people facing the same problem in order to benefit from practical and moral support. At Health Link, when an enquirer asks for information about a chronic condition, they are generally also provided with information about a relevant support group or organization.

"ILLNESS" INFORMATION VERSUS "HEALTHY LIFESTYLE" INFORMATION

Kempson[22] has concluded that "All the previous research seems to indicate that the prime area in which people want information is related to specific diseases." At Health Link, a record has been made of every topic about which the librarian was asked to find material for the 54.6 percent of users seeking specific information between March 1985 and July 1989. This percentage represents a total of 14,468 specific requests covering 450 subjects. During this time, 59 percent of the specific requests were classed as "Information for coping with an illness" and 41 percent were classed as "Information for a healthier lifestyle." The total number of requests in the "Illness" category (8,554) is made up of many small totals. Many subjects (e.g., Marfan's syndrome, Primary sclerosing cholangitis, or Psoriatic arthritis) are requested infrequently. The records reveal the wide diversity of topics which are requested at Health Link and the need for a broadly based service. The total number of requests in the "Lifestyle" category (5,914) comprises a few large totals (e.g., Weight reduction, Stress management, and Nutrition).

These records agree with reports from other consumer health information services that the majority of requests are for information relating to specific diseases and conditions. Because Health Link is situated in a large teaching hospital, it is perhaps surprising that requests for information relating to diseases and conditions comprise only 59 percent of specific requests. Over the years, there appears to have been a decline in the number of requests in the "Illness" category and an increase in the percentage of requests for wellness information on certain topics such as cholesterol, nutrition, stress management, and weight reduction. This trend suggests an increasing awareness of health promotion and self-care (*See* Tables 21-1 and 21-2).

TABLE 21-1: "Illness" Information Versus "Healthy Lifestyle" Information

% OF THE TOTAL NUMBER OF
SPECIFIC ENQUIRIES

Topic	*	85-86	86-87	87-88	88-89	Total
Illness	67	63	62	55	56	59%
Lifestyle	33	37	38	45	44	41%

* March to June 1985 — limited opening

TABLE 21-2: Specific Requests for Some Common Health Promotion and Self-Care Topics

Topic	*	85-86	86-87	87-88	88-89	Total
Cholesterol	1	155	339	421	308	1,224
Nutrition	12	134	148	277	326	897
Stress Management	9	63	143	113	107	435
Weight Reduction	3	38	122	112	120	395

* March to June 1985 — limited opening

Ten topics accounted for 45 percent (6,586) of all specific requests for information. These topics are listed in Table 21-3. The volume of enquiries relating to cancer, diabetes, coronary heart disease, stroke, and arthritis reflects the morbidity statistics and the prevalence of these illnesses in the community.

TABLE 21-3: Top Ten Topics Since March 1985

	Total	%
Cholesterol	1,224	8.4
Cancer	1,065	7.4
Diabetes	960	6.7
Nutrition	897	6.1
Coronary Heart Disease	474	3.3
Stress Management	435	3.0
Pregnancy/Childbirth	420	2.9
Weight Reduction	395	2.7
Stroke	372	2.6
Arthritis	344	2.4
TOTAL		45.5%

The data reveal that when a health topic is targeted for a campaign in the media there is a noticeable increase in the number of enquiries related to that topic. However, after a peak in 1986–87, there has been a decline in the number of people looking for information about AIDS, which perhaps reflects a disinclination by the public to learn any more about the disease.

Kempson[23] reports that during the March 1986 survey period at Lister Hospital Health Information Service at Stevenage, Hertfordshire, 37 percent of enquiries from the public and 22 percent of enquiries from health-care staff related to medication or drugs. Health Link statistics record only 69 enquiries (0.47 percent) related to medication. However, when providing information about an illness or treatment, the resources often include information about medication (e.g., Parkinson's disease and Levodopa); the statistics only record the occasions when an enquirer has requested information about a medication by name. It would appear that the users of Health Link are not very interested in the benefits or side-effects of the substances prescribed to them. Perhaps this is further evidence of the consumer health information movement being in its infancy in Australia.

Health Link appears to be closer in character to consumer health information services in the United Kingdom than in the United States. To date, we have not been asked about two types of information which appear to be important elsewhere. Rees[24] has defined these as "Access-related information," which enables the enquirer to assess the availability, quality, and cost of health care, and "Medical ethics-related information," which tackles the dilemmas brought about by modern medical technology, such as the value of saving the life of a very premature baby who might grow up to have limited quality of life. There is more emphasis on seeking information which relates to an individual's health status than information which assists the individual to obtain maximum benefit from the health-care system.

CONCLUSION

The experience gained at Health Link since 1985 confirms that a consumer health information service needs to provide a wide range of printed medical and health-related resources in easy-to-understand language and to be able to direct enquirers to support services and self-help groups. It has been observed that inpatients comprise only a small proportion of those seeking information, that the majority of people come with a specific request, and that although the majority of enquirers are seeking illness-related information there is an increasing number of requests for lifestyle information.

ACKNOWLEDGMENTS

No account of Health Link would be complete without an acknowledgement of the preparatory work which was done within the Westmead Hospital community by a group of people who wanted to turn the concept of a health information centre into a reality. These were Judy

Barker (Social Work Student Supervisor), Deirdre Degeling (Head, Health Promotion Unit), Dr. John Dowsett (Director of Teaching and Research Resources), Brenda Heagney (Westmead/AMA Librarian) and Rosalind Spencer (Health Education Officer, Department of Paediatrics). My personal thanks also goes to my husband, Associate Professor Roland Bryant who has supported my role at Health Link in many large and small ways.

REFERENCES

1. *Health Insurance Survey March 1986.* Canberra: Australian Bureau of Statistics, 1986.

2. *Information Bulletin No. 3.* Canberra: Australian Institute of Health, 1988.

3. *Australian Budget Paper No. 1.* Canberra: Australian Government Publishing Service, 1988.

4. *Australian Health Expenditure 1970–71 to 1984–85.* Canberra: Australian Institute of Health, 1988.

5. *Information Bulletin No 3.* Canberra: Australian Institute of Health, 1988.

6. *Deaths Australian 1986.* Canberra: Australian Bureau of Statistics, 1987.

7. *Australian Health Survey 1977–78 Chronic Conditions.* Canberra: Australian Bureau of Statistics, 1980.

8. *Handicapped Persons Survey 1981.* Canberra: Australian Bureau of Statistics, 1984.

9. Beck, E.J. *The Enigma of Aboriginal Health.* Canberra: Australian Institute of Aboriginal Studies, 1985.

10. Davis, Alan and George, Janet. *States of Health: Health and Illness in Australia.* Sydney: Harper and Rowe, 1988. 102.

11. Hicks, N. "The Community in Community Health" in Potter, J.D. and Hodgson, A.M.A. *Working Papers in Community Health.* Adelaide: ANZSERCH/APA, 1982.

12. Grant, C. and Lapsley, H.M. *The Australian Health Care System.* Australian Studies in Health Service Administration, Monograph No. 64. Sydney: School of Health Administration, University of New South Wales, 1989.

13. Jacques, B. "Investors Move into Medicine." *Australian Business.* 13, August 1986. 16–19.

14. Davis, Alan and George, Janet. *States of Health: Health and Illness in Australia.* 203.

15. Rees, A.M. "Health Information and Medical Consumerism" in Rees, A.M. and Hoffman, C., eds. *The Consumer Health Information Source Book.* 3rd ed. Phoenix, AZ: Oryx Press, 1990. 10.

16. *Encyclopedia of Associations: Vol. 1: National Organizations of the U.S.* Martin, Susan B. and Koek, Karin, eds. 22nd ed. Detroit: Gale, 1987.

17. Dunnell, K. and Cartwright, A. *Medicine Takers, Prescribers and Hoarders.* London: Routledge and Kegan Paul, 1972.

18. Elliot-Binns, C.P. "An Analysis of Lay Medicine." *Journal of the Royal College of General Practitioners.* 23, 1973. 255–64.

19. Williamson, J.D. and Danaher, K. *Self Care in Health.* London: Croom Helm, 1978.

20. Cunningham-Burley, S. and Irvine, S. "'And Have You Done Anything So Far?' An Examination of Lay Treatment of Children's Symptoms." *British Medical Journal.* 295, 1987. 700.

21. Marshall, J.G. "McMaster University Health Sciences Library and Hamilton Public Library, Hamilton, Ontario" in Rees, A.M., ed. *Developing Consumer Health Information Services.* New York: Bowker, 1982.

22. Kempson, E. *Informing Health Consumers: A Review of Consumer Health Information Needs and Services.* London: College of Health and The British Library, 1987. 19.

23. Kempson, E. *Informing Health Consumers: A Review of Consumer Health Information Needs and Services.* 52, 56.

24. Rees, A.M. "Health Information and Medical Consumerism" in Rees and Hoffman, eds. *The Consumer Health Information Source Book.* 1–13.

CHAPTER 22
Developing Consumer Health Information Services in New Zealand

Jill Harris

Many New Zealanders today wish to take a more active role in their health care, and in planning and monitoring public health services. Librarians and health professionals report an increasing demand for information to make this possible. Changes in the health-care system during the last decade can be seen as both a consequence and an encouragement of these trends.

THE NEW ZEALAND HEALTH-CARE SYSTEM

For the past 50 years health care in New Zealand has been funded and provided by government, private, and voluntary agencies interacting with one another.

The Public Sector

The government meets an estimated 80 percent of total health spending.[1] Funded through general taxation, the Department of Health provides for free hospital treatment for all, and free dental treatment for those under 18 years of age. Through a system of health benefits it subsidises health care provided by private medical practitioners, private hospitals, and some voluntary agencies. Pharmaceuticals, diagnostic services, physiotherapy, home nursing, artificial aids, and other services are also subsidized. The government helps to fund the training of health professionals, is responsible for public health measures through local body government, and partly funds the Accident Compensation Corporation, which provides a comprehensive system of treatment and compensation and programs for accident prevention for virtually all individuals resident in or visiting New Zealand.

The Private Sector

Operating in the private sector are medical practitioners (both general and specialist), dentists, pharmacists, radiologists, physiotherapists, podiatrists, chiropracters, naturopaths and other alternative healers, private hospitals and nursing homes, and health-care schemes provided by private companies and organizations. An increasing number of New Zealanders now carry private health insurance to pay for health care provided by the private sector. They are concerned about much-publicised shortcomings in the public health system, dissatisfied with the lack of choice, desirous of securing refunds on medical bills, and unable or unwilling to put up with long waiting lists for surgery and other services in public hospitals. Insurance is available through nonprofit friendly societies and private insurance companies, of which the Southern Cross Medical Care Society is by far the largest, holding approximately 80 percent of all policies. Almost one-half of all New Zealanders have joined medical insurance schemes. Many medical practitioners, in fact, believe all New Zealanders should pay for visits to the family doctor through compulsory health insurance, with the government paying the premiums of the very poor.

The Voluntary Sector

The large number of voluntary organizations ranges from national branches of international organisations like the Red Cross Society to small self-help groups which cater to people with particular illnesses, as well as their caregivers. The scale of their activities varies widely—some run hospitals and fund research and extensive educational programs, while others provide support and information from minimal funds. Many are encouraged and assisted by grants from the government.

RECENT CHANGES IN THE HEALTH-CARE SYSTEM

The emphasis in government health spending has been on providing sickness services. Two-thirds of the health budget has been spent on hospital-based services and less than 2 percent on health promotion.[2]

However, in 1983 the Area Health Boards Act was passed, signalling a restructuring of the health service. Hospital boards, elected by the community to administer public hospitals, were to be integrated with Department of Health district offices to form area health boards with much wider responsibilities for the health of the community. This process was completed by the end of 1989. Area health boards must now concern themselves with coordinating the planning of all the public, private, and voluntary health services in the area, with health promotion and preventative as well as curative services, community health initiatives as well as professional programs.

COMMUNITY PARTICIPATION ENCOURAGED

Facilitating community involvement in planning and providing health care is seen as an important responsibility of area health boards. Community health committees and service development groups are provided for in the Area Health Boards Act. Community participation is one of the five principles of health care set out in the New Zealand Health Charter released by the Minister of Health in December 1989.[3] Another publication, issued by the Department of Health for use by both the public and area health boards, spells out just how this involvement is to be managed.[4]

The devolution of operational responsibility for health services from the Department of Health to area health boards has been accompanied by more stringent requirements for accountability in the use of public funds. Faced with rising health-care costs, the government commissioned two reviews to examine the equity and efficiency of public expenditure on health benefits[5] and public hospitals.[6] The review of public hospitals, in particular, criticised poor management and lack of accountability. Both reviews presented options for the greater privatisation of health services.

A PUBLIC HEALTH SYSTEM UPHELD

Despite these options, the views of medical practitioners and the rapid increase in private health insurance, the Health Charter makes clear the government's commitment to a public health service:

> The objective is to maintain a nationwide publicly funded health system. . . .Essential health care will be universally accessible, in a manner that is acceptable to both individuals and the community, taking into account the cost that the community and the country can afford.[7]

Two major inquiries in 1988 contributed to the new climate of health services accountability. An inquiry into forensic psychiatric services[8] attributed a number of prison suicides to the refusal of psychiatric hospitals to admit prisoners with serious psychiatric disorders. Bureaucratic neglect, buck-passing and lack of hospital board accountability were highlighted.[9]

In 1987, allegations were made in the June issue of *Metro* (a popular Auckland monthly magazine) of the failure to inform patients at Auckland's National Women's Hospital adequately about their medical condition and management, and to obtain their informed consent to participating in an experiment in the management of cervical cancer.[10] A judicial inquiry, created to investigate the allegations, found that the women had indeed not been informed. The "Cervical Cancer Inquiry" raised issues of accountability and peer review in the medical profession and hospital administration, and affirmed patients' rights—particularly to information. Judge Cartwright, who headed the inquiry, stated in her report: "I have come to consider the patient is entitled to all relevant information. . . "[11] She also recommended the establishment of a health commission to protect health consumer rights, and the appointment of patient advocates in public hospitals. Ensuring adequate public access to health information is to be an important part of these positions.

PUBLIC DEMAND AND NEED FOR HEALTH INFORMATION

One result of these changes in health services funding and delivery has been a growing need and demand by the public for better access to consumer health information.

The Evidence for the Need and Demand: Surveys

Various surveys over the last 15 years have attempted to gauge public satisfaction with access to health and sickness information. A patient opinion survey carried out at Wellington Public Hospital in 1974[12] asked 230 patients recently discharged from general, medical, and surgical wards whether they felt they knew enough about their illness and treatment. One in four said they did not. A more recent hospital survey carried out nationally,[13] although not specifically measuring satisfaction with information, showed that 5 percent of the 330 subjects who had used public hospital services in the last three years did not feel they had been kept informed of their progress. It is also possible that some of the 15 percent who found public hospital staff overworked (the main complaint expressed) felt this had affected the amount of information they were given.

A further survey at Wellington Public Hospital was carried out by the author in 1988 to determine the level of satisfaction with information about medical conditions and treatment felt by a group of 274 hospital outpatients or their caregivers. Forty-six percent said they wanted to know more about illness and 39 percent more about treatment. Nearly two-thirds of further comments made by the respondents confirmed this wish for more information. Although it cannot be assumed that all of these people would actively seek more information, some certainly would—15 percent of the comments indicated a commitment to taking personal responsibility for health care, including acquiring information.[14]

Recent surveys of community opinion have also indicated a wish and need for more health and sickness information. The Auckland Division of the New Zealand Medical Association recently carried out a market survey on the view of general practitioners held by 300 Auckland residents. Respondents listed as the most important features of the ideal general practitioner: (i) a doctor who listens; (ii) a doctor who explains things adequately; and (iii) a doctor who spends sufficient time with you.[15] Such attributes were seen by McCormick to be part of the "augmented product" as opposed to the "core product" (accurate diagnosis and adequate prescribing), which general practitioners should be marketing. The survey also found that the adequacy of doctors' explanations of problems to their patients was one of the three main gaps experienced between ideal and reality.

A survey of 135 New Zealand asthmatics[16] showed that 20 did not know they had asthma; almost half had a very limited or no knowledge of the nature of their illness; many were confused about their drug therapies, especially the use of corticosteroids; and one in four did not know what they would do in the event of a severe attack. The authors concluded that the high asthma mortality rate in New Zealand may be compounded by such ignorance.

The demand for health and sickness information in Wellington Public Library was measured by the author in 1988. The survey found that 7.4 percent of information requests and 25.2 percent of reserves in the Science and Technology Department of the Central Library, and 6.2 percent of total Central Library nonfiction book returns, were health-related. In the Library's branches the corresponding figures were 10.6 percent for subject inquiries, 15.1 percent for nonfiction reserves, and 6.5 percent for nonfiction issues.

Other Evidence of Health Information Need

The Women's Health Movement

Health initiatives taken by women in recent years have been widespread and extensive, if somewhat fragmented. The inauguration, in 1989, of Women's Health Councils in two of the country's largest cities (Auckland and Wellington) indicate increasing strength and coordination. The need for health information has always been central to the women's health movement, which has been described as "an information based phenomenon."[17] Two recent publications emphasize this. *Women's Health in New Zealand: 1985–1988* states that almost all the issues and topics dealt with by a Health Department committee on women's health raised the need for health education and appropriate health information. The report states "there is a dearth of readily accessible and appropriate information on women's health." It argues that:

> The need for a clearinghouse for some of the excellent material currently available is urgently needed. Much verbal information is given to women when they are not well and needs to be reinforced by written material.[18]

The second publication evaluates three government-funded women's health centers. The provision of health information to women is seen as one of the most important functions of the centers, which have all started their own libraries of books, journal articles, and pamphlets.[19] They were frequently contacted for information, including information about other helping agencies. The centers were deemed a success because they met a need for information that is difficult to obtain from a single traditional source, especially about alternative health-care options.

The Self-Help Movement

The same determination to take control of one's own health is evident in the many health self-help groups in the community. Whether they are large and well-funded, like the Heart Foundation, or small and struggling, self-empowerment through the sharing of information, experience, and social support is a common aim. Of particular significance are self-help initiatives taken by Maori people, such as the extension of Maori language kindergartens into health centers for Maori of all ages.[20] A report into Maori standards of health[21] makes it clear that the health services do not benefit Maori to the same extent as non-Maori and such self-help initiatives indicate a bid for greater equity.

A national organisation called Open Forum for Health Information of New Zealand Association Incorporated has as its primary function to collect, evaluate, and disseminate information to the 8,500 people on its mailing list. Its scope includes both orthodox and complementary therapies.

Increasing Community Responsibility for Health Care

The Department of Health has signalled its intention to transfer greater responsibility for health care—particularly of the elderly and chronically ill—from institutions to the community. Recent incidents in which facilities for intellectually handicapped children have been threatened with closure have raised alarm because of the lack of community resources to pick up the job of caring for the children. Despite assurances from the minister of health that the resources will be provided, there is doubt that the resources—including information—are in fact available.

The Search for Information through Citizens' Advice Bureaux

Many people already seek information on the care of sick and disabled family members from Citizens' Advice Bureaux. The 1988/89 national statistics show that 33,693 inquiries were received from the public about health services and support groups, illnesses (particularly addictive ones), care of the elderly, and accident prevention and compensation. These inquiries comprised 8.3 percent of the 403,588 inquiries received in all categories, and are a slight increase on the previous year's 8.1 percent.

Emerging Medical Consumerism

Medical consumerism in New Zealand is a relatively new phenomenon. It has been somewhat stifled in the past by the lack of consumer choice in the largely state-funded health system. "The current system does little to foster the goals of giving users greater choice, more participation and more responsibility," says the review of health benefits.[22] There are signs, however, of an emerging health consumer movement, stimulated perhaps by that very lack of choice. In his review of public hospitals, Gibbs refers to public dissatisfaction with health services and their lack of responsiveness to the consumer. "This criticism of lack of choice and control is growing," he warns, and adds that: "Other concerns relate to the nature of information available to patients. . . to place them in a position where they can make fully informed choices. . . . "[23]

The health benefits review also refers to an emerging health consumerism: "Consumer involvement is being demanded by a more informed and articulate population with greater awareness of their rights."[24] It recognises the need for information for health consumers: "We support efforts by users to be better informed about many aspects of the health services. . . . Access to and use of such information will allow health care users to be more involved in the management of their own health care. . ."[25]

This association between consumer empowerment and information is reinforced in a policy document produced for the Policy and Communications Unit of the Department of Health. *Having a Say in Health* begins:

> The task [for the document] was to propose some practical ways to make the health system and its workers more responsive to consumers, to consider accountability mechanisms and complaints systems and suggest improvements which would provide consumers with more support, information and voice.[26]

Concluding that "The present system was found not to be working for consumers,"[27] the paper suggests how it could be improved. Its fourth recommendation states: "That Health Department units and area health boards support co-ordinated approaches to set up consumer health information services in local libraries."[28]

The Response of the Medical Profession to Health Consumerism

The medical profession is also aware of the growing consumerism—an awareness no doubt heightened by the unfavorable publicity generated by the Cervical Cancer Inquiry. The presentation of a paper entitled "The Marketing of General Practice"[29] at the annual conference of the Royal New Zealand College of General Practitioners certainly suggests such an awareness. It would appear from this paper that general practitioners are sensitive about their public image and responsive to public pressure for a different kind of doctor who:

> answers questions patiently and provides anticipatory guidance. The relationship is adult to adult and greater responsibility for the outcome of care is shifted to the patient.

A series of pamphlets for the public is being written for the New Zealand Medical Association by a Christchurch doctor on matters which affect the public perception of the medical profession. This is a further indication of sensitivity about image.

A Health Commission for New Zealand

Possibly the clearest signal of the emerging consumerism is the proposed establishment of a health commission as recommended by the Cervical Cancer Inquiry. Reporting on the proposal, the Working Party on the Establishment of the Health Commissioner(s) states in a postscript:

The members of the working group believe however that the concept of a national Health Commissioner, in conjunction with local patient advocates, will provide an important new means by which health consumers are able to have their concerns addressed.[30]

MEETING THE NEED FOR HEALTH INFORMATION

There are many sources of health information in the community for those with the know-how, confidence, and perseverance to seek them out. In the survey of information needs and resources of outpatients and their caregivers at Wellington Public Hospital, up to 16 significant sources were mentioned, although 80 percent of the sample had used no more than six.[31] The hospital doctor was clearly of primary importance, followed by the family doctor. Friends, family and neighbours, health support organisations, and magazines and newspapers figured prominently among the commonest nonprofessional sources of information. Eighteen percent of the 274 respondents and 14.5 percent of those receiving treatment (N=249) had used a library for information about illness and treatment.

The Library Response

Public libraries, medical and nursing libraries, the Department of Health libraries, technical institute libraries, the National Library of New Zealand, and many small libraries attached to health support organisations and women's health centres are all involved in responding to the public demand for health and sickness information. This occurs partly through direct public access and, for professional libraries, through the country's interloan network as well.

Public Libraries

Public libraries, appropriately, play the largest part in this service. However, as the surveys of Wellington Public Library and Wellington Public Hospital outpatients showed, although the Library's health collections appear to be well used, they were not a significant source of information for hospital outpatients or their caregivers.[32]

Health Sciences Libraries

The four main medical libraries serving schools of medicine and teaching hospitals do not receive a large number of inquiries direct from the public, although their resources are drawn on by public libraries through interlibrary lending. All were prepared to allow the public to use their facilities, though they varied in how much assistance they were willing to give. They point out that primary users have priority where resources and services are limited. Some attempts have been made by hospital libraries or departments to set up small collections of material suitable for the public but no major, specialised service exists anywhere in the country.

Two significant initiatives, however, have emerged in the last year. In Christchurch, representatives of the Christchurch Citizens' Advice Bureau, Canterbury Public Library, the Technical Institute Library, Canterbury Medical Library, and the Christchurch School of Medicine met to discuss the "large number of health-related inquiries and requests for information" they were receiving. A questionnaire sent to 200 community health groups (78 responses) showed strong support for a new consumer health information service. In June 1989, a firm proposal for a service based on the public library was submitted to various funding bodies. This application was not successful.

In Wellington, after an approach from a local medical librarian, the Wellington Area Health Board set up a working party to consider the establishment of a health information service for patients and the public in the region. At its first meeting in February 1990 it affirmed the need for wide community consultation and took steps to distribute a questionnaire to community groups, seeking their views on the need for such a service.

Further Library Response to the Demand

In recognition of the need for better public access to health and sickness information, a one-day seminar—largely for public librarians—was organised as an adjunct to an Australasian medical librarians' conference held in Auckland in November 1989. The seminar, attended by some 30 participants from New Zealand and Australia, was taught by Professor Alan Rees. A small group meeting after the seminar concluded that:

1. There is a need and growing demand for consumer health and patient information in New Zealand.
2. Most of the information is now available in New Zealand, but it is often difficult to access.
3. The main need now is for the development of consumer health collections in public libraries and hospitals, and also basic collections in general practitioners' surgeries and health centers. Cooperative schemes should be encouraged, with the emphasis on finding local solutions to issues of funding and location.
4. Medical library collections will still be needed as a back-up for the more unusual subjects or in-depth inquiries.
5. Public libraries have a problem identifying materials to acquire.
6. Free and inexpensive pamphlet material, available from health support agencies, is difficult to track down and keep up-to-date.
7. A simple, centralised distribution system for pamphlets to supply libraries and health centres could be helpful.
8. It is difficult to distinguish good from fad in commercially published material.

9. There may be a need for a national reviewing service for consumer health information—local selection to take account of local conditions and treatment methods would be desirable.
10. Support needs to be given to health professionals in fulfilling their important role in providing consumer health information.
11. Multilingual literature and publications in nonprint formats are also needed.[33]

Information on Health Support Agencies

Health support agencies are included in directories and databases of community organisations compiled by major public libraries and other organisations. However, because they are notoriously hard to keep track of, the Department of Health Library is developing a database of health self-help groups not funded by the government for inclusion in its computerised Health Sciences Network.

CONCLUSION

People have a right to feel in control of their lives and to make sense of their experience. When their well-being is threatened by ill-health—their own or somebody else's—they often feel a loss of control and do not understand what is happening to them. Information is an important component in coping with this uncertainty and in regaining equilibrium.

Maintaining a healthy lifestyle and a healthy environment is also part of feeling in control of one's life and destiny, and once again information forms an important part of achieving this goal. Patients are partners with their doctors and as health consumers expect to challenge community health leaders in allocating scarce health resources. These choices require new information services.

The librarian is one of a team of persons whose job it is to provide information. The doctor or nurse who first explains, the health educator who points to cause and effect, the family member or friend who talks it through, the other patient who shares similar experiences, the woman in the magazine article who narrates her story, and the librarian who locates the pamphlet or book written in everyday language—are all colleagues in the important tasks of helping people cope with illness or stay healthy and act as responsible members of society.

There is growing interest in New Zealand in providing consumer health information services. Most of the initiatives taken so far involve just such a team effort. It remains to be seen, however, whether the efforts of determined enthusiasts can prevail against the present severe financial constraints on health spending in New Zealand.

REFERENCES

1. [Scott, Claudia]. *Choices for Health Care: Report of the Health Benefits Review.* Wellington: Health Benefits Review Committee, 1986. 17.
2. New Zealand. Department of Statistics. *New Zealand Official Yearbook 1988–89.* 93rd ed. Wellington: Government Printing Office, 1988. 295.
3. Clark, Helen. *New Zealand Health Charter, in a New Relationship: Introducing the New Interface Between the Government and the Public Health Sector.* Wellington: [Government Printing Office], 1989.
4. Caird, Ray. *A Guide to Getting Involved: Area Health Boards and Community Participation.* Prepared for the Department of Health, Wellington, New Zealand. Wellington: Department of Health, 1989.
5. [Scott, Claudia]. *Choices for Health Care: Report of the Health Benefits Review.*
6. [Gibbs, Alan]. *Unshackling the Hospitals: Report of the Hospital & Related Services Taskforce.* Wellington: Hospital and Related Services Taskforce, 1988.
7. Clark, Helen. *New Zealand Health Charter, in a New Relationship: Introducing the New Interface Between the Government and the Public Health Sector.* 1.
8. [Mason, Kenneth Hector]. *Report of the Committee of Inquiry into Procedures Used in Certain Psychiatric Hospitals in Relation to Admission, Discharge or Release on Leave of Certain Classes of Patients.* [Wellington: Government Printing Office], 1988.
9. Brookes, Barbara. "The New Health Service in New Zealand." *The Hastings Center Report.* July/August 1989. 13–15.
10. Bunkle, Phillida and Coney, Sandra. "An Unfortunate Experiment at National Women's Hospital." *Metro.* June 1987. 46–65. See also Coney, Sandra. *The Unfortunate Experiment.* Auckland: Penguin, 1988.
11. [Cartwright, Silvia]. *Report of the Committee of Inquiry into Allegations Concerning the Treatment of Cervical Cancer at National Women's Hospital and into Other Related Matters.* [Wellington: Government Printing Office], 1988. 136.
12. Salmond, G.C., Powell, Gaylia D., Gray, Alice, and Barrington, Rosemary. *A Patient Opinion Survey: Wellington Hospital—1974.* Special Report Series, no. 49. Wellington: Department of Health, Management Services and Research Unit, 1977.
13. Chetwynd, S. Jane. "Satisfaction and Dissatisfaction with Public and Private Hospitals." *New Zealand Medical Journal.* 101(853), September 14, 1988. 563–66.
14. Harris, Jillian J. *Informing the Public About Health and Sickness: The Role of Libraries.* A Masters thesis from Victoria University of Wellington, New Zealand, in progress for completion in 1990.
15. McCormick, Ross. "The Marketing of General Practice," Paper presented to the conference of the Royal New Zealand College of General Practitioners, Wellington, 1989.
16. Sinclair, Barbara L., Clark, David W.J., and Sears, Malcolm R. "How Well Do New Zealand Patients Understand and Manage Their Asthma?" *New Zealand Medical Journal.* 100, November 11, 1987. 674–77.
17. Landwirth, Trudy K. "The Women's Health Movement: An Information Based Phenomenon." *The Serials Librarian.* 12 (3/4), 1987. 89–105.
18. *"Women's Health in New Zealand 1985-1988."* Report of the Women's Health Committee to the Board of Health. [Wellington: Government Printing Office], 1988. 24.

19. Norris, Pauline, Maskill, Caroline, Morrell, Vivienne, Brander, Penny, Barnett, Pauline, and Bunnell, Julie. *Profiling Women's Health Centres: An Evaluation of a Primary Health Care Initiative.* Discussion Paper 4. Wellington: Department of Health, Health Services Research and Development Unit, 1989.

20. Pomare, Eru W. and de Boer, Gail M. *Maori Standards of Health: A Study of the Years 1970–1984.* [Wellington]: New Zealand Department of Health and the Medical Research Council, 1988.

21. Pomare, Eru W. and de Boer, Gail M. *Maori Standards of Health: A Study of the Years 1970–1984.*

22. [Scott, Claudia]. *Choices for Health Care: Report of the Health Benefits Review.* 102.

23. [Gibbs, Alan]. *Unshackling the Hospitals: Report of the Hospitals & Related Services Taskforce.* 11.

24. [Scott, Claudia]. *Choices for Health Care: Report of the Health Benefits Review.* 12.

25. [Scott, Claudia]. *Choices for Health Care: Report of the Health Benefits Review.* 122.

26. Nuthall, J.J. *Having a Say in Health.* Wellington: Department of Health, Policy and Communications Unit, 1988.

27. Nuthall, J.J. *Having a Say in Health.* 3.

28. Nuthall, J.J. *Having a Say in Health.* 24.

29. McCormick, Ross. "The Marketing of General Practice."

30. *Report of the Working Party on the Establishment of the Health Commissioner(s).* Wellington: Department of Health, 1989.

31. Harris, Jillian J. *Informing the Public About Health and Sickness: The Role of Libraries.*

32. Harris, Jillian J. *Informing the Public About Health and Sickness: The Role of Libraries.*

33. Mosley, Isobel. "Consumer Health Information in New Zealand." *Library Life.* 133, February 1990. 9.

INDEX

by Linda Webster